High Blood Pressure Lowered

Naturally –

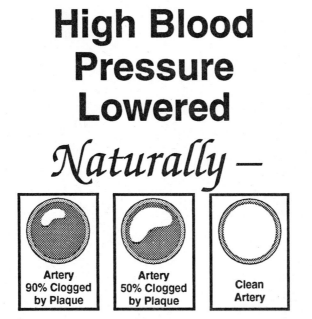

| Artery 90% Clogged by Plaque | Artery 50% Clogged by Plaque | Clean Artery |

Your Arteries Can Clean Themselves!

High Blood Pressure Lowered

Naturally –

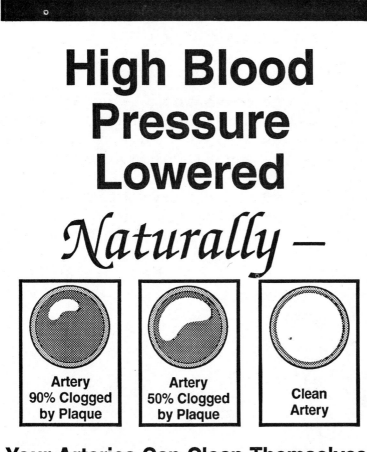

Artery
90% Clogged
by Plaque

Artery
50% Clogged
by Plaque

Clean
Artery

Your Arteries Can Clean Themselves!

By the Editors of FC&A

FC&A Publishing
103 Clover Green
Peachtree City, GA 30269

Publisher: FC&A Publishing
Editors: Linda M. Sciullo and Sherryl D. Wade
Production: Carol L. Parrott
Cover Design: Diane Dunn
Printed and bound by Banta Company

Fourth printing December 1995

ISBN 0-915099-68-3

✳️ Table of Contents

Chapter 32: Menus Designed to Lower High Cholesterol 457

Notice:

This book is for information only. It does not constitute medical advice and should not be construed as such. We cannot guarantee the safety or effectiveness of any drug, treatment or advice mentioned. Some of these tips may not be effective for everyone.

A good doctor is the best judge of what medical treatment may be needed for certain conditions and diseases. We recommend in all cases that you contact your personal doctor or health care provider before taking or discontinuing any medications, or before treating yourself in any way.

Your body, you know, is the temple of the Holy Spirit, who is in you since you received Him from God. You are not your own property. You have been bought and paid for. This is why you should use your body for the glory of God.

1 Corinthians 6:19-20

But I will restore you to health and heal your wounds, declares the Lord.

Jeremiah 30:17a

✳ ‖ Introduction

High blood pressure, also known as hypertension, is the single most common risk factor for heart, blood vessel and kidney disease in the United States today. It is estimated that approximately 50 million, or one in every four, adults in the United States have some form of high blood pressure.

The number of people who actually have been properly diagnosed with high blood pressure is smaller, probably around 30 to 40 million people.

High blood pressure is a subtle condition, often with no obvious signs or symptoms in its early stages. Unless you get annual checkups and have your blood pressure checked regularly, you could be suffering from mild to moderate high blood pressure and not even realize it.

High blood pressure causes long-term damage in the heart, kidneys and blood vessels even in the early stages, before you know that your blood pressure is high. (For an explanation of the new classification of blood pressure levels, please see page 20.)

Although it is rarely listed on death certificates as the cause of death, high blood pressure (even mildly elevated blood pressure) can lead to strokes, heart attacks, congestive heart failure, kidney failure and blindness.

Men and women of all ages experience an increased risk of these complications if they have high blood pressure, and this risk increases with age. In addition, the higher your blood pressure, the greater your risk of developing serious, even life-threatening, complications.

The introduction of the National High Blood Pressure Education Program in 1972 and other similar education programs in the last 20 years has resulted in more people seeking medical attention, diagnosis and treatment for high blood pressure.

This increased awareness and public effort to fight high blood pressure has resulted in a 50-percent drop in the number of deaths from coronary heart disease (the number one cause of death in the United States), as well as a 57-percent fall in the number of deaths from strokes.

The purpose of this book is to help you understand what high blood pressure is, the effects it can have on your body, what lifestyle changes you can make to lower high blood pressure if you already have it, and the types of drugs used to treat it when lifestyle changes aren't enough.

In addition to describing how to lower high blood pressure, this book will provide tips on how to prevent high blood pressure from developing, especially among groups of people who are at high risk.

These groups include African-Americans, people with family histories of high blood pressure, people with a "high-normal" blood pressure, people with high cholesterol levels and

people whose lifestyles put them at risk for developing high
blood pressure.

Lifestyle risk factors include high salt intake, diets high
in fat and calories, excessive drinking of alcoholic beverages,
lack of physical exercise and vitamin deficiencies.

A study reported in a leading medical journal shows that
you can cut your risk of ever developing high blood pressure
by making moderate changes in your lifestyle.

The study involved 201 male and female volunteers who
were slightly overweight, ate salty foods, smoked, drank several alcoholic drinks a day and rarely exercised. All of them
had blood pressure in the high-normal range but, otherwise,
they were all healthy.

These prime candidates for high blood pressure agreed
to work on better nutrition and to shoot for four goals:

❑ lose at least 10 pounds

❑ reduce daily salt intake to less than one-tenth of one
ounce

❑ cut back to no more than two alcoholic drinks a day

❑ exercise for 30 minutes three times a week

Smokers who participated in the study were advised to
quit smoking, and the researchers encouraged the study participants to stick to a low-fat diet recommended by the American Heart Association.

For five years, the participants, ranging in age from 30
to 44, kept food diaries, visited their doctors regularly, were
given blood and urine tests, and had their blood pressures
checked periodically.

Three-quarters of them exercised faithfully, mostly walking, jogging and cycling. One out of four met the weight-loss goal, but fewer than two in 10 reduced salt intakes.

All said they averaged no more than two drinks a day. They cut their daily calorie intake by an average of 800 calories, a drop of 30 percent. They cut back modestly on saturated fat and cholesterol.

During the same period, doctors kept track of another, similar group that took no special dietary, weight-loss or exercise measures.

After five years, the researchers found that this group had double the rate of high blood pressure as the changed lifestyle group.

Some members of the changed lifestyle group developed high blood pressure, but the researchers found that the improved nutrition and exercise routines had delayed the onset of the high blood pressure for a year or more in most cases.

Those who lost the most weight experienced the most benefits. And, unfortunately, smokers were nearly four times as likely to develop high blood pressure as nonsmokers.

One in five people in the group that didn't make any lifestyle changes developed high blood pressure during the five-year trial, compared with one in 11 in the changed lifestyle group. That proved true even though most people in the changed lifestyle group did not reach their original goals. Just the emphasis on healthy eating and regular exercising helped lower blood pressure.

Such modest changes in lifestyle could slash the risks of heart disease and stroke in one million people with high-normal blood pressure over the next five years.

The researchers recommend that doctors start aiming for the prevention of high blood pressure by nutritional means in addition to prescribing drugs to fight the disease.

But there is also good news for people who have already been diagnosed with high blood pressure. Blood pressure can often be lowered naturally without taking blood pressure medications.

According to a university study, over 85 percent of patients with high blood pressure were able to stop taking their medication by changing their lifestyle, and their blood pressures were lower than when they were taking drugs.

Many of the people who participated in the study also found that their blood cholesterol levels dropped an average of 26 percent by the end of the study.

These findings were confirmed by a new four-year study by the University of Minnesota. The researchers at the university also found that people with mild high blood pressure who had been taking prescription blood pressure lowering drugs could maintain lower blood pressure without drugs by losing weight and reducing salt and alcohol.

While drugs have helped lower blood pressure in many people, doctors are concerned about possible adverse side effects.

In the study, 189 men who had mild high blood pressure were divided into three groups.

The first group stopped taking prescription drugs and received nutritional counseling. They learned the importance of controlling their weight, increasing physical activity and reducing their intake of sodium and alcohol.

The second group discontinued drug therapy but did not receive any nutritional counseling. Group three continued taking their blood pressure medication.

Four years after the study began, almost 40 percent of group one participants had normal blood pressures without taking drugs, the researchers reported. But 95 percent of groups two and three had to return to, or continue with, drug therapy.

The nondrug, nutrition group lost an average of 5 to 10 pounds and kept the weight off during the four years. Their salt intake was reduced by 36 percent, and the amount of alcohol they consumed also was reduced.

However, the other groups gained weight and showed no change in their salt and alcohol intakes.

Group one also had improved levels of cholesterol, potassium and uric acid in the blood, an unexpected but pleasant side effect, the doctors noted.

The results of these studies and numerous other similar studies suggest that there are many natural, healthy things you can do to lower your high blood pressure, even if you are already taking blood pressure medications.

Working closely with your doctor, you can begin living a healthier lifestyle that will lead to lower blood pressure and, therefore, lower your risk of heart, blood vessel and kidney diseases.

However, the key is working closely with your doctor. You should never stop taking your medication on your own without your doctor's consent. This can cause very serious problems. Work with your doctor.

As you begin to eat more healthily, exercise more regularly and start lowering your blood pressure naturally, your doctor will be able to wean you off the medications slowly to avoid problems from suddenly stopping all medications.

1 | Understanding Blood Pressure

B lood pressure refers to the pressure inside the blood vessels. Without a certain base pressure, blood couldn't circulate through the vessels. This means that tissues and organs in the body wouldn't get the vital oxygen and nutrients they need to keep functioning.

Your blood pressure doesn't always stay the same. It changes from moment to moment and from day to day, depending on your body's activities and daily needs.

For example, when you're asleep or comfortably watching television, your heart rate will be slow and steady, and your blood pressure will be low.

However, when you're exercising, angry or frightened, your heart will beat much faster and harder, which results in higher blood pressure.

The circulatory system and how it works

To get the most accurate picture of what blood pressure

is, you need to start with the heart. The heart is a muscular organ made up of four separate chambers: the right atrium, the right ventricle, the left atrium and the left ventricle.

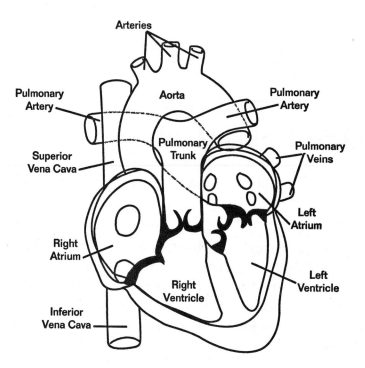

Blood travels through each of these chambers into about 60,000 miles of soft, elastic tubes called blood vessels. Blood vessels in a healthy person are elastic so they can stretch and expand to allow blood to flow through them with each heartbeat.

Vein

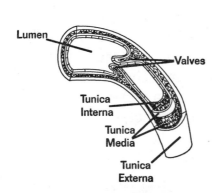

Lumen

Valves

Tunica Interna

Tunica Media

Tunica Externa

There are four main types of blood vessels: arteries, arterioles (small branch of an artery), capillaries and veins. The arteries are some of the largest and most muscular vessels in the body.

These hearty vessels deliver oxygen and nutrients in the blood to the body's various organs. Most arteries have relatively thick muscular walls that are capable of stretching to accommodate the pulses of blood from the heart. Arteries are divided into three categories based on their size and certain other characteristics:

❑ large or elastic arteries, such as the aorta, leading straight out from the heart
❑ medium-sized or muscular arteries, also known as distributing arteries
❑ small arteries, which are usually less than two millimeters (mm) in diameter, often referred to as arterioles

All arteries are made up of three tissue layers: the tunica interna, the tunica media and the tunica externa. The tunica interna is the innermost layer of tissue in the arteries. It is made up of endothelial cells and connective tissue. It directly surrounds the opening in the vessel where the blood flows, known as the lumen of the vessel.

The tunica media is located in the middle of the vessel wall. It is a muscular layer of tissue, containing muscle tissue and elastic tissue. And, the tunica externa is the outermost layer making up the arteries. This layer contains nerve fibers and thin nutrient vessels.

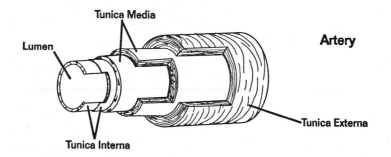

The large arteries have especially muscular tunica media layers. These vessels can range from several centimeters to only a few millimeters in diameter.

The larger arteries are especially susceptible to the buildup of cholesterol and other fatty material in the artery walls, a process known as atherosclerosis. This buildup leads to a narrowing of the vessel chamber (lumen), which can contribute to high blood pressure.

The arterioles are small, thick-walled muscular vessels that are largely responsible for regulating blood flow throughout the body.

Contraction and relaxation of the muscles in these vessels allow them to regulate blood flow. Depending on the situation, arterioles can direct more or less blood flow to different organs or muscles for optimal functioning.

The degree of contraction of these vessels not only regulates the amount of blood flow to organs and muscles, but it also affects the pressure in the larger arteries that lead into the arterioles.

When the arterioles are tightly constricted and not allowing much blood through, the pressure in the larger arteries that supply those arterioles begins to increase. This is much like the pressure that builds up in a water hose when you turn the water on but clamp the end of the hose so water cannot escape.

High blood pressure is usually caused by these important vessels. The state of contraction of the arterioles is usually increased in high blood pressure, and the increased resistance to blood flow in these vessels results in increased pressure in the large arteries.

From the arterioles, the blood vessels continue to divide into smaller and smaller branches to reach the smallest vessels, the capillaries. The diameter of the capillary lumen is just large enough to allow the blood cells to pass through.

Capillary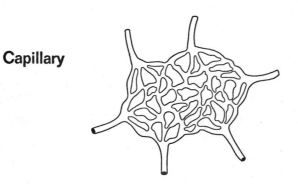

It is at the capillary level that the oxygen and nutrients carried in the blood cells travel across the vessel walls into the tissue to nourish the cells. Likewise, the waste material from the cells travels back into the capillary to be transported away for disposal.

The capillaries are connected to more tiny vessels known as venules. These vessels have larger lumens, but thinner muscular walls compared with arteries.

Although there is less muscle tissue in the walls of the venules compared with arteries, the muscle in venule walls can still contract and relax. The rhythmic contraction and relaxation helps to transport blood back to the heart and lungs where it can pick up more oxygen and nutrients.

The tiny venules begin joining together to form larger veins. The larger veins eventually merge into the two largest veins in the body: the superior vena cava and the inferior vena cava, which return blood directly to the heart.

What's happening in your body when you have high blood pressure

The circulatory system works efficiently to provide blood, oxygen and nutrients to every cell in the body. The blood vessels carry out their different jobs to result in a well-tuned system.

However, changes in some of the vessels can result in dramatic changes throughout the entire circulatory system.

High blood pressure causes structural changes in the arterioles and medium-sized muscular arteries. The changes are referred to by scientists and doctors as hypertrophy and hyperplasia.

Hypertrophy refers to an increase in the size of an individual cell. When all the cells making up a muscle undergo hypertrophy, the whole muscle gets larger. Hypertrophy is what happens to muscles of body builders: The individual cells get larger, resulting in a larger muscle.

Hyperplasia, on the other hand, refers to an increase in the number of cells that make up a muscle or other tissue.

The actual size of the individual cells does not change much. This is what happens as children's muscles grow as they age: The actual number of muscle cells increases, resulting in a bigger muscle.

High blood pressure causes both hypertrophy and hyperplasia of the muscle cells in the middle layer of the arteries and arterioles. These changes are accompanied by hypertrophy and hardening (known as fibrosis) of the inner layer.

All these changes result in a narrowing of the lumen of the blood vessels, which worsens the already existing resistance to blood flow in the vessels.

Blood pressure is determined by a combination of how much blood the heart pumps as well as how high the resistance in the arterioles is.

The amount of blood the heart pumps (known as cardiac output) is controlled by factors such as heart rate, the physical state of the heart muscle (whether it's a healthy muscle or a weak muscle), and the influence of various chemicals and hormones in the body.

The resistance in the arterioles (known as peripheral resistance) is controlled mainly by the nervous system and certain chemicals in the blood that can cause dilation or constriction of the muscular walls of the arterioles.

In most people with essential hypertension, these blood pressure controlling factors are somehow out of whack. For example, some scientific studies show that many people with essential hypertension have a normal arteriole resistance, but an increased cardiac output, which results in higher blood pressure.

Other people, however, have normal cardiac output but increased vascular resistance. This also results in higher blood pressure levels. The reasons why these people have increased cardiac output or increased peripheral resistance are not always clear.

Scientists have discovered, however, that later in the course of high blood pressure, most people have elevated arteriole resistance, regardless of which risk factors might have caused it.

Although scientists are still trying to discover why the arterioles constrict to cause higher blood pressure, they feel certain that risk factors such as heredity, age, gender, obesity and high cholesterol all contribute to the process.

Another factor in the development of high blood pressure is how the kidneys respond to blood pressure and salt. The relationship between blood pressure and salt (sodium chloride) normally provides a nearly perfect way for the kidneys to help control blood pressure.

Under normal circumstances, the kidneys can either hold onto extra salt when the body needs higher blood pressure, or they can flush out extra salt if the body needs to lower blood pressure.

However, some people have kidneys that do not respond this way to help control blood pressure.

The kidneys might have decreased sensitivity to excess sodium chloride in the blood, or the kidneys could have increased sensitivity to chemicals and hormones in the blood that stimulate them to hold extra salt.

Either situation leads to increased salt retention and elevated blood pressure. And to make matters even more complicated, the kidneys can stimulate the release of a chemical known as angiotensin, which acts on the arterioles and causes them to constrict and raise blood pressure.

In normal situations, this is a safety system designed to keep the blood pressure from ever falling to dangerously low levels. However, when the kidneys are not responding like they should to blood pressure or sodium load in the blood, that extra angiotensin can result in blood pressure elevations that are too high.

Although doctors and researchers are still trying to discover all the causes and influencing factors behind high blood pressure, they have learned a great deal about the effects of high blood pressure.

Elevated blood pressure does not cause a person to feel bad for many years, but it slowly takes its toll on the body. High blood pressure eventually affects almost every organ in the body, but its effects on the heart, brain and kidneys account for the greatest amount of illness and death.

What are the symptoms of high blood pressure?

The symptoms of high blood pressure are usually silent in the early stages. Many people have high blood pressure for years and don't realize it. That's why high blood pressure is so dangerous. It can do a lot of damage before you even know you have it.

The only way to find out if you have high blood pressure is to have your blood pressure measured by your doctor or other health care worker. You should have your blood pressure checked at least once every year.

Although the early stages of high blood pressure are silent, many health problems might begin to show up in people who have had high blood pressure for a long time.

Symptoms such as depression, ringing in the ears, fainting spells, difficulty breathing, swelling of the legs, flushing of the face, headaches, tension, dizziness, nosebleed or blurred vision may be experienced by some people.

How is blood pressure measured?

Blood pressure is usually taken with an arm-pressure cuff,

called a sphygmomanometer, which comes from two Greek words that mean pulse measurement. When your doctor or other health care worker takes your blood pressure, it is recorded as two separate numbers: for example, 120/80 (120 over 80).

The first (or top) number refers to systolic pressure, or the pressure which is produced as the heart contracts to pump blood out into the body.

The second (or bottom) number refers to diastolic pressure, or the pressure which remains in the blood vessels as the heart relaxes to allow blood to flow into the pumping chamber (the left ventricle of the heart).

Both of these numbers are important to your doctor because they give him a great deal of information about the health of your cardiovascular system (the heart, arteries, arterioles, capillaries and veins).

The systolic pressure is important because it tells the maximum amount of pressure placed on your arteries. The diastolic is equally important, telling the minimum pressure on your arteries.

The harder it is for the blood to flow through your vessels, the higher both numbers will be.

Blood pressure is measured in millimeters of mercury, abbreviated as mm Hg, for example 120/80 mm Hg. Mercury is used as a standard because it is much heavier than blood or water (13.6 times heavier), and its rises and falls accurately show the rises and falls in blood pressure.

Mercury was first used to measure blood pressure by Jean Leonard-Marie Poiseuille in Paris in 1828, and it continues to be used for blood pressure measurement today.

When someone takes your blood pressure with a standard sphygmomanometer, it is called an indirect measurement. It is known as indirect (rather than direct) because the instrument is measuring the pressure in the cuff rather than directly measuring the pressure of the blood in the vessel itself.

Using this method, a cuff containing an inflatable bladder is wrapped around your upper arm, with the middle of the bladder placed directly over the brachial artery, the large artery in your arm.

This bladder is connected to a needle-valved rubber bulb by a piece of rubber tubing. Air is pumped into the cuff by squeezing the rubber bulb. As the bulb is pumped and the bladder begins to fill with air, the pressure in the cuff goes up.

This pressure is shown on the calibrated tube of mercury. The bladder is pumped up until it stops the flow of blood in your arm. Using a stethoscope placed over the brachial artery on the arm, the person taking the blood pressure listens to the sound of blood pulsing through the artery.

When that pulsing sound stops, the examiner knows that the cuff has been pumped up enough to stop blood flow in that artery.

At that point, the examiner turns the valve on the bulb to begin slowly releasing air from the bladder. As the valve is turned and the air begins to escape from the cuff, blood is able to flow through the artery again, and the first pulse sound is heard through the stethoscope.

The sharp tapping or knocking sounds generated by the blood pulsing through the artery are known as Korotkoff sounds. The height of the mercury or the number on the gauge is noted when the first pulse is heard. This is the systolic level.

As the air continues to be released from the cuff, the pulse sounds get stronger, then fade. When they finally fade away, another steady sound is heard. This is the sound of the blood flowing through the veins. The number on the gauge at this point is your diastolic pressure.

The American Heart Association describes the sounds that

you hear while taking blood pressure as five distinct phases:

Phase 1: Pressure level (mercury level) at which you hear the first, faint clear tapping sounds as blood begins flowing through the artery again (systolic blood pressure — the top number).

Phase 2: Time during which the bladder is deflating when you can hear murmur or swishing sounds.

Phase 3: Sounds become more crisp and increase in intensity.

Phase 4: Time when the crisp sound changes to a muffled sound. This phase represents diastolic blood pressure in children.

Phase 5: Pressure level (mercury level) when the last sound is heard. This represents the diastolic blood pressure in adults.

Electronic or digital gauges have replaced the traditional column of mercury in most new blood pressure measuring devices.

Automatic blood pressure monitors, where a cuff is automatically inflated around your arm at regular intervals and the blood pressure noted, also are becoming popular. Automatic monitors, known as ambulatory monitors, can be worn throughout the day and provide accurate blood pressure readings under different conditions, like working, sleeping and resting.

The most accurate way of measuring blood pressure is having a catheter inserted into an artery. The catheter's electronic signal is recorded, and the blood pressure is measured. This type of blood pressure measurement is known as direct measurement.

It measures the pressure directly in the blood vessel rather than indirectly through a blood pressure cuff. This method is sometimes used in people with hardening of the arteries to get more precise readings.

Recording the full range of blood pressure, including the systolic highs and the diastolic resting pressure, may be the next step in diagnosing high blood pressure. A new monitor being developed at the Technion-Israel Institute of Technology in Haifa, Israel, will eliminate the need for the arm cuff and stethoscope.

The experimental monitor uses a small wristband that is more comfortable than a cuff, according to its developers. And the reading will be taken in just one second, compared with more than a minute needed for present monitoring.

Sensors in the new monitor will give doctors a printout of waves of blood pressure, providing more information than current techniques.

A similar method, which records the sounds of the blood pulsing through the veins in a continuous wave of blood pressure levels, is now being researched at the Cardiovascular Center of Cornell University Medical College.

Rather than having only the high (systolic) and the low (diastolic) readings, the waves will show a continuous reading of all the blood pressure levels on a printed graph.

The new classification of blood pressure levels

There are ideal ranges of blood pressure for different groups of people. Normal blood pressure readings are based on average blood pressures for different age groups.

Generally, blood pressures increase as people get older. A blood pressure reading, for example, of 139/89 might be considered normal for someone over 50 but too high for a younger person.

In the past, doctors and other health care workers classified high blood pressure as mild, moderate or severe. However, the Joint National Committee on Detection, Evaluation and Treatment of High Blood Pressure did not feel that some of these terms were strong enough to convey the true seriousness and impact of high blood pressure.

For example, many people who discovered that they had mild high blood pressure didn't get too concerned, because it just didn't sound serious or life-threatening.

Remember, even mild high blood pressure can cause long-term, life-threatening damage to your blood vessels, heart and kidneys. With that in mind, the Joint National Committee recently developed a new way to classify high blood pressure.

Classification of Blood Pressure for Adults 18 Years and Older			
Systolic, mm Hg (Top Number)	Diastolic, mm Hg (Bottom Number)	Classification	Follow-Up Recommendations
130 or lower	85 or lower	Normal	Recheck in two years
130 -139	85 - 89	High Normal	Recheck in one year, and begin some simple lifestyle modifications to avoid high blood pressure
140 - 159	90 - 99	Stage 1	Recheck in two months
160 -179	100 - 109	Stage 2	See doctor within one month
180 - 209	110 - 119	Stage 3	See doctor within one week for treatment
210 or higher	120 or higher	Stage 4	See doctor immediately

Use the higher classification when the systolic and diastolic pressures fall into different categories, as well as the recommendations for having your blood pressure checked.

The new classification system no longer uses the traditional terms mild, moderate, severe and very severe. Instead, the new system, listed on the previous page, is based on four stages of high blood pressure and levels for normal and high-normal blood pressures.

This new classification of blood pressure describes stages of blood pressure. All stages of high blood pressure are associated with an increased risk of serious, life-threatening heart, blood vessel and kidney diseases. And, the higher the blood pressure, the greater the risk.

High blood pressure stage 1, previously known as mild high blood pressure, is the most common form of high blood pressure among adults.

This mild form of high blood pressure is responsible for a large proportion of the illnesses, disabilities and deaths associated with high blood pressure. Mild high blood pressure simply isn't as mild as people used to think.

All four stages of high blood pressure are serious and can cause long-term problems. If your blood pressure falls in these ranges, see your doctor for his advice.

The category of high-normal blood pressure is included in the new classification system because people with blood pressure in this range are at an increased risk of developing definite high blood pressure (and the resultant diseases) compared with people who have normal blood pressure.

Almost 30 million Americans have blood pressure levels in this range. These people should have their blood pressures checked regularly, and they should begin lifestyle changes that will lower their risk of developing high blood pressure.

The Joint National Committee considers a normal and ideal blood pressure to be one with a systolic pressure of less than 130 mm Hg and a diastolic pressure of less than 85 mm

Hg. Some people have blood pressure values far below these normal values.

These lower blood pressure readings are generally completely normal. However, if your blood pressure is below 90/60, you should talk with your doctor.

2 | The Dangers of High Blood Pressure

High blood pressure can affect almost every organ in the body. It is the single most important risk factor for the development of heart disease and stroke, and it can lead to other serious health problems, such as kidney disease, aneurysms, loss of vision and memory loss.

Coronary artery disease

Of all the serious and even life-threatening side effects of high blood pressure, coronary artery disease is by far the most common.

Coronary artery disease kills more people in the United States than any other illness.

We know that the heart is the organ responsible for pumping blood to the rest of the body to provide oxygen and nutrients vital for sustaining life.

However, even though the heart pumps blood 24 hours every day, the blood that flows through its four chambers does not provide the heart muscle itself with those vital nutrients. That's where the coronary arteries come into play.

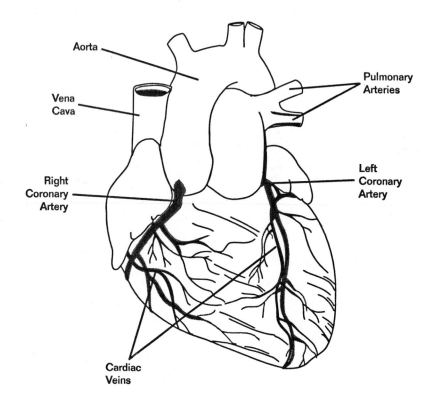

Aorta

Pulmonary
Arteries

Vena
Cava

Right
Coronary
Artery

Left
Coronary
Artery

Cardiac
Veins

The coronary arteries are the vessels that supply the heart muscle with blood, oxygen and nutrients. These arteries are filled with blood from the left ventricle.

The cardiac veins empty that blood right back into the heart for reprocessing with the rest of the blood from the body.

As long as these arteries stay clean and do not get clogged, the heart muscle usually stays pretty healthy. However, when these vessels begin to narrow and get blocked, the heart muscle gets damaged.

This damage can occur suddenly, which usually results in a heart attack. But the damage can occur slowly over a long period of time, which can lead to congestive heart failure.

Coronary artery disease usually is caused by a combination of high blood pressure and atherosclerosis, also known as hardening of the arteries. Atherosclerosis typically begins when fatty streaks form in the inner linings of the elastic arteries throughout the body.

Although these fatty streaks can be found in any artery in the body, they are most commonly found in the aorta (the main artery leading out from the heart), the coronary arteries (the arteries that feed the heart muscle), and the cerebral arteries (the arteries that supply blood to the brain).

Autopsies show that fatty streaks can begin in the aorta as early in life as infancy. These buildups are frequently found in the smaller coronary arteries by the time children become teen-agers.

The fatty streaks may develop into atheromas, small raised plaques of mushy cholesterol, fat and foam cells on the inner walls of the arteries. The plaques start out as small elevations. Over time, however, they enlarge as more cholesterol and other fatty material is deposited.

At first, these atheromas are sparsely distributed throughout the arteries, but, as the disease progresses, they become more and more numerous. Sometimes, they even cover the entire inner surface of some of the affected arteries.

As the plaques grow, they start to come together and cause a narrowing of the lumen of the vessel, which seriously constricts the flow of blood within the arteries. They also begin to push into the middle layer of the arteries.

By this time, the atheromas contain muscle tissue as well

as cholesterol, lipids and other fatty material. Scar tissue eventually begins to grow under and on top of the fatty plaque.

This scar tissue may become hardened by deposits of calcium. This process is why scientists refer to the disease as hardening of the arteries.

At this point, the arteries have reached an advanced state of disease. The flow of blood may be severely constricted by hard, chalky plaque, which may not shrink even with the best of care.

Coronary artery disease refers to the state in which these atheromas have built up in the coronary arteries to the point that blood flow to the heart muscle is decreased because of the narrowed vessels.

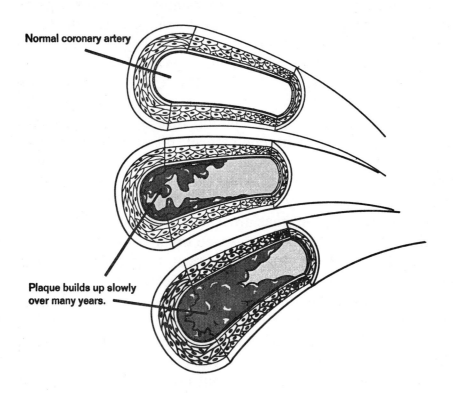

Normal coronary artery

Plaque builds up slowly over many years.

High blood pressure speeds the development of athero-sclerosis. The hardened arteries, in turn, increase the blood pressure.

Many scientists still wonder which came first: the high blood pressure or the atherosclerosis. But no matter which one came first, they both work together to increase the risk of heart attacks from coronary artery disease.

Blood traveling through the narrowed, hardened vessels at high pressure and high speed can often cause part of an atheroma to break off and be washed away with the blood.

If this little piece of plaque gets lodged in a narrowed stretch of a coronary artery, it can block the flow of blood to that portion of the heart muscle. This is called myocardial ischemia. (The word "myocardial" refers to the heart muscle and the word "ischemia" means that the blood flow to that tissue is blocked.)

If blood flow is blocked long enough, the cells in that portion of the heart muscle begin to suffer from what scientists refer to as hypoxia. This means that the muscle is not getting enough oxygen.

The cells in the heart (and everywhere else in the body) need oxygen to survive. If the blood flow is not returned to the hypoxic heart muscle in a matter of minutes, the cells begin to die or infarct. When enough cells die to cause a portion of the heart muscle to die, the result is a myocardial infarction or heart attack.

The seriousness of the heart attack depends upon how large a portion of the heart muscle was damaged. If only a small section of the heart muscle was damaged from the myocardial infarction, there's a good chance of survival.

If, however, one of the larger coronary arteries that supplies a large section of heart muscle was blocked, the heart attack could damage enough of the heart muscle to result in death. Obviously, immediate medical attention is needed to ensure the best possible outcome from a heart attack.

If you think you are having a heart attack, call for emergency help immediately. Coronary intensive care units in larger hospitals are well-equipped to handle heart attack emergencies.

Sometimes, when a piece of an atherosclerotic plaque breaks off and gets caught in a narrowed stretch of a coronary artery, the blood flow is not completely blocked. It may only cause a partial blockage of blood flow. This partial blockage might upset the normal rhythm of the heartbeat.

The heart may stop beating in a normal way and go into a series of ineffective, twitching contractions known as fibrillation. (This also can occur during or after a heart attack.) Fibrillation often can be stopped by an electrical shock given through the wall of the chest by an electronic defibrillator. After defibrillation, the heart may recover its normal beat.

Knowing the warning signs of a heart attack may save your life, especially if you do not delay in seeking medical help. Some heart attacks are called silent heart attacks because there is no advance warning.

However, many heart attacks are not unexpected because the victim has suffered, perhaps for years, from chest pain (angina pectoris).

This chest pain referred to by doctors as angina frequently occurs while a person is physically active. The problem is that the coronary blood vessels supplying the heart muscle are hardened and narrowed from high blood pressure and atherosclerosis. This makes it harder for the blood to get through and supply the heart muscle.

While a person is physically active, the heart has to pump more blood to supply the muscles in the body. As the heart pumps faster, it needs more blood and oxygen from the coronary arteries. Unfortunately, the hardened, narrowed coronary arteries cannot accommodate the extra blood needed by the heart.

When this happens, the active heart muscle gets low on blood and oxygen, resulting in pain. This pain is similar to the pain runners feel in their leg muscles during a long run when the leg muscles need more blood and oxygen.

When someone experiences this kind of chest pain, he needs to stop and rest. As he rests, the heart stops beating so fast. And since it doesn't need as much blood and oxygen, the pain eases.

However, some people need to take a medication known as nitroglycerin to help relieve the chest pain. Doctor-prescribed nitroglycerin (often referred to simply as nitro) causes the coronary arteries to relax and expand. This allows more blood to get to the heart muscle, relieving the chest pain.

Since people with high blood pressure are at increased risk for having a heart attack, be sure you know the symptoms:

- heavy pressure or a choking or squeezing sensation in the center of the chest
- chest pain that may radiate down one or both arms, across the back or up the neck
- shortness of breath
- an unexplained sensation or feeling of fear
- perspiration
- nausea
- dizziness or lightheadedness
- weakness or a fainting sensation
- angina pain that lasts for more than a few minutes

All of these symptoms don't have to be present to indicate that you are having a heart attack, and the chest pain does not necessarily have to be crushing. Sometimes, the pain a person experiences with a heart attack is not as severe as they expect it to be.

In fact, some people who have suffered from heart attacks and lived to tell about it describe the pain as a feeling of heartburn that just wouldn't go away.

If you develop symptoms like that or any of the other symptoms, call for medical help immediately. It could mean the difference between life and death. Do not wait and hope the pain will go away. The longer you wait to go to the hospital after a heart attack, the worse your chances of living through it.

Heart failure

Heart failure occurs when the heart is unable to pump enough blood to meet the requirements of the body. Many cases of heart failure are the direct result of high blood pressure.

About 75 percent of high blood pressure victims develop heart failure, and only 50 percent of patients survive five years after heart failure is detected.

High blood pressure is the leading cause of left ventricular hypertrophy, a major risk factor for heart failure. Remember that hypertrophy is what happens when cells increase in size. Left ventricular hypertrophy is an increased size of the muscular portion of the left ventricle of the heart due to enlarged muscle cells.

Like any muscle cells in the body, the muscle cells in the heart will hypertrophy (grow larger) when they constantly have to work harder, as they do when you have high blood pressure.

The heart has to work harder to pump blood into the narrowed, hardened arteries that result from high blood pressure and atherosclerosis. This all results in a larger left ventricle, just as more bench-presses result in bigger arm muscles in a weight lifter.

At first, this larger muscle seems to be better at pumping blood to the body. But over time, a hypertrophied left ventricle becomes a significant risk factor for heart failure. Unlike most of the other muscles in the body, the heart muscle has a limited ability to increase in size.

The larger the heart muscle is, the harder it is for the coronary arteries to supply it with enough oxygen and nutrients. As the left ventricle increases in muscle mass, the space within the ventricle where blood collects to be pumped to the body gets smaller.

As that space gets smaller, the heart has less and less ability to pump enough blood to supply the body with blood, oxygen and nutrients. And as the heart wall gets thicker, it gets stiffer. This makes it harder to fill with blood and then

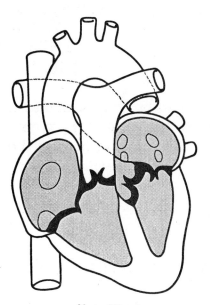

Normal Heart

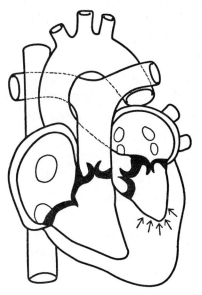

Left Ventricular Hypertrophy

pump it out to the body.

With many cases of left ventricular hypertrophy due to high blood pressure, the heart may maintain an adequate output of blood for many years, even decades.

However, as the heart wall thickens over time, it becomes more and more difficult for it to keep up with the body's demands.

Left ventricular hypertrophy is more prevalent in patients with blood pressures of 160/95 mm Hg or higher. However, even milder cases of high blood pressure (such as 140/90 or higher) over time can result in left ventricular hypertrophy. The risks also increase with age.

In the Framingham Heart Study, 3 to 7 percent of adults under 50 years of age were found to have left ventricular hypertrophy. That figure went up to 12 to 40 percent in the over-50 population.

Studies show that black people with high blood pressure are twice as likely to have left ventricular hypertrophy as white people with similar blood pressures.

When doctors diagnose a case of congestive heart failure, they usually specify whether it is left-sided heart failure or right-sided heart failure.

The right side of the heart receives the oxygen-depleted blood from the body and sends it to the lungs for oxygen. The blood then flows into the more muscular left side of the heart, which pumps the oxygenated blood from the lungs out to the rest of the body.

Left-sided heart failure (which often, but not always, results from left ventricular hypertrophy) is frequently caused by high blood pressure.

As the left side of the heart begins to fail and is unable to pump enough blood to meet the needs of the body, the vessels that lead directly into the left side of the heart begin to feel the bad effects. Those vessels are found in the lungs.

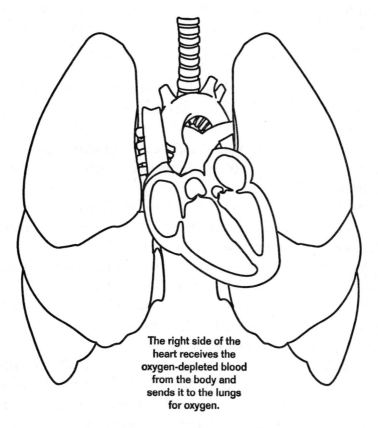

The right side of the
heart receives the
oxygen-depleted blood
from the body and
sends it to the lungs
for oxygen.

With progressive left-sided heart failure, the right side of the heart is still pumping blood to the lungs even though the left side of the heart can't keep up with it. As this happens, more and more blood gets backed up in the vessels of the lungs.

This results in increased pressure within the blood vessels of the lungs (known as the pulmonary vessels). The increased pressure in the smaller, delicate capillaries that line all of the lungs eventually causes some of the blood to leak out of the capillaries into the lung tissue.

Fluid accumulating in the lung tissue causes shortness of breath. At first, this breathlessness (which doctors refer to as dyspnea) is only noticeable while lying down, especially at night.

People suffering from this often wake up in the middle of the night gasping for air. That breathless feeling is quickly relieved by sitting up on the side of the bed or by walking around. As the situation worsens, breathing while lying down becomes more difficult. Some people eventually need to sleep sitting up in a chair.

As the fluid continues to build up in the lung tissue, it becomes more difficult to breathe while standing up, and the situation becomes worse with activity.

People who were once healthy find themselves having to sit and catch their breath after walking up just one flight of steps or out to the mailbox. And, as the left-sided heart failure gets worse and worse, these people find it increasingly hard to catch their breath even while sitting still.

In addition to breathlessness, cough is another common complaint of people suffering from left-sided heart failure. Sometimes, in severe cases of heart failure, the coughing may raise frothy, blood-tinged sputum (a discharge from the respiratory tract).

Over time, left-sided heart failure affects more than just the lungs. Because the left side of the heart is not able to pump enough blood to meet the oxygen and nutritional needs of the body, certain vital organs begin to suffer damage.

The kidneys, for example, need a substantial blood flow in order to function properly. When they don't get enough blood, they begin to release a chemical known as renin, which indirectly stimulates the body to hold on to excess sodium.

This, in turn, results in higher blood pressure, which

makes the problem even worse. Because of the decreased blood flow to the kidneys, the kidney tissue becomes damaged and could eventually lead to kidney failure.

The brain also is affected by left-sided heart failure. The brain needs more blood flow and oxygen than any other organ in the body.

Long-term lack of oxygen due to left-sided heart failure can lead to symptoms such as irritability, loss of attention span, forgetfulness and other mental problems. Fortunately, these mental problems are only seen in severe, life-threatening cases of heart failure.

Finally, long-term, left-sided heart failure eventually begins to affect the right side of the heart and can lead to right-sided heart failure.

The increased pressure and buildup of blood from the left side of the heart and the lungs inevitably produces an increased burden on the right side of the heart. The major organs affected by right-sided heart failure are the liver, spleen, kidneys and brain.

As the blood from the heart gets backed up because of the left-sided heart failure, the right side of the heart loses its ability to pump blood from the body into the lungs.

This causes the blood to be stalled in the veins leading back to the heart. This causes a buildup of blood in the liver, which results in an enlarged liver. If not relieved soon, the enlarged liver begins to suffer cell damage and can release substances into the blood that are damaging to the brain and other organs.

Sometimes, this can lead to massive swelling of the abdomen. This situation requires immediate medical attention.

The spleen also becomes enlarged in right-sided heart failure. And, as blood begins to pool in the veins in the legs and feet, they begin to swell. In fact, ankle and leg swelling, also called edema, is a characteristic of congestive heart failure. And, right-sided heart failure also has a negative influence on the brain, resulting in some of the same symptoms as left-sided heart failure.

Heart failure as a result of high blood pressure is a serious illness that can range in severity from a simple case of occasional breathlessness to life-threatening brain damage.

Heart failure can occur for other reasons but high blood pressure is considered one of the top contributing factors.

Stroke

Strokes are the third leading cause of death in most industrialized countries. People with high blood pressure or a personal or family history of heart disease or stroke, diabetics, men, smokers, and women smokers taking oral contraceptives are at high risk of having a stroke.

A stroke is similar to a heart attack, except it occurs in the brain. When high blood pressure and atherosclerosis cause hardening and narrowing of the blood vessels that supply blood to the brain, a portion of an atheroma (or plaque) can break off and clog up one of the narrowed vessels in the brain.

When this occurs, the portion of the brain that was supplied by the clogged artery gets deprived of oxygen and nutrients. If that blockage lasts several minutes, those brain cells become damaged and can even die, just as the heart muscle cells do in a heart attack.

This type of stroke, caused by a blocked vessel, is known as an occlusive stroke. And just as a heart attack is referred to as a myocardial infarction, a stroke is often referred to as a cerebral infarction.

A stroke that is not caused by a blocked blood vessel is called a hemorrhagic stroke. Instead, it is caused by a blood vessel that begins to leak blood into the surrounding brain tissue. Hemorrhagic strokes can occur for a variety of reasons, but high blood pressure is a factor in many cases. The blood leaking into the surrounding, sensitive brain tissue can cause brain cell damage.

And this vessel leakage can result in insufficient blood flow to other areas of the brain, causing brain cell damage there as well.

The problem with brain cells and nerve cells is that they cannot repair themselves or reproduce like other cells in the body. For example, when a bone is broken, new bone cells are produced to help repair the damage and patch up the broken portion of the bone.

Similarly, a skin wound results in new cells that will fill in the wound and repair the damage. However, if the brain is injured by being deprived of blood, the brain cells get damaged or die and cannot be replaced. As a result, much of the damage caused by a stroke is permanent.

If the right side of the brain is damaged by a stroke, the victim could be paralyzed on the left side and experience a loss in perception and memory.

If the left part of the brain is damaged, the victim could be paralyzed on the right side and have difficulty with speech and remembering words.

It may take years for high blood pressure to weaken and damage blood vessels, but a stroke can happen within seconds without warning. However, about 10 percent of strokes are preceded by transient ischemic attacks or TIAs.

A transient ischemic attack occurs when blood flow is interrupted in some part of the brain for a short period of time, usually without causing long-term damage.

Transient ischemic attacks are sometimes called "little strokes" because the symptoms are similar to a stroke, but they last only for a few minutes. TIAs should be considered a warning for a stroke, says the American Heart Association. People who have experienced one of these temporary blockages of blood flow to some part of the brain are nearly 10 times more likely to suffer a paralyzing stroke than those who haven't had a TIA.

Controlling high blood pressure can reduce your risk of stroke. Researchers have found that as blood pressure is decreased, the risk of stroke is decreased.

If you are at high risk for stroke, you should learn the early warning signs and be prepared to report them to your doctor immediately.

Here are some of the signs of a stroke, as identified by the American Heart Association:

- ❏ sudden change in vision, like a flash of blindness, double vision or dimness of vision, particularly in one eye
- ❏ sudden difficulty with speech, including loss of ability to speak or trouble talking or understanding speech
- ❏ unexplained or unusually severe headaches or dizziness, especially when associated with other mental or neurological signs
- ❏ sudden change in mental abilities
- ❏ impaired judgement
- ❏ sudden numbness, weakness or tingling sensations of the face, arm and leg, usually on one side of the body
- ❏ sudden change in personality
- ❏ any symptoms, such as paralysis, that seem to occur only on one side of the body.

If you experience any of these symptoms, call your doctor and get medical help immediately. Since 38 percent of all stroke victims die within a month, the 30 days following a stroke are critical. Yet, according to the American Heart Association, nearly half the people who survive the first month are still living seven years after their stroke.

Kidney disease

Every ounce of blood that flows through the body passes through the kidneys several times throughout the day to be filtered of certain substances and impurities that can be flushed out in the urine.

Without the kidneys, these waste products would build up to toxic, or poisonous, levels in the blood, a life-threatening situation that requires emergency medical attention.

The blood flows into the kidneys through the renal arteries into structures known as glomeruli. The glomeruli are a complex web of capillaries where the majority of things that

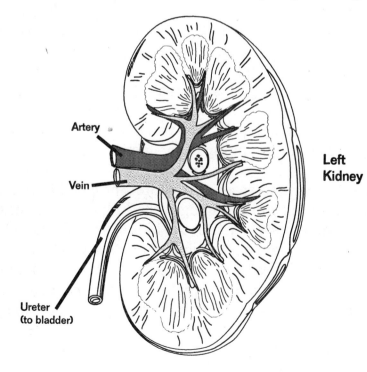

Artery

Vein

Ureter
(to bladder)

Left
Kidney

are filtered from the blood are removed. From the glomeruli, these waste products are passed along through a network of pipes known as tubules.

The tubules provide a location where the body can reabsorb substances (such as vitamins) that were originally headed towards elimination as urine.

The remaining waste products then pass into a collecting system, then on to the bladder, eventually to be flushed away as urine.

Over time, high blood pressure can damage the kidneys. It causes the renal arteries to constrict and become tighter and more narrow, which reduces the blood flow to the kidneys. The kidneys need large quantities of blood in order to work well.

In order to increase the amount of blood flow, the tubules reabsorb more salt and water, which results in increased blood pressure. Even though the kidneys' actions are meant to help the blood flow, the increased blood pressure only serves to worsen the problem.

As the already high blood pressure gets even higher, the blood vessels and tubules within the kidneys are damaged by the high pressure within the vessels. The high blood pressure can cause a hardening of the glomeruli found throughout the kidneys.

This further decreases the amount of blood that can get into the kidneys, which damages the kidneys even more. As more and more vessels within the kidneys are damaged, they become less efficient at filtering out waste products.

Once the kidneys begin to function below normal, waste products are not properly excreted. With salt and other normally excreted products remaining in the kidneys, they continue to malfunction. When the kidneys become damaged, they cannot be repaired.

Once the kidneys can no longer filter the blood, the waste products build up to a toxic level, a condition called uremia.

At this point, kidney dialysis or a kidney transplant is necessary to prevent the waste products in the blood from accumulating to dangerous, life-threatening levels. In some cases, death occurs before dialysis or transplantation can occur.

The bottom line is this: Uncontrolled high blood pressure can eventually result in severe and irreversible kidney damage.

Aneurysms

The rapid, turbulent blood flow that often accompanies high blood pressure can sometimes damage the lining of the arteries. If that damage is not adequately repaired, the artery wall can become weak and fragile at the site of the damage.

The weakened portion of the artery wall then responds to the continued high blood pressure by ballooning out. This is called an aneurysm.

The ballooned portion of the vessel wall can be anywhere from a few millimeters (about one-eighth of an inch) in diameter to many centimeters (several inches) in length. The dangerous thing about an aneurysm is that it can begin to leak or burst at any time, resulting in life-threatening blood loss from the damaged artery.

There are several different kinds of aneurysms, classified by their appearance.

A saccular aneurysm is a sphere-shaped bulge on one side of an artery, due to a weak area on one side of the vessel. Its diameter can reach up to 20 centimeters.

When all the walls of a blood vessel dilate more or less equally, it's called a fusiform aneurysm. The swelling is

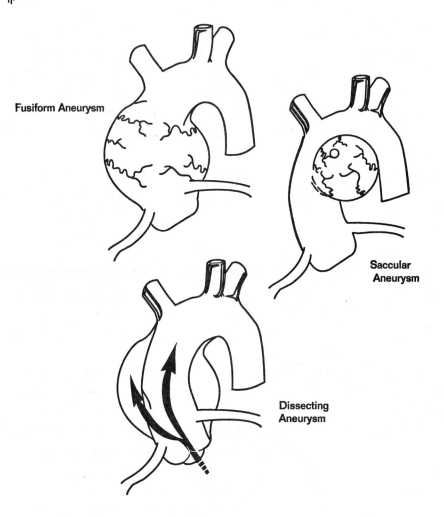

Fusiform Aneurysm

Saccular
Aneurysm

Dissecting
Aneurysm

shaped like a tube.

A dissecting aneurysm, on the other hand, occurs when blood escapes from the lumen of the artery and gets in between two layers of the blood vessel wall. The pressure of the blood in between these two layers creates a cavity within the vessel wall.

Aneurysms can occur in any artery in the body, but there are some locations that are more commonly involved than others. For example, a berry aneurysm is a small saccular aneurysm that affects a vessel in the brain. It's usually no larger than one or two centimeters in diameter.

Dissecting aneurysms most frequently affect the aorta soon after the vessel leaves the heart and travels down the chest into the abdomen. Large, saccular aneurysms are very common in the portion of the aorta located in the abdomen and in the arteries that supply blood to the legs.

People with aneurysms less than six centimeters in diameter rarely suffer from rupture of the weakened vessel wall. However, over 50 percent of the aneurysms larger than six centimeters in diameter will rupture within 10 years.

Berry aneurysms within the brain are usually very small because the vessels there are so small. Unfortunately, when they do rupture, they can cause very serious complications, and even death.

Dissecting aneurysms form suddenly, within minutes, and can have disastrous results. In fact, if a dissecting aortic aneurysm is not treated immediately, the risk of death is very great. Many doctors believe that over 90 percent of the cases of dissecting aneurysm are directly related to high blood pressure.

Once aneurysms form in blood vessels, they will never go away. Fortunately, modern medicine allows skilled vascular surgeons to surgically remove the damaged portions of the blood vessels to avoid the dangerous chance of the aneurysm bursting. Much simpler, and much less risky, is avoiding the development of aneurysms by avoiding or appropriately managing high blood pressure.

Loss of vision

High blood pressure also forces the small blood vessels in the eyes to thicken and narrow. If the capillaries in the eyes begin to deteriorate due to lack of blood, tunnel vision or blindness can result.

The relationship between uncontrolled high blood pressure and loss of vision has been verified. Doctors are now aware of the importance of regular eye checkups when treating people with elevated blood pressure.

Memory loss

High blood pressure is something that many people would like to forget. According to some recent scientific studies, high blood pressure will allow you to do just that, forget.

James A. Blumenthal, a psychologist at Duke University Medical Center in Durham, North Carolina, and a group of researchers recruited 100 people between the ages of 29 to 59 years to test the effects of high blood pressure on memory. Of the 100 volunteers, 68 of them had blood pressure between 140/90 and 180/105 mm Hg. The remaining volunteers had blood pressure levels around 110/70 mm Hg.

All of the study participants completed eight tests that involved different aspects of memory. After everyone took the tests, the researchers discovered that the people who suffered from high blood pressure did not perform as well in certain areas of the test.

The researchers are still not certain whether this memory loss will show up in other areas of daily living.

3 ║ Are You At Risk?

Scientists estimate that one out of every four people in the United States has high blood pressure. And out of those people who have high blood pressure, 90 to 95 percent of them are suffering from essential hypertension, high blood pressure with no known, specific cause.

Although scientists have not yet found the specific causes of essential hypertension, they have learned that some factors can increase a person's risk of developing hypertension.

Some of the risk factors that seem to predispose a person to developing essential high blood pressure cannot be avoided or changed.

For example, scientists have found that being male, African-American or elderly or having a family history of hypertension are all risk factors for developing high blood pressure. These are traits that no one can change.

The good news, however, is that many of the other risk factors associated with high blood pressure can be changed or avoided. Avoiding those risk factors gives people the opportunity to lower their risk of ever developing high blood pressure.

Some of the risk factors that can be avoided include obesity, high-salt diets, high-fat diets, lack of exercise, smoking and drinking too much alcohol.

The rest of this chapter will give you a thorough explanation of the risk factors for high blood pressure that can't be changed.

Family history

Doctors and scientists who are experts in the field of blood pressure have found that a tendency to develop high blood pressure seems to run in families.

That means that if your parents or other close blood relatives have high blood pressure, you have a greater chance of developing high blood pressure compared with someone whose close blood relatives have normal blood pressure. And it seems that the more relatives you have who suffer from high blood pressure, the greater your risk of developing high blood pressure.

Children who have one parent with high blood pressure have a greater chance of developing the disease than children with no family history of high blood pressure, but when both parents have high blood pressure, the odds are even greater.

Check out your family's health history. Finding a history of high blood pressure in your immediate family does not mean that you will definitely develop high blood pressure, but you do have an increased risk.

Some good news for people with family histories of high blood pressure is that a new genetic screening test might eventually make it possible to identify people at risk for high blood pressure before clinical signs of disease appear. Researchers in California and Michigan have discovered genetic markers which signal increased risk for high blood pressure and atherosclerosis (hardening of the arteries).

Dr. Phillipe Frossard, project director at California Biotechnology, has identified 14 markers for hypertension so far, focusing on genes involved with regulating blood pressure.

At Cornell University Medical Center, a link between the markers and high blood pressure is being studied in 70 people with high blood pressure and 30 people with normal blood pressure levels.

Frossard believes that genetic testing to predict high blood pressure in people with no symptoms will become routine within the next few years.

Not only will accurate prediction of high blood pressure and atherosclerosis enable doctors to truly practice preventative medicine, Frossard says, but also the prescribed treatment will be more effective if the doctor knows what genetic defect is causing the problem.

In separate research, Dr. Brian Robinson at St. George's Hospital in London found that a basic hereditary cell defect might be the cause of high blood pressure in about half of the people who develop it.

He found that some people with high blood pressure have an abnormal reaction to calcium in their muscle cells. Robinson hopes to be able to identify who has these cell defects and how their blood pressure can be properly regulated.

If you have a family history of high blood pressure, you should pay special attention to the risk factors that you can control, such as body weight, diet and exercise habits.

Race

As many as 50 million people in the United States are

coping with high blood pressure every day. And that 50 million is made up of more African-Americans than white Americans.

Researchers are not sure what causes the difference, but high blood pressure is usually more severe, starts earlier in life, and usually leads to more severe complications in African-Americans.

For example, African-Americans have about two times more strokes, 10 to 18 times more kidney failure and three to five times more heart failure related to high blood pressure compared with white Americans. High blood pressure and its related diseases are among the major causes of death among African-Americans.

In fact, as many as 30 percent of all deaths in black men with high blood pressure and 20 percent of all deaths in black women with high blood pressure are directly related to high blood pressure.

There also is a high prevalence of obesity, cigarette smoking, diabetes and salt-sensitivity among African-Americans. These additional risk factors for high blood pressure add to the seriousness of the situation.

Because of their increased risk from race alone, it becomes particularly important for African-Americans to avoid as many risk factors as possible.

One theory that attempts to explain racial differences in rates of high blood pressure has to do with where our ancestors came from.

People with ancestors from the tropics, where salt is often lacking and fluid loss from perspiration is high, are more likely to have a salt retention gene than people whose ancestral home was outside the tropics. This salt retention gene, when it is present in any race, causes the body to retain fluids and increase blood pressure.

Other theories blame socioeconomic factors, lack of access to medical care and dietary influences for the higher rates of high blood pressure among African-Americans. However, some scientists believe that the difference rests on a more biological cause.

One of the scientists who is trying to prove biological differences, David Calhoun, M.D., assistant professor of medicine at the University of Alabama at Birmingham, recently conducted a study of black and white Americans and how they respond to stress.

The study focuses on the response of the sympathetic nervous system, the part of the central nervous system that controls blood pressure and heart rate. The sympathetic nervous system reacts to stress or danger by speeding the heart rate and increasing blood pressure, the well-known "fight or flight" reaction

Over time, this reaction to stress seems to cause wear and tear on the blood vessels and heart, which is associated with high blood pressure, heart disease and strokes.

The team of researchers recruited volunteers to participate in the study and divided them into four separate groups: African-Americans with and without family histories of high blood pressure and white Americans with and without family histories of high blood pressure.

In order to measure how the body and blood pressure react to stress, Dr. Calhoun and his colleagues used the "cold stress test" in which the volunteers in the study placed one hand in ice-cold water for two to three minutes while the researchers measured their nerve impulses.

The researchers discovered that African-Americans with family histories of high blood pressure had the greatest response to the stress of the cold water.

This group had the highest rise in heart rates and blood

pressures compared with the other three groups.

In addition, the researchers found that the group of African-Americans without a family history of high blood pressure had stress responses (heart rate and blood pressure changes) that were generally higher than the responses in both groups of white volunteers.

The researchers warn that these results do not mean that African-Americans have greater responses to stress in general.

However, the results are intriguing enough to encourage the scientists to look further into how stress might influence blood pressure among white and black people.

A separate team of scientists from the University of Medicine and Dentistry of New Jersey — New Jersey Medical School in Newark think that the mineral calcium might be involved in the higher rate of high blood pressure among African-Americans.

Calcium is an important component of the muscle cells throughout the body, and when the level of calcium in the muscle cells is high, the muscle contracts. (One cause of high levels of calcium in your cells is not getting enough calcium in your diet. See Chapter 12, "The Calcium Advantage," for more information.)

When the muscles in the blood vessel walls contract, blood pressure in those vessels goes up. The New Jersey researchers think that black and white people might process calcium differently, causing the difference in the rates of high blood pressure.

Their studies seem to indicate that this calcium theory is legitimate. However, the researchers stress that calcium metabolism is just one portion of a larger puzzle. Factors such as obesity, family history and diet are other components that are equally important in solving the blood pressure puzzle.

The following chart shows the estimated rates of high blood pressure in black and white Americans, based on the final report of the 1984 Joint National Committee on Detection, Evaluation and Treatment of High Blood Pressure.

Rate of High Blood Pressure in Black and White Americans

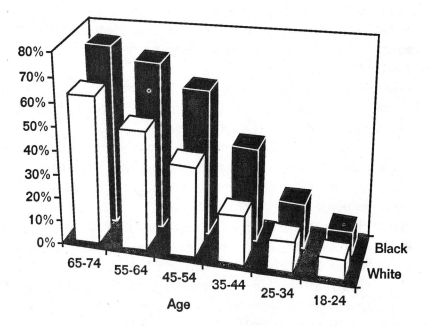

Gender

When people think about high blood pressure and who gets it, most folks envision a middle-aged, overweight man who eats too much, drinks too much, smokes too much and doesn't exercise enough.

And although it is true that men fitting that description are strong candidates for developing high blood pressure, anyone can have high blood pressure.

Just as family history and racial background influence a person's risk of developing high blood pressure, gender is another unchangeable risk factor for high blood pressure.

Men, just due to the nature of their makeup, have a greater risk of developing high blood pressure than women, up to a certain point, that is.

From adolescence through age 54, men have a much greater risk of developing high blood pressure compared with women of the same age.

However, scientists have recently discovered that women past the age of 54 have a greater incidence of high blood pressure than men of the same age.

Apparently, the female hormone estrogen seems to have a protective effect against heart disease and high blood pressure. Women enjoy this fringe benefit from their natural hormones until the age of menopause.

In addition to hormones influencing the risk of high blood pressure in women, a group of scientists from the Long Island Medical Center in New York also suspect that some women might inherit a particular gene that could predispose them to developing high blood pressure.

The scientists are calling this gene the human estrogen receptor (ER) gene.

It seems that a variant or mutant form of the ER gene might be responsible for increasing a woman's chances of developing high blood pressure.

In an effort to shed more light on their gene theory, the New York researchers gathered 88 women who volunteered to be tested for the variant ER gene.

Through the use of a complicated procedure (known as allele-specific oligonucleotide hybridization) the scientists were able to isolate the individual genes from the blood samples given by the volunteers.

After careful research, they discovered that the women who had the normal form of the gene experienced high blood pressure at an incidence similar to the general population (around 12 to 32 percent).

However, the women who tested positive for the variant ER gene had an alarming 48 percent incidence of high blood pressure.

The scientists suspect that the variant ER gene is related to the marked difference in incidence of high blood pressure among the 88 volunteers.

Although women experience an increased risk of developing high blood pressure after the age of 54, overall, men still have a greater risk of high blood pressure.

In fact, an estimated 33 percent of men between the ages of 18 and 74 suffer from high blood pressure, whereas only 27 percent of women in that same age category suffer from high blood pressure.

Age

The older a person is, the more likely he is to develop high blood pressure. But that doesn't mean that children, teens and young adults don't have high blood pressure.

Admittedly, high blood pressure is much more common in older adults.

Some sources suggest that around 60 percent of all adults over the age of 65 suffer from high blood pressure. However, only 21 percent of men aged 25 to 34 and 20 percent of women aged 35 to 44 suffer from high blood pressure.

The following chart illustrates the prevalence of hypertension in different age groups:

Prevalence of Hypertension* By Age

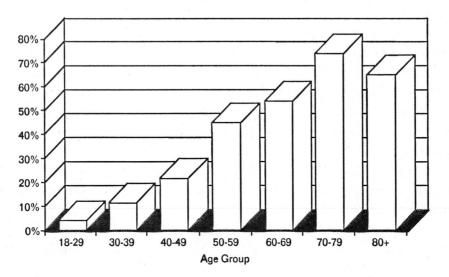

*   Hypertension defined as the average of three blood pressure measurements greater than or equal to 140/90 mm Hg on a single occasion or reported taking of antihypertensive medication, among noninstitutionalized civilian adults, 1988-91

Children and teens

Even though high blood pressure is usually a disease of older Americans, high blood pressure in children and teens must not be overlooked.

Dr. Andrew G. Aronfy, a Fellow of the American Academy of Pediatrics (F.A.A.P.), writes: "Until about 10 to 15 years ago, most pediatricians did not own a blood pressure cuff. In those days, the practice of pediatrics stopped at puberty, and blood pressure measurements were not part of a routine physical examination.

"During the past decade all that has changed. Other doctors started telling pediatricians that many young adults had high blood pressure, and they wondered when it started. When they asked pediatricians for blood pressure readings on their former patients, most pediatricians were embarrassed to confess they had never checked it.

"Secondly, new discoveries about high blood pressure and coronary artery disease revealed that some cases may be strongly influenced by heredity. The tendency toward these diseases can be detected even in early childhood with high blood pressure readings and relatively simple blood tests, such as serum cholesterol and triglycerides.

If a hereditary pattern seems to be developing, proper diet, exercise and lifestyle throughout the child's life may help reduce the inherited dangers.

"The most common cause of high blood pressure in children is kidney disease. (This is known as 'secondary hypertension.') A high blood pressure reading in a child may be a 'tip-off' that the child needs to be referred to an expert in nephrology to determine if kidney disease is present.

"There are other causes of high blood pressure in children. They are rare, and they are usually related to abnormal hormone production which can be caused by a tumor.

"For all these reasons, all children should have their blood pressure routinely checked from the time they are about 3 years old. If there is a history of high blood pressure or heart disease in the family, children should also have regular appropriate blood tests."

The following chart lists normal blood pressure readings for children ages 3 to 18 according to the Report of the Second Task Force on Blood Pressure Control in Children — 1987.

To be diagnosed with high blood pressure, your child would have to get a higher-than-normal reading on three separate occasions. Only four points higher than normal may put a young child in the "significant hypertension" category.

Approximate Normal Blood Pressure Readings in the Young

If Age Is	Normal Reading is Approximately
3 – 5 years	108/70 or less
6 – 9 years	114/74 or less
10 – 12 years	122/78 or less
13 – 15 years	130/80 or less
16 – 18 years	136/84 or less

As Dr. Aronfy stated, many cases of significant or severe childhood hypertension have identifiable, underlying causes, such as kidney disease. When these underlying illnesses or conditions are treated and eliminated, the secondary high blood pressure usually resolves.

The higher the blood pressure reading and the younger the child, the greater the possibility that an underlying condition is causing the elevated blood pressure.

In teens, elevated blood pressure values might signal the use of alcohol, cocaine, crack or other addictive substances. Diet pills, cold medicines and birth control pills also can elevate blood pressure in teens and adults.

Discontinuation of the medications (or alcohol and drugs) usually results in the blood pressure levels returning to normal.

Children and teens, on the other hand, who only have slight or occasional elevations of blood pressure might be at risk for future heart and blood vessel diseases, and they are more likely to suffer from high blood pressure and heart disease as adults.

In fact, one study conducted at the Department of Epidemiology at the University of Pittsburgh examined the changes and causes of blood pressure in about 200 teen-agers beginning around the year 1957.

The researchers followed the changes in these men and women for 30 years, and they found that most of the study participants who had high blood pressure as teens also suffered from it as adults.

Similarly, they discovered that most of the subjects who had healthy blood pressure readings in high school managed to maintain a healthy reading, even 30 years later (only 18 percent of the study participants developed high blood pressure).

The mild or occasional elevations of blood pressure seen in children and teens are often strongly linked to hereditary causes, with evidence of other cases of high blood pressure found within the family.

For accurate readings, children usually require a smaller blood pressure cuff. The widest cuff that will give an accurate reading will comfortably encircle the arm without extending below the elbow.

If you are monitoring your family's blood pressure at home and have questions about the size cuff you are using on your children, you can check with your doctor or other health care provider to see if you need a smaller cuff for more accurate measurements.

The elderly

Some studies indicate that approximately 60 percent of

people over the age of 65 have high blood pressure. In this group, as in other age groups, high blood pressure is a well-established and significant risk factor for the development of cardiovascular disease, congestive heart failure, kidney disease and stroke.

The diagnosis and treatment of high blood pressure are more complicated in older adults because many of them are suffering from other illnesses (such as diabetes, arthritis, osteoporosis and gout).

Additionally, many senior adults are taking different medications for various other illnesses, and the addition of high blood pressure medications (antihypertensives), or even simple dietary changes to help lower their blood pressures, could have dramatic effects on their well-being. Elderly people are more sensitive to the effects of dietary changes and medications than younger people.

For example, a 50-milligram antihypertensive tablet might lower a young person's blood pressure only a few points, whereas that same 50-milligram dose could drop an elderly person's blood pressure to dangerously low levels. This makes it difficult to treat high blood pressure aggressively in the elderly.

Authorities on heart and artery disease only recently began to acknowledge the unique aspects of high blood pressure in the older population and, as is often the case with such changes of direction in medicine, there is debate among medical leaders on how to treat the disorder.

According to Dr. W. McFate Smith, Professor of Epidemiology, University of California School of Public Health, Berkeley, mild high blood pressure in the elderly has been virtually ignored.

Many authorities believed that high blood pressure was a physiological consequence of aging which was necessary to carry nutrients and oxygen to vital organs like the brain. Lowering blood pressure could be counterproductive, they argued. A more recent concern was the possible adverse effects of drug treatment.

In contrast to these views, scientific evidence suggests high blood pressure is a significant risk factor for the elderly.

Even a nominal rise in blood pressure in the elderly will lead to a higher occurrence of strokes, scientists believe.

It took some time for researchers to establish the benefits of effective therapy among the elderly.

The early literature, which studied stroke survivors and attempted to evaluate the influence of high blood pressure on stroke recurrence, provided inconsistent and conflicting information on the value of therapy, Dr. Smith noted.

However, he pointed out, well-controlled clinical trials published in the last decade without exception show a reduction in the risk of stroke and suggest reduction in death rates because of high blood pressure therapy.

Dr. Abrams, a researcher in the area of blood pressure and the elderly, says both the effects of aging and high blood pressure on the cardiovascular system and the kidneys should be taken into account when prescribing treatment.

According to Dr. Abrams, the major age-related heart and artery changes are stiffening of the arterial system (hardening of the arteries) which can lead to a progressive rise in systolic blood pressure.

This falsely elevated blood pressure measurement is often referred to as "pseudohypertension." In this condition, the blood pressure measurement is falsely elevated because the brachial artery is so rigid from the effects of atherosclerosis (hardening of the arteries) that it cannot be compressed by the blood pressure cuff.

This condition can be confirmed when you can feel the radial artery (in the wrist) even though the blood pressure cuff is inflated to pressures high enough to stop the blood flow.

In addition to putting elderly people at risk for getting antihypertensive medications unnecessarily, this atherosclerotic condition can result in thickening of the muscle in the wall of the heart, a condition known as "ventricular hypertrophy" (enlarged heart), frequently seen in old age.

Along with family history, racial background and gender, the aging process is one of those unchangeable risk factors associated with high blood pressure.

The older you get, the greater your chances of developing high blood pressure. Although no one can change that fact, young and older people alike can eliminate some of the other changeable risk factors associated with high blood pressure.

4 | Getting It Checked

If you have normal blood pressure (less than 130/85), you should have your blood pressure measured once every two years, although once every year is better.

On the other hand, if your blood pressure is in the high normal range (130/85 to 139/89), you should have it checked at least once every year.

If you have one or more risk factors for high blood pressure, many doctors recommend that you have your blood pressure checked every six months, even if your blood pressure is currently normal.

Those risk factors include a family history of high blood pressure, obesity, high cholesterol, high triglycerides, sedentary lifestyle, African-American race, male sex, high-salt diet, high-fat diet and use of birth control pills and other medications that can raise blood pressure.

Any one of these risk factors should prompt you to write a reminder on the calendar to have your blood pressure checked at least every six months.

Blood pressure checks every six months are sufficient for people who do not have high blood pressure.

However, those people who have high blood pressure need to follow a more rigorous schedule of follow-up blood pressure checks. Refer to the chart in Chapter 1 for recommendations on how quickly you should visit a doctor after a high blood pressure reading.

If you are already seeing a doctor for diagnosed high blood pressure, disregard the chart's recommendations and follow your doctor's advice about follow-up visits.

Everyone, including teen-agers and children, should be tested for high blood pressure, with regular follow-up measurements. Remember: The only way to detect high blood pressure is to measure it.

Who should take your blood pressure?

Many people are ready and willing to have their blood pressure checked regularly, but they are uncertain about where to go to have it measured.

If you visit your doctor a few times each year, you shouldn't have any trouble monitoring your blood pressure. Most doctors will check your blood pressure at every office visit.

Many doctors even encourage their patients to stop by the office for blood pressure measurements anytime during office hours without having to make an appointment. The nurse can take your blood pressure and record it on your chart.

However, not everyone has a family doctor or goes to a doctor regularly. Fortunately, you don't need to go to a doctor's office every time you want to measure your blood pressure.

Many sports centers, pharmacies and supermarkets have blood pressure monitoring machines that you can use free of charge. It only takes a minute or two to get your blood pressure reading.

Although these devices might not be quite as accurate as the blood pressure cuff at your doctor's office, they work fine for a rough estimate. Try one the next time you visit your pharmacy or supermarket.

In addition to supermarkets and pharmacies, many fire stations have personnel and equipment for measuring blood pressure. The firemen or emergency medical technicians are usually more than happy to measure your blood pressure. In fact, some fire stations actually advertise this service to the public and encourage anyone to stop by for a quick check.

County health departments also are perfect places for regular blood pressure measurements for anyone in the county. These services are usually free of charge for county residents.

People with busy schedules or strange work shifts often find it difficult to make special trips for blood pressure readings. In those cases, it might be easier or more practical to purchase a blood pressure device to use at home.

Your doctor or pharmacist can tell you where you can buy a standard sphygmomanometer for home blood pressure measurements.

Most medical supply stores even carry electronic blood pressure devices. These electronic measuring devices are usually battery operated and are a bit easier to operate than the standard sphygmomanometers.

With electronic devices, you don't have to inflate and deflate the cuff and try to listen with the stethoscope all at the same time.

The machine does all that for you. Either way, standard or electronic, home devices allow the convenience of quick and frequent blood pressure checks without ever having to leave your home.

At the doctor's office

Before your doctor examines you for any reason, he will take a thorough medical history. The doctor or nurse might ask you a list of questions or you might be asked to fill out a detailed questionnaire. Either way, a good medical history includes the following topics:

- ☐ Family history of high blood pressure, heart disease, heart attacks, strokes, blood vessel diseases, diabetes and cholesterol problems
- ☐ Symptoms that you have experienced (such as headaches, dizziness, shortness of breath, chest pain) that might suggest high blood pressure, heart disease, kidney disease or diabetes
- ☐ High blood pressure during a particularly tense time or during pregnancy
- ☐ Weight gain, smoking habits, drinking habits and exercise habits
- ☐ Overview of your diet, such as salt intake and fat and cholesterol intake
- ☐ Extra factors that might influence your blood pressure and health, such as stressful family or job situations
- ☐ Medications (such as blood pressure medication, steroids, birth control pills) you are currently using, including over-the-counter drugs (such as appetite suppressants, aspirin, cold medications, nasal decongestants)

If your doctor doesn't ask you some of these questions, feel free to volunteer the information. It will help him design a better health plan for you.

After your doctor has a full medical history, he'll begin the exam. Listed below are some techniques for taking blood pressure measurements. The guidelines listed below are recommended by the Joint National Committee on Detection, Evaluation and Treatment of High Blood Pressure. Following these guidelines will provide the most accurate measurement of your blood pressure:

> ➤ Sit in a comfortable position and support your arm on a table or desktop at heart level. Roll up your sleeve so your arm is bare.
> ➤ Don't have caffeine (coffee, soft drinks) or smoke cigarettes within 30 minutes of the measurement.
> ➤ Sit quietly for about five minutes before your blood pressure is measured.

The doctor or other health care worker taking your blood pressure should use an appropriately sized cuff. The cuff should completely encircle the arm.

Another measurement should be taken two minutes after the first one, and the two values averaged together. However, if those two measurements differ by more than 5 mm Hg, additional readings are necessary.

Based on your medical history, the doctor might measure your blood pressure as you lie down, stand and sit. The doctor also might take two measurements, one on each arm. These different positions provide more information that the doctor might need in special cases.

At home

Because of the false elevation in blood pressure readings attributed to anxiety in the doctor's office, many doctors are now encouraging their patients with high blood pressure to monitor their own levels and record them at home.

They are using home monitoring for people who have not actually been diagnosed with high blood pressure, but who might be borderline hypertensive (high-normal blood pressure, according to the new classifications).

After recording their own blood pressure values several times a day for a few weeks, the patients bring their blood pressure diary to each checkup.

This way, the doctor can evaluate the blood pressure based on the normal daily blood pressure, rather than on an inflated blood pressure reading taken during a stressful visit to the doctor's office.

In most cases, blood pressure readings are higher in the doctor's office than they are at home. Doctors at the New York Hospital — Cornell University Medical College conclude that home readings are lower and more accurate and reflect the overall level of blood pressure more reliably than office readings.

And many doctors feel that home monitoring can provide more useful information simply because the pressures are recorded more frequently at home.

A home blood pressure diary might contain around 30 readings over a two-week period, whereas there might only be three or four measurements if the person had to stop by the office for measurements over the same two-week period.

James Lynch, director of the Psychophysiological Clinic at the University of Maryland Medical School, urges people to measure their blood pressure levels at home, at work and during different stressful situations.

All readings should be recorded with any unusual circumstances noted. Knowing your blood pressure levels helps you learn your own reactions to stress and learn which everyday activities increase your blood pressure.

Home monitoring itself can be a factor in lowering your blood pressure. A study in Seattle showed blood pressure levels lowered by 10 mm Hg or more in 43 percent of people when they monitored their blood pressure levels at home.

The researchers suspect that people who are measuring their blood pressures at home become more accustomed to regular blood pressure monitoring and react to it with less stress.

The researchers also believe that regular monitoring increases awareness of blood pressure. This can help people with high blood pressure remember they have a serious medical problem and make lifestyle changes to improve their health.

Home monitoring techniques

If you have your own sphygmomanometer, follow the techniques listed below. All sphygmomanometers will come with instructions, but here are a few tips you can use no matter what type you buy:

1 Sit down next to a table. The tabletop should be at the level of your heart.

2 Using either arm, roll your sleeve up well above the elbow. Make sure the rolled sleeve is not tight.

3 Rest your arm on the table with the palm facing up and your hand relaxed.

4 Position the deflated cuff in the middle of the upper arm (over the biceps). This will cover the brachial artery. Secure the cuff snugly on the arm with the Velcro on the cuff. Be sure to use a cuff that will completely encircle your arm.

5 Feel for the radial pulse in your wrist. The radial pulse is located on the thumb side of the wrist, right above where the wrist actually bends.

6 After finding your radial pulse, inflate the blood pressure cuff using the bulb. Keep inflating until you can no longer feel the radial pulse. The cuff will feel very tight on your arm, but it should not be painful. Notice the measurement on the mercury gauge at this point. That measurement will be in the general vicinity of the systolic blood pressure.

7 Rapidly deflate the cuff completely without taking further measurements. Wait about 1 to 2 minutes before proceeding.

8 After waiting a few minutes, place the head of the stethoscope over the brachial artery just above the crook of the elbow, making sure the stethoscope isn't rubbing against the cuff.

9 Inflate the cuff again to a point where the needle on the mercury gauge is about 30 mm Hg above the point where you lost the radial pulse earlier.

10 Now, slowly begin releasing the air in the cuff while listening to the blood flow in the artery through the stethoscope. The pressure should drop at the rate of 2 to 3 mm Hg per second. If you deflate much faster or slower than this, you will not get an accurate reading.

11 When the air pressure in the cuff is slightly lower than the blood pressure in the artery, the blood will begin to flow through the artery again. This will sound like a faint, clear tapping. As soon as you hear that tap-

ping noise, record the pressure on the mercury gauge.
This is your systolic pressure.

12 The tapping noise will get louder and more intense as
you continue to let the air escape from the cuff. Then
the sounds will become fainter and eventually completely disappear. When the sounds completely disappear, record the measurement on the mercury gauge.
This is your diastolic pressure.

13 After you have recorded your diastolic pressure, rapidly deflate the cuff the rest of the way until the cuff
is empty.

14 Record the blood pressure with the first number (systolic pressure) written over the second number (diastolic number). For example, 125/85.

15 Wait a few minutes, then repeat the process beginning with step 9. Average the two systolic numbers
together, then average the two diastolic numbers together. This new averaged number is your blood pressure.

If you are having difficulty taking your blood pressure,
ask a health care professional to help you with your technique. Practice taking someone else's blood pressure and soon
you'll feel more comfortable taking your own.

Causes of inaccurate readings

Measuring blood pressure is a simple process, but you
must be sure your reading is accurate. False high readings
can lead to unnecessary drug treatment, and false low readings can result in delays in treatment.

In order to avoid making mistakes in taking blood pressure measurements, you need to be aware of the most common errors.

Many cases of inaccurate blood pressure measurements can be blamed on the equipment used to take the measurement: the sphygmomanometer and the stethoscope.

One of the most common equipment errors involves the size of the blood pressure cuff. Cuffs that are too large for the arm will give a false low reading, and cuffs that are too small will falsely elevate the reading.

In fact, in a recent study on blood pressure readings, doctors found that cuffs that were too small for the subjects' arms produced diastolic blood pressure readings (the bottom number) that averaged 10 points higher than the true reading from a properly sized cuff. Those results often lead to inappropriate medical treatment.

Although the majority of adults can use the regular blood pressure cuff and get an accurate reading, children and obese adults usually need special cuffs to ensure proper measurements.

The American Heart Association recommends that the bladder of the blood pressure cuff used, when turned lengthwise, should encircle 40 percent of the subject's arm. In other words, the short-length side of the rectangular-shaped cuff should almost go halfway around the arm.

If it covers more than half the arm, the cuff is too large. Likewise, if it does not cover 40 percent of the arm, the cuff is too small.

Inaccurate blood pressure measurements from incorrectly sized cuffs occur most frequently in overweight adults with large arms rather than in children.

This is because most children have their blood pressure measured in pediatric offices, which are equipped with child-sized cuffs.

However, many doctors' offices are not equipped with blood pressure cuffs that are big enough for large or overweight adults. These people generally need to use a special cuff which is over 6 inches wide.

Other blood pressure equipment errors can result from using damaged equipment. For example, it is important that the air vents at the top of the mercury column be open and unobstructed for the gauge to work correctly.

Also, the needle in the mercury gauge must settle at the zero mark on the gauge before each pressure measurement. If the needle is above or below zero before taking a measurement, the reading will be incorrect. Leaking equipment and uncalibrated gauges also can produce inaccurate blood pressure readings.

Fortunately, most health care organizations have written policies concerning regular assessment and maintenance of mercury sphygmomanometers. If you have purchased your own equipment, contact the manufacturer if you have any problem with the equipment or want periodic maintenance checks.

The stethoscope also can contribute to inaccurate blood pressure measurements. For example, the size of the rubber tubing on the stethoscope can influence the measurements.

Although the length of the tubing (from the ear pieces to the bell) does not affect the sounds, using narrow tubing instead of larger tubing will result in better sound transmission so you can hear the lower frequency sounds more easily.

Any stethoscope used for measuring blood pressure should have a bell-shaped portion instead of just a flat-surfaced diaphragm.

Using the bell portion of the stethoscope (rather than the flat diaphragm side) will yield more accurate results. The bell portion allows you to pick up low frequencies more eas-ily.

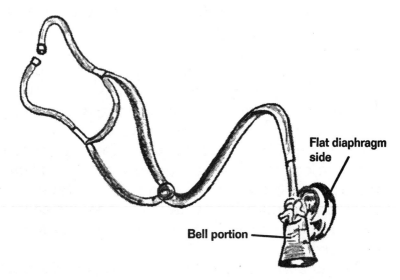

In addition to using the correct side of the stethoscope, it is equally important to operate the stethoscope correctly. If the stethoscope is pressed into the arm with too much force, the diastolic blood pressure reading can be as much as 10 percent too high. For an accurate reading, the stethoscope needs to be pressed against the artery with firm, but gentle, pressure.

Raising your arm above the level of your heart while measuring your blood pressure will often result in a reading that is lower than the true measurement.

In the same way, letting the arm hang down at your side can result in a false low reading due to the forces of gravity at work.

Your arm should be supported on a table. If you hold your arm out straight, muscle contractions can falsely elevate your blood pressure.

Blood pressure measurements also vary greatly based on

whether you are standing, sitting or lying down. The most accurate way to measure blood pressure is for you to sit down with your arm resting comfortably on a table that is level with your heart.

Physical exercise also can affect your blood pressure levels. Exercising right before a blood pressure measurement (like climbing the steps to the doctor's office) will yield a false high measurement.

You should always sit down and rest quietly for at least five minutes before having your blood pressure measured. This will allow your blood pressure to return to the level that is most representative of your blood pressure under normal circumstances.

Your immediate environment can influence your blood pressure reading, too. For example, hot or cold temperatures can directly affect blood pressure.

If you are hot and sweaty, your blood pressure reading will be lower than usual due to your blood vessels dilating in response to the heat. Cold weather, on the other hand, will cause your blood vessels to constrict, which can elevate your blood pressure.

The time of day also seems to affect blood pressure levels. Due to the body's natural circadian rhythms, most people tend to have higher blood pressure early in the day compared to late afternoon and evening. An early morning elevated reading might not be an accurate picture of your true blood pressure.

Smoking and drinking caffeinated drinks within 30 minutes of a blood pressure measurement might result in a false high reading. Stress, pain, anxiety and discomfort can all result in false elevations of blood pressure.

Medications you are taking can alter blood pressure readings. Diet pills, cold medicines and birth control pills are among the most common offenders. And don't talk while having your blood pressure measured. This can sometimes result in false high readings.

Blocked arteries or other problems in the arm (especially among the elderly) may cause inaccurate blood pressure readings. In fact, Dr. Frank H. Messerli, a blood pressure specialist, reports that hardening of the arteries in the elderly often causes high, inaccurate blood pressure readings.

Dr. Messerli discovered that people over 65 with hardened arteries had higher blood pressure when monitored with a blood pressure cuff rather than using a needle inside the arteries.

The reason is because more pressure has to be exerted in the cuff to temporarily stop blood flow in the hardened, pipe-like brachial arteries.

For an accurate diagnosis of mild high blood pressure in the elderly with possible hardened vessels, blood pressure measurements should be taken in both arms and both readings should be recorded, stating which arm was used for each measurement.

Then, if the readings are similar, the right arm can be used for future monitoring. Also, take three or four separate readings over as long as six months to get a more accurate picture of your true blood pressure.

Interestingly, the position of your sleeves does not seem to affect the blood pressure reading. A recent study at Duke University showed that blood pressure measurements were similar whether taken on bare skin or through clothing.

However, most people find it easier to position the cuff on the upper arm and the stethoscope over the artery if the sleeve is rolled up out of the way.

The final source of blood pressure measurement errors is the person operating the equipment. If the operator has inadequate knowledge about how to take an accurate blood pressure reading or uses an improper or sloppy technique, inaccurate measurements will probably occur.

Occasionally, health care workers who are running behind schedule will take blood pressure readings too hastily to be accurate. A hurried, improper technique almost always yields false results.

Being familiar with these common mistakes will help you adjust your technique and limit the errors you might make while taking your own blood pressure.

'White coat hypertension'

There are times when health care workers follow every guideline for taking blood pressure measurements without making a single error and still come out with inaccurate readings.

Many people who have been diagnosed with high blood pressure have actually been wrongly diagnosed. Their blood pressure was indeed elevated when the health care worker took it, but that elevated blood pressure was not their true blood pressure.

Their true blood pressure was much lower than the measurement the doctor got — a phenomenon known as white coat hypertension.

In a recent study, researchers from Canada found that one out of every four people who seemed to have high blood pressure had a falsely elevated reading.

Dr. Nicholas Birkett, the study's chief researcher, speculates that those people experienced white coat hypertension, an artificial elevation of blood pressure that can be caused by anxiety about being in a doctor's office, clinic or hospital. This anxiety caused their blood pressure to be unusually high during the doctor's visit, sometimes without the people even realizing their own anxiety.

However, when blood pressure was taken twice more on two separate occasions in the Canadian study, the people were found to have normal blood pressure levels.

Dr. Birkett's findings about white coat hypertension have been confirmed by investigators at New York Hospital - Cornell University Medical Center.

These Cornell researchers compared blood pressure measurements obtained by doctors with readings taken by an automatic 24-hour arm recorder which volunteers wore during the day.

For people with high blood pressure and those with normal blood pressure, the highest blood pressure recorded was the one taken by the doctor — the person with the white coat.

Blood pressure levels taken by a nurse were lower, and the levels recorded on the automatic 24-hour recorder worn at home were even lower.

Dr. Jeffrey H. Ferguson, clinical instructor in family medicine at Indiana University School of Medicine, came up with similar results in a separate study. He and a team of researchers gathered 60 volunteers for a comparison study of blood pressure measurements taken in the doctor's office with those taken from a 24-hour blood pressure monitoring device.

Of the 60 volunteers in the study, 17 had normal blood pressures and 43 were already taking medications for high blood pressure.

After measuring the volunteers' blood pressures several times in the doctor's office and recording the blood pressures measured by the continuous 24-hour monitor, the researchers found that some people get nervous and anxious enough at the doctor's office to cause a rise in their blood pressure levels.

Among the 17 volunteers without a history of high blood pressure, 12 demonstrated elevated blood pressures when the measurements were performed in the doctor's office. However, only three were found to have occasional episodes of high blood pressure on the 24-hour monitoring devices.

Similarly, among the 43 volunteers with histories of high blood pressure, the researchers found that as many as 36 had higher blood pressure readings in the doctor's office compared with the readings from the 24-hour blood pressure monitor.

Dr. Ferguson suggests that the "white coat" phenomenon can affect anyone — young or old, male or female, with or without a prior history of high blood pressure.

Researchers from the Cornell University Medical Center suggest that women are most likely to be misdiagnosed as having high blood pressure when their levels are taken by a male doctor.

Apparently, blood pressure levels are more accurate when taken by a technician instead of a doctor, but the Cornell researchers aren't sure why.

Dr. Thomas G. Pickering, one of the researchers, suggests that the doctor is seen as more of an authority figure and causes more anxiety than a technician.

The researchers conclude that many women, especially younger women, who are diagnosed with high blood pressure are misdiagnosed. They really have normal blood pressure levels. Having a woman doctor or technician take the blood pressure measurement can give a more accurate reading.

Dr. Lawrence Krakoff, of the Mount Sinai Medical Center, often uses ambulatory 24-hour blood pressure monitors which can be worn throughout the day to provide accurate readouts under different conditions, like working, sleeping and resting.

Fifty percent of his patients with mild high blood pressure have lower blood pressure levels when an ambulatory 24-hour blood pressure monitor is used, Dr. Krakoff explains.

5 ‖ Benefits of Weight Loss

When you weigh too much, you're used to hearing every health problem you have blamed on the extra pounds you carry. Go to the doctor with a backache, he'll tell you to lose weight. Having stomach pains? The doctor says, "Lose weight." Diabetes? Heart disease? Kidney stones? "Lose weight." "Lose weight." "Lose weight."

You may be tired of hearing it, but here we are again. Being overweight is probably the main cause of high blood pressure. The heavier you are, the higher your blood pressure will be.

If you're determined to get your weight under control, here are some encouraging numbers to get you motivated:

❑ A recent scientific study showed that people with Stage 1 (mild) high blood pressure (140-159 over 90-99) who lost just 10 pounds were able to stop taking medicine to control their blood pressures.

❐ Another study showed that overweight people who lose up to 20 pounds can lower their systolic and diastolic blood pressure levels by 15.8 and 13.6 mm Hg.

❐ A third study involved nearly 800 overweight people with Stage 1 (mild) high blood pressure. Half the group dieted and half didn't. Some people received a hypertensive medication, and others received a placebo (a fake, harmless pill). The people who lost 10 pounds or more had an average diastolic reduction of 12 points, whether they were taking the blood pressure drugs or the placebo.

❐ A different research team found that with every seven pounds lost, the systolic blood pressure level will drop seven points and the diastolic will drop four points.

So that's the good news. The bad news, you already know: For most people, losing weight is tough. More people are overweight now than ever before.

And once you've lost weight, keeping it off is another matter. Nine out of 10 people who lose weight gain it all back within five years.

People who manage to lose weight fast, three or more pounds a week, almost always gain it back within the next year.

Traditional diets don't work for most people. Fortunately, there's a middle ground between endless bouts of crash dieting and simply giving up, indulging in ice cream every night and watching our blood pressures soar.

It's called weight management and it includes normal, healthy eating and moderate exercise. We'll tell you the basic 10 steps, then it's your turn to experiment and find out what works for you.

Your ideal weight

How heavy is too heavy? Most medical professionals describe obesity as being 20 to 40 percent heavier than your ideal weight. However, health professionals warn that even 10 pounds over your ideal weight is still overweight.

You probably already have a good idea what your ideal weight is. It's the weight at which you feel fit and healthy. You have plenty of energy and feel good about yourself. Your clothes fit comfortably, and you know you look your best. However, there is a safe and healthy range of weight that depends on your height, sex and age. See the chart on the following page.

Remember to be realistic with your weight-loss goals. Being overweight is dangerous, but so is being underweight.

Potbellies get your pressure cooking

Consider where you carry your weight when you're determining your ideal weight. Extra weight around your waist is worse for your blood pressure than extra weight in the hips and buttocks. Some researchers refer to the body shapes as "apple-shaped" and "pear-shaped."

It's better to be shaped like a pear (heavy in the hips and buttocks) than to be shaped like an apple (heavy around the waist and trunk).

Studies show that a waist-to-hip ratio greater than .85 in women and .95 in men increases the risk of high blood pressure and its associated diseases. To determine your own waist-to-hip ratio, use a flexible measuring tape and write down your waist and hip measurements.

Simply divide the waist measurement by the hip measurement. For example, 25 inches (waist measurement) divided by 37 inches (hip measurement) equals .68 waist-to-hip ratio.

Suggested Weights for Adults

Height	Weight (pounds)	
	19-34 Years Old	35 Years Old and Over
5'0"	97-128	108-138
5'1"	101-132	111-143
5'2"	104-137	115-148
5'3"	107-141	119-152
5'4"	111-146	122-157
5'5"	114-150	126-162
5'6"	118-155	130-167
5'7"	121-160	134-172
5'8"	125-164	138-178
5'9"	129-169	142-183
5'10"	132-174	146-188
5'11"	136-179	151-194
6'0"	140-184	155-199
6'1"	144-189	159-205
6'2"	148-195	164-210
6'3"	152-200	168-216
6'4"	156-205	173-222
6'5"	160-211	177-228
6'6"	164-216	182-234

Note:
- ❏ The height is without shoes. Weight is without clothes.
- ❏ The higher weights in the ranges generally apply to men, who tend to have more muscle and bone. The lower weights more often apply to women, who have less muscle and bone.

No 'crashing' allowed

You've figured out how many inches and pounds you'd like to lose — the first part of weight management. Now, don't think about it. Dwelling on an ideal weight will probably make you feel miserable and guilty whenever you eat a bite.

All you need to think about is gradually switching your lifestyle to low-fat eating and regular exercising. You're ready for Weight Management Rule Number 2: No "crash dieting" allowed.

Forget the old rigid diets that restricted you to a list of acceptable foods and an extremely low number of calories each day. With the traditional diet, you get so hungry and feel so deprived that you can't think logically about food.

You have uncontrollable cravings for high-fat foods, and you can't resist giving in to eating binges. In fact, scientific studies have found that animals on a severely restricted diet choose more fatty foods once they are taken off the diet.

After you go on an eating binge, you feel so guilty that you hardly eat anything for a couple of days and start the cycle all over again.

These starvation diets also slow down your metabolism and make your fat cells more resistant to losing their stored fatty energy reserves.

With weight management, you eat three healthy, low-fat, high-carbohydrate meals a day plus between-meal snacks. You won't feel deprived, hungry or anxious about the food you eat. You can reduce the amount of fat in your food without bringing on an eating binge, and you'll still have enough energy to exercise.

Slow weight loss is safe and healthy, but still consult your doctor before you begin if you are pregnant, over 60 years old and need to lose 20 pounds or more, or have an immediate family member who has had a heart attack or diabetes.

Know how much you're really eating

Do you think you "eat like a bird" but you never lose weight? Weight Management Rule Number 3 is you must keep tabs on your true food intake. You may be eating more and exercising less than you think.

After studying 90 overweight people for two weeks, researchers found that every one of them underestimated the amount of food they ate and overestimated how much they exercised.

As many as 80 percent of us underestimate the number of calories we eat, sometimes by as much as 800 calories a day. One possible reason for this is that some of us don't accurately judge how much food we put on our plates.

In the study, the diet-resistant participants (people who had a long history of dieting without losing weight) consumed nearly twice as many calories as they thought and exercised approximately one-fourth less than they estimated.

The root of the problem appears to be denial. Researchers speculate that denial may stem from pressures caused by a lifetime of unsuccessful dieting and from society's prejudice against people who can't control their weight.

The pressure to fix their weight problem may have affected their ability to think objectively about calorie intake and output.

When some of the diet-resistant participants stuck with a truly low-fat diet, they lost weight.

If you are trying to lose weight, you may want to weigh and measure the food you eat so you'll be able to accurately judge serving sizes. This is especially important for high-fat foods. Use the charts on the following pages to figure out how many calories you can eat to sustain your ideal weight.

Level of Activity:

Extremely inactive, or sedentary (Example: No aerobic exercise in the course of a week)
Moderately active, or light activity (Example: Aerobic exercise 2-3 times a week)
Active, moderate exercise and/or work (Example: Aerobic exercise 4-5 times a week)
Extremely active, heavy exercise and/or work (Example: Aerobic exercise 6-7 times a week)

Calories Needed Daily By Men To Sustain Weight

Height	Ideal Weight	Extremely Inactive	Moderately Active	Active	Extremely Active
5'2"	118	1,298	1,534	1,770	2,124
5'3"	124	1,364	1,612	1,860	2,232
5'4"	130	1,430	1,690	1,950	2,340
5'5"	136	1,496	1,768	2,040	2,448
5'6"	142	1,562	1,846	2,130	2,556
5'7"	148	1,628	1,924	2,220	2,664
5'8"	154	1,694	2,002	2,310	2,772
5'9"	160	1,760	2,080	2,400	2,880
5'10"	166	1,826	2,158	2,490	2,988
5'11"	172	1,892	2,236	2,580	3,096
6'0"	178	1,958	2,314	2,670	3,204
6'1"	184	2,024	2,392	2,760	3,312
6'2"	190	2,090	2,470	2,850	3,420
6'3"	196	2,156	2,548	2,940	3,528
6'4"	202	2,222	2,626	3,030	3,636

Note:
These ideal weights are estimates and may be better suited for younger people.

Level of Activity:

Extremely inactive, or sedentary (Example: No aerobic exercise in the course of a week)
Moderately active, or light activity (Example: Aerobic exercise 2-3 times a week)
Active, moderate exercise and/or work (Example: Aerobic exercise 4-5 times a week)
Extremely active, heavy exercise and/or work (Example: Aerobic exercise 6-7 times a week)

Calories Needed Daily By Women To Sustain Weight

Height	Ideal Weight	Extremely Inactive	Moderately Active	Active	Extremely Active
4'11"	95	1,045	1,235	1,425	1,710
5'0"	100	1,100	1,300	1,500	1,800
5'1"	105	1,155	1,365	1,575	1,890
5'2"	110	1,210	1,430	1,650	1,980
5'3"	115	1,265	1,495	1,725	2,070
5'4"	120	1,320	1,560	1,800	2,160
5'5"	125	1,375	1,625	1,875	2,250
5'6"	130	1,430	1,690	1,950	2,340
5'7"	135	1,485	1,755	2,025	2,430
5'8"	140	1,540	1,820	2,100	2,520
5'9"	145	1,595	1,885	2,175	2,610
5'10"	150	1,650	1,950	2,250	2,700
5'11"	155	1,705	2,015	2,325	2,790
6'0"	160	1,760	2,080	2,400	2,880

Note:
These ideal weights are estimates and may be better suited for younger people.

Remember, if you weigh 160 pounds but you want to weigh 130 pounds, you have to eat like a 130-pound person.

Keep a food log of what, how much and when you eat each day. You'll be able to see exactly where your calories and nutrition are coming from and how you can change your eating habits.

It also may be helpful for you to keep an exercise journal. A journal may help keep you motivated and will help you acurately judge your activity level. You may be surprised how much you can eat if you are very active.

Weigh yourself once a week and record it in your food journal. Daily fluctuations in weight are not reliable, but weighing yourself weekly will allow you to evaluate whether or not your program is working.

Know what you're eating

Many times when you read about dieting, you are bombarded with information about calories, carbohydrates, fats and protein. What is even more confusing are the different ways these items are combined in different diets.

Sometimes diet books advocate reducing calories without saying which calories to reduce. Every day you could conceivably eat a hot fudge sundae and very little else. But what would that do to your health? To lose weight, you should eat more complex carbohydrates and fewer fats.

The fourth part of weight management is defining your dieting terms.

> ***Calorie*** — Scientists would say that one "kilocalorie" is the amount of heat needed to raise the temperature of one kilogram of water one degree centigrade. In popular usage, however, the technical term kilocalorie has been shortened to the more familiar and more popu-

lar calorie.

We use calorie to mean the amount of energy produced by food when utilized by the body. In other words, it is a way to measure the amount of energy that a food will produce in the body.

If a calorie is not used up during normal activity, it is stored in some form in the body for later use. If the amount of calories burned is consistently more than the amount of calories eaten, weight loss will result.

Carbohydrates — Carbohydrates are energy-producing foods, such as sugars, starches and cellulose. Carbohydrates are typically divided into two types.

The first type includes simple and double carbohydrates, such as honey and refined sugars. The second type consists of complex carbohydrates, such as the starches found in whole grains.

Simple sugars are easily digested and enter the bloodstream rapidly. This may cause difficulty for individuals who have trouble controlling the effects of sugar in the body, like diabetics. In most people, simple carbohydrates will cause sudden peaking and dropping of blood sugar levels, which could lead to a craving for food and a net loss of energy.

Complex carbohydrates require prolonged action by digestive enzymes before the body can use the energy from these foods. The effects of complex carbohydrates on the body are much more gradual, and they are unlikely to lead to surges and drops in blood sugar levels and overeating.

Fats — For all their bad reputation, fats do play an important role in a healthy body. Also called lipids, fats are the most highly concentrated source of energy in the body. One gram of fat will produce about nine calories for the body's use or storage.

Fats also are important because they are necessary for the body to utilize vitamins A, D, E and K, as well as calcium. They also protect vital organs and help to insulate the body from changes in the surrounding environment.

Too much fat in your diet will lead to excessive weight gain. Such an excess also will slow digestion. And too many saturated fats, the types that are solid at room temperature, may lead to high levels of cholesterol and heart disease.

Protein — Protein is of vital importance for good health. Protein forms the body's building blocks for muscles, blood, skin, internal organs and hair. It is necessary for both the formation and regulation of hormones.

When proteins are digested, they are broken down into simpler units known as amino acids. The body can use amino acids only when they appear in certain combinations. These combinations are readily available in most meat and egg products. The right combination may be created by combining certain food products. For example, to create a complete protein using a food from the grain family (such as oats), it must be paired with a legume (such as peas). But too much protein will lead to weight gain. Extra protein in the body can be converted by the liver and stored in body tissues as fat.

Controlling your appetite

Never feeling deprived is the key to controlling your appetite, says Weight Management Rule Number 5. You should never starve yourself or even skip meals. You should schedule snack times in your day, too. If you let yourself get very hungry, you're much more likely to overeat.

But even if you eat sensibly, it's hard to adjust when you're cutting back on your food intake. Try these time-proven techniques to control your appetite:

- ❑ Squeeze your earlobe for one minute before eating. This acupressure technique may help curb your appetite.
- ❑ Drink grapefruit juice, low-salt tomato juice or unsweetened lemonade as an appetizer before your meal. If you allow 20 minutes before you eat, the acid in the juice will help you feel full, and you will be able to eat less. Drink the juice of a whole lemon squeezed into a glass of water, twice a day, for another natural appetite suppressant.
- ❑ Brushing your teeth frequently may help reduce snacking. Your teeth and mouth feel so good that you don't have the desire to eat. And the Good Wellness Program for Weight Management suggests placing a bottle of mouthwash in front of your refrigerator door. If you stray into the kitchen looking for something to eat, you will have to move the mouthwash first. Rinsing with the mouthwash will help satisfy your cravings without consuming any calories.
- ❑ Serve a salad or low-calorie soup with most meals. They will fill you up, and you will eat smaller portions.
- ❑ Serve your meals on smaller plates so they will look fuller.
- ❑ Put the food on the plates away from the table. If you bring serving dishes to the table, you will be more tempted to have additional helpings.
- ❑ Keep food out of sight. Get all the candy, potato chips and gooey cinnamon rolls out of your house and don't

buy any more. If your kids can't live without them, tell them to put them in their rooms under lock and key or stash them at a friend's house. If you decide to eat a cookie or some ice cream every once in a while, buy single servings.

❑ Keep healthy snacks available. Try cutting up celery, carrots, broccoli, cauliflower, radishes and whatever other vegetables you like and leaving them in your refrigerator. Buy plenty of fruit. It provides quick and easy snacks. Place no-calorie drinks at eye level.

❑ Before beginning your diet, write a list detailing your reasons for following a healthy eating plan, including health problems you are trying to prevent. Keep the list handy for moments when your willpower is weak.

Breaking bad habits

Some bad habits are hard to break, especially when food is involved. Here are some habits that put on those extra pounds we carry:

➤ *Gulping down food.* Put your utensils down after each bite. It takes several minutes for the stomach to tell the brain that it is full, so eating slowly will help you realize you're full before you overeat.

➤ *Eating food out of the original container.* Take out an appropriate serving and return the container to its proper place. By eating directly out of the container, you are more likely to eat too much.

➤ *Eating everything on your plate.* Try to leave something on your plate. In some Oriental countries, this is considered a high compliment because it shows that you have had plenty to eat. If you have been taught to clear your plate and not to waste food, learning to leave a small portion on your plate will be good for you.

➤ *Drinking a diet soda so you can eat a candy bar.* Many doctors even recommend avoiding products with artificial sweeteners. In an American Cancer Society study of 78,000 dieters, people using artificial sweeteners gained more weight than people not using substitutes. The people thought they were cutting back by using the artificial sweeteners, and they didn't limit their calories overall. Artificial sweeteners may even increase or maintain your desire for sweets.

➤ *Eating a big lunch and dinner even when you're not hungry.* If you satisfy your hunger pangs with a small, healthy snack when you get home from work, eat smaller portions for dinner. That's what skinny people do. The same goes for your kids: Let them eat when they're starving (like right after school), and don't force them to clean their plates at mealtimes. Choose what they eat, but not when or how much.

➤ *Saving calories through the day so you can binge at night.* Eat a healthy breakfast, a hearty lunch and a small dinner. You'll lose weight if you eat all your daily calories in your morning meal, but you'll gain weight if you eat that meal at night. Most binge eaters eat very little for breakfast and lunch, then stuff themselves in the evening. If you eat normally throughout the day, you won't feel so much like bingeing at night.

Researchers at Tulane University found that people who ate their last meal at least eight hours before they went to sleep lost between five and 10 pounds a month. The participants did not change the amount of food they ate, or the number of calories, just the time of day it was eaten. Eating most of our daily calories early in the day seems to allow the food to be used to produce energy. Therefore, fewer calories are left over to change into fat.

➤ *Watching television while eating meals.* Sit down and really enjoy what you are eating.

➤ *Rewarding yourself with food or using food to fight stress or depression.* Rather than using food as a release or reward, buy yourself a gift or treat yourself to a favorite activity.

➤ *Going grocery shopping when you are hungry.* If you are hungry, you will be tempted to buy more, and you are more likely to buy high-calorie foods. Make a shopping list of things you need and stick to it.

10 healthy eating habits

These rules are designed to help you make healthy food choices rather than restricting you to a list of certain foods. If you are not allowed to have a specific item, you will probably crave that food. Here are some good overall eating habits to help you with the seventh part of weight management:

- ❐ Eat more vegetables and fruit (at least five to six servings a day) and smaller portions of meat, especially red meat. You should eat no more than 5 or 6 ounces of meat a day. (A three-ounce serving of meat looks about like a stacked deck of cards.)
- ❐ When you do serve meat, make sure it's lean and trim away any excess fat. Lean meats are skinless, white poultry, pork loin, flank steak and ham. Don't fry your meat. Bake or broil it instead.
- ❐ Try steaming your vegetables or sautéing them in

chicken broth instead of butter or oil. Flavor cooked vegetables and fish with lemon or lime juice and herbs instead of butter or margarine.

❐ Eat plenty of high-fiber foods like whole-grain products, beans and vegetables.

❐ Use a low-calorie, soft-spread margarine as an alternative to butter. It contains less saturated fat, and you may use less because it spreads easier.

❐ Switch to lower calorie foods and calorie-reduced products. See Chapter 25 for low-fat substitutions to replace high-fat foods.

❐ Remember to count the calories in your beverages. Most soft drinks and fruit-flavored beverages are loaded with calories and have very little nutrition to offer in return.

❐ Switch from mayonnaise and egg sauces to nonfat yogurt and low-fat cottage cheese. The yogurt and cottage cheese can produce a creamy base for many sauces with far less fat and calories than mayonnaise.

❐ Reduce or eliminate high-calorie nuts and nut products, including peanut butter.

❐ Never use canned fruit products that have been packaged in heavy syrup. Use fresh fruit or fruit that has been packed in its own unsweetened juice.

If you do splurge and eat high-fat for a day, don't let guilt drive you away from your healthy eating plan. Read over your reasons for being on the diet in the first place, and pick up again where you left off.

Social eating

One of the main reasons diets fail is that dieters don't get the support they need from family and friends. Weight Management Rule Number 8 is to get people on your side. Talk with your family and friends about how they can help encourage and support you as you try to lose weight.

Here are some hints on eating when you're out of the house or around others.

☐ Learn to say no without feeling guilty. Don't let someone force you into eating.

☐ Before attending receptions and parties, eat a small, very-high-fiber meal. If you are full, you will be less likely to overeat. Plus, the high-fiber might help reduce your taste for fat-filled foods.

☐ Alcohol contains a lot of calories with no nutritional value. Alcohol consumption also is a contributing factor in high blood pressure.

☐ If you must have dessert, try sharing it with one or two other people. A small sample may satisfy your craving for a sweet.

☐ If you eat at a cafeteria, like a school lunchroom, check with the food services manager to see if low-calorie meals can be ordered.

☐ When flying or traveling by train, request a low-calorie meal at least 24 hours in advance of your departure.

Boosting your metabolism

Until now, scientists have thought that people who lose weight through low-calorie diets ended up in a catch-22 situation: Losing weight slows down the body's resting metabolic rate. Your resting metabolic rate is the amount of energy needed to maintain basic body functions, such as breathing and heart beat.

A slower metabolic rate is your body's way of functioning

normally with a smaller amount of food.

The problem is that a slower metabolism makes it easier to gain weight and harder to keep off those unwanted pounds. Exercise, however, can help restore a healthy metabolism.

One reason is that lean muscles use more calories than other body parts, so you boost your resting metabolism when you build muscles. You'll burn extra calories even when you're just sitting around.

People who lose weight by combining a low-calorie diet and exercise will experience a drop in their metabolism at first. In fact, the exercise may even increase the initial drop. But after a few weeks of this routine, the metabolism springs back to a level that is normal for their lower body weight.

The new metabolism will be slightly slower than the original metabolism. However, the new metabolic rate is perfect for the new body weight.

Dieters should not be concerned about a plunging metabolic rate. As long as you exercise, your metabolic rate will stabilize at a healthy level that will suit your new, thinner body.

Other ways dieters benefit from exercise: It gives you more energy, boosts your self-esteem and even reduces your desire for fatty foods.

Avoiding the gimmicks

Dieters are bombarded every day with weight-loss gimmicks. Follow Weight Management Rule Number 10 — Don't fall prey to these:

> ➤ *Products that promise to reduce or remove fat in one specific body area.* Except for specific exercise or cosmetic surgery, one part of your body cannot be reduced while the rest remains the same.

➤ *Body wraps.* The only weight loss that body wraps provide is the loss of sweat which is just temporary. Using body wraps can be harmful because they allow the body's temperature to increase.

➤ *Diet pills.* Do not use over-the-counter appetite suppressants. One common ingredient, phenylpropanolamine hydrochloride (PPA), has been found to cause high blood pressure even at the doses recommended for weight loss. Anyone with diabetes, heart disease, thyroid disease or high blood pressure should avoid products containing PPA.

Some weight-loss programs are gimmicks, but others can be enormously successful. You need support from others when you're trying to lose weight. Weight-loss programs also can be great sources of information on health and nutrition. But you need to consider several things before you enroll.

First, decide what will work best for you: a program that meets three days a week or just once a month, a program that meets in the mornings or evenings, an inexpensive program or a costly one.

One rule-of-thumb to remember is this: Don't judge a weight-loss program based on the success stories that they publish or advertise. These success stories don't always reflect the true success of the program as a whole.

Instead of listening to success stories, try to get the following information:

❒ How many people who enroll in the program actually complete it?

❒ How many of the people who enrolled and finished the program lost the amount of weight they wanted to?

❒ How many who lost their desired amounts of weight

kept it off for one, two and five years after the program?

❒ Have many people experienced any kind of emotional, mental or physical problems related to the program?

If the program you are looking at does not have this information available, you might be able to find it in some published studies. Ask your local librarian to help you locate this information.

After getting the answers to those first questions, it's time to begin looking into the more specific details of the program. Take time to find out about the following:

❒ Does this program require you to buy and use its food, or can you prepare your own meals using food you buy at the grocery store?

❒ Does the exercise program require you to use specialized equipment from its program, or can you learn the proper exercises and then do them at home or at your own private health club?

❒ How does this program blend together a mix of diet, exercise and behavior modifications? Is there a good mix of all three, or are one or two areas stressed more than the others?

❒ Does this program combine counseling with the weight-loss program? If so, is it a group setting or individual counseling? If it is group counseling, will there be open or closed groups? (Open groups allow people to drop out or join randomly. Closed groups start with a small group of people and don't add newcomers, even if some drop out.)

❒ If this program does provide counseling, how are the counselors trained? Are they professionals with the appropriate educational degrees, or were they trained at a weekend seminar?

☐ Does this program offer any type of continuing education, such as classes on nutrition, preparing healthy
meals and exercise safety? If so, are the teachers properly trained?

☐ Does this program stress long-term behavior changes
that will help you keep the weight off and live a
healthier life, or does it focus on quick weight-loss gimmicks?

☐ Do you set your own weight-loss goals, or do program
directors help you decide how much weight to lose?

Take time to ask questions. Each of these factors will
impact the success or failure of your weight-loss plan. It's
important to get all the information you can on the program
you're thinking of joining.

Protecting your teens

Don't think your kids are safe from the health consequences of being overweight because they are young. Overweight teen-agers are more likely to have high blood pressure when they are older. Plus, they are at increased risk of
heart disease, cancer, arthritis and gout.

The American Heart Association explains that the blood
vessels of obese teen-agers change from flexible tubes into
hardened pipes that carry less blood.

Apparently these changes can be reversed by losing weight
while still in the teen-age years. Waiting until adulthood to
try to lose weight and reverse the hardening of the vessels is
less successful.

According to the study, up to 25 percent of all adolescents
in the United States are overweight and are at risk for developing the adult consequences of adolescent obesity. Check

with your pediatrician to see if your children are classified as overweight. If they are, the doctor will be able to place them on a safe and healthy diet to help them lose the appropriate amount of weight for their heights and ages.

Don't try to place your children on diets without a doctor's advice. Children need a healthy, well-balanced diet for proper growth and development. Fad diets run the risk of being poorly balanced in essential nutrients, which could be more damaging to a child than obesity.

Special cautions for dieting seniors

Older people get the fat end of the deal when it comes to food. You know you're not eating any more than you used to, but you keep putting on extra pounds.

You've got three strikes against you:

➤ The rate your body burns calories (your metabolic rate) decreases about 2 percent every 10 years.
➤ Your body makes less protein as you get older. Protein burns calories. Since your body is making less protein, you need less calories than before.
➤ You are probably less active and get less exercise than when you were younger.

It's OK to be a few pounds heavier than you were in your 20s. Many older people are too thin. That's also a health risk. If you're 40 or 50 pounds overweight, you're increasing your risk of heart disease, diabetes, cancer and arthritis. You'll improve your health even if you lose only 10 or 15 pounds.

Here are some special cautions for dieting seniors:

❑ You may want to ask your pharmacist to help you choose a good multi-vitamin/mineral supplement.
❑ Try to get about 70 grams of protein a day. You can get

this much from five or six ounces of lean meat and two large glasses of skim milk. Grains, fruits and vegetables also are good sources of protein.

❒ Make sure you take in 1,200 to 1,500 milligrams of calcium a day. Women over 60 and men over 70 often have trouble absorbing calcium. Older people often avoid dairy products because of lactose intolerance. If you're lactose intolerant, dairy products may cause intestinal gas and stomach cramps. You may need lactase-treated milk (Lactaid) or Lactaid tablets. You probably should take a calcium supplement if your multi-vitamin/mineral tablet doesn't provide calcium.

❒ Buy dairy products that have vitamin D added to them or help your body produce vitamin D by spending 15 minutes a day in the sun. Vitamin D helps your body absorb calcium.

❒ Drink plenty of fluids while dieting, especially if you're also taking diuretics.

❒ Exercise regularly to keep your muscles toned and your weight down. You don't automatically lose muscle and gain fat as you get older.

Good exercises for seniors include stretching, walking, low-impact aerobics, water aerobics, swimming and cycling. If you can't move very well, do leg lifts and arm exercises while you are sitting or lying down. Even if one arm or leg is painful to move, exercise the other one. See Chapter 6 for more information on exercising to lose weight and lower your blood pressure.

6 ‖ Exercise for Health

Very few of us can honestly say that regular exercise is a part of our life. Most of us have given up on the idea of exercise. A few others are in the middle of a "crash exercise program." We are frantically and vigorously working out every day, hating every minute of it, and, in a few months, we'll be watching television during our scheduled workout hour — exercise nothing but a distant memory.

Nonexercisers have up to a 50 percent increased risk of high blood pressure compared with more active people. Regular aerobic exercise, on the other hand, can help reduce systolic blood pressure levels by as much as 10 mm Hg.

Plus, exercise helps reduce your risk of heart disease, diabetes, arthritis, constipation, insomnia, stroke and osteoporosis, the brittle bone disease. It also can increase mental alertness, help you cope with stress, increase your self-esteem and reduce depression.

The good news is that you don't have to be an Olympic

athlete to enjoy the benefits of exercising. In fact, if you begin a hard exercise program that you don't enjoy, you're probably not going to keep it up.

You can lower your blood pressure with only moderately intense physical activity. Walking briskly 30 to 45 minutes three to five times each week is a perfect aerobic exercise.

But what if you are working up a sweat but not losing any weight? Will you still benefit from the exercise? Absolutely. The protective effects of exercise on blood pressure are completely independent of weight loss. In fact, you might actually gain a few pounds as you transform fat into muscle.

Of course, most of us could stand to lose a few pounds, and, unless we begin eating more, we will slowly but surely lose weight when we exercise. For example, walking only 20 minutes three times a week uses 300 calories per week.

How exercise beats high blood pressure

Scientists are still studying exactly how exercise lowers blood pressure. Some hormones and chemicals, such as epinephrine, cause blood pressure to rise when released into the bloodstream. Exercise decreases many of those substances. Also, regular exercise improves your heart's ability to pump blood.

Since the heart is a muscle, it must be exercised like any other muscle to become stronger. If it is exercised regularly, its strength increases. If not, it becomes weaker. Although some people believe that strenuous work harms the heart, scientific research has found no evidence that regular exercise is harmful for the normal heart.

A strong heart muscle can pump a greater amount of blood with fewer strokes per minute. For example, the average person has a resting heart rate of between 70 and 80 beats per minute, while a trained athlete may have a resting heart rate in the low 50s or even in the 40s. A strong heart requires less force and effort and, therefore, less pressure to move blood through your body.

Exercise speeds up the removal of a type of fat known as triglycerides from the bloodstream, too, says new research from Rockefeller University. After a meal, triglycerides can flood the bloodstream and deposit part of their load onto the walls of arteries.

That sets the stage for atherosclerosis (hardening of the arteries), high blood pressure and a heart attack. The study showed that even after a high-fat meal, regular exercise can reduce levels of triglycerides in the blood by one third.

Exercise can work better than drugs

A recent medical study conducted in Maryland suggests that adding high blood pressure drugs to an exercise program might be unnecessary, at least in mild cases of high blood pressure. According to the study results, the natural way does the job as well as or better than drugs.

The Maryland doctors studied men with high blood pressure averaging 145/97 mm Hg. None of the men exercised regularly. They put one group of men on an antihypertensive medication known as a beta-blocker and a second group on a calcium-channel blocker. The third group received only a placebo, a fake, harmless pill with no medical effect.

Three times a week, the men performed 20 minutes of aerobic exercises, either stationary cycling, walking or jogging. They also lifted weights for 30 minutes on a 20-station weight-training circuit.

After 10 weeks, average blood pressure had fallen 14 points systolic and 13 points diastolic to 131/84. More significantly, the drop occurred whether or not the men were taking blood pressure medicine.

Exercise alone accounted for the improvement, the researchers concluded. In addition, the men experienced a drop in total cholesterol and LDL cholesterol levels. As added benefits, the men lost a little weight and increased their overall strength by an average of 25 percent.

Just a little exercise goes a long way

Since the late 1950s, Martha L. Slattery, a researcher at the University of Utah Medical School, has been studying the health history and leisure time physical activity of 3,043 white, male railroad workers whose jobs ranged from strenuous physical activity to desk work. Their leisure time physical activities were classified as light, moderate or intense.

Light activity ranged from walking for pleasure to bowling or raking the lawn. Ballroom dancing and gardening were considered part of the moderate activities, while backpacking, jogging and snow shoveling, among others, were classified as intense activities.

Death rates from diseases of the heart and blood vessels were 30 percent lower for the men who used 1,000 or more calories a week in leisure time physical activity. That is the equivalent of spending 30 minutes a day in some moderately intense activity, such as playing softball or weeding the garden.

In other words, desk jockeys and couch potatoes get a great deal of added protection against heart attacks and other diseases just by hoeing weeds in the yard or taking a brisk walk several times a week.

According to Dr. Steven Blair, director of epidemiology at the Institute for Aerobics Research in Dallas, you don't need to be as fit as an athlete to get the benefits of exercise.

Many experts believe that timesaving technology has decreased our activity levels, especially at home.

Do you use the remote control to change television channels? Use a riding lawn mower? An electric snow blower?

Electric garage door opener? Conveniences such as these are turning Americans into couch potatoes.

Dr. Blair concludes that most men and women could reduce their risk of heart disease with the addition of very modest exercise. He recommends walking as the exercise that is easiest to mold into your lifestyle.

The best workout for you

Regular aerobic exercise, 20 to 60 minutes at a time three to five times a week, is the key to lowering your blood pressure. Spurts of activity can actually be harmful to a nonactive person, so you should exercise on a regular basis and build up slowly to a steady pace.

Walking is usually recommended by doctors as the best exercise for people who are just getting started. Walking can help lower high blood pressure and improve your fitness level.

If you don't like to walk, try swimming, cycling on a stationary bike, rowing, cross-country skiing, aerobic dancing or water aerobics. These are only a few of the many aerobic activities you might find enjoyable.

Don't feel guilty because you're not jogging or exercising strenuously every day. The regular jogger who lifts weights five times a week does not get more cardiovascular benefits than the regular walker.

A National Exercise for Life Institute report says that although the person who exercises heavily might be more fit, the light exerciser gets exactly the same cardiovascular benefits.

Walkers lose body fat and improve good HDL cholesterol levels just like joggers. In fact, a longer, less intense workout is actually more effective at burning fat than a short, tough exercise routine.

According to some authorities, your body can only burn off fat when you exercise aerobically or "with air." In other words, your activity should raise your heart rate from 60 to 80 percent of its maximum rate.

After exercising at this level for 20 minutes, your body will begin to consume fat for fuel. On the other hand, if your workout pushes your heart rate above 85 percent of the maximum level, this is considered anaerobic or "without air" exercise.

At this point, your body automatically switches over to the higher test fuels, carbohydrates and protein, leaving the fat right where you don't want it.

Measuring your exercise intensity

Moderate exercise means that you are maintaining your heart rate at 40 to 60 percent of your maximum heart rate. Exercise intensities greater than 60 percent are called vigorous or intense. Researcher Steven N. Blair, of the Cooper Institute of Aerobics Research, states that how much you exercise is more important than how hard you exercise.

To maximize your aerobic benefits from exercising, it's best to find your target heart rate (the exercise intensity you want to achieve) and maintain it for at least 20 minutes.

❏ Start with the number 220:   220
❏ Subtract your age (50, for example):   -50
❏ The answer is your maximum heart rate   170
❏ Multiply your max. heart rate by 0.6:
(Low end of the target range for vigorous exercise; 60 percent)   x 0.6
     102

❏ Multiply your max. heart rate by 0.8:   170
(High end of the target range for vigorous exercise; 80 percent)   x 0.8
     136

You can use this equation to figure out your target heart rate, or, to make things simpler while you are exercising, use the exercise intensity chart on this page. All you need is a watch with a second hand. Use your index finger and middle finger to count your pulse at your wrist or at your neck, just below your jaw, for 10 seconds, then use the chart to discover how hard you are exercising.

For instance, a 50-year-old woman who counts 20 beats in 10 seconds is exercising at 70 percent intensity.

Exercise Intensity Guidelines

Heartbeats Per 10 Seconds for Women

Percentage of Maximum Heart Rate	20 years	30 years	40 years	50 years	60 years	70 years
90%	30	29	27	26	24	23
80%	27	25	24	23	21	20
70%	23	22	21	20	19	18
60%	20	19	18	17	16	15

Heartbeats Per 10 Seconds for Men

Percentage of Maximum Heart Rate	20 years	30 years	40 years	50 years	60 years	70 years
90%	29	29	28	27	26	26
80%	26	25	25	24	23	23
70%	23	22	22	21	20	20
60%	20	19	19	18	18	17

You need to check your heart rate regularly while you are exercising. If you are a beginner, always work at the lower end of your range. Only those already physically fit should attempt to achieve the 80 percent rate.

Lower the intensity of your workout if your heart rate gets too high by keeping your arms down and your feet close to the ground or floor.

After you've exercised for several weeks and your heart gets stronger, you may need to increase the duration of your exercise time to maintain the heart rate you want.

If you want to exercise at the high end of your target range, make sure you warm up first. Warming up allows your blood vessels to dilate and eases the increase in blood pressure.

Walking guidelines

You don't need a gym membership to start walking. Most people can start right outside their front door, or in a shopping mall when the weather is poor.

In fact, you may want to avoid walking on an official walking track. You spend so much time making turns that you can aggravate your joints. If you must walk on a track, change direction halfway through.

Walking on grass isn't a good idea, either. The uneven surface can cause a fall or an injury. Stick to the sidewalk or street. You'll want to walk three to five times a week, for at least 20 minutes at a time. If you haven't been walking and you feel out of shape, work your way up the following steps.

Step 1	One mile
Step 2	One mile in 20 minutes
Step 3	One and one-half miles in 30 minutes
Step 4	Two miles in 40 minutes
Step 5	Two miles in 30 minutes
Step 6	Three miles in 60 minutes
Step 7	Three miles in 45 minutes

It may take you several months to reach Step 7. Anytime you feel sore or achy, go back down a step.

Does one mile seem too far for you? Here's another way to measure your progress: Count telephone poles. You can start by walking from one telephone pole to the next. Your goal every day is to add one telephone pole to your walk.

How to get your upper body in action

Walking is an excellent exercise, but it can leave your upper body weak. Sports physicians are now recommending exercise that uses both the legs and the arms.

Window washers, farmers and orchestra conductors, all people who use their arms daily, seem to have an increased life expectancy.

But doctors suggest that people with high blood pressure should avoid lifting heavy weights and isometric exercises. Isometrics are exercises that involve muscle contractions while the joints remain in place, like squeezing the hand against a fixed object such as a tennis ball.

The strain of lifting heavy weights and isometrics can cause your blood pressure to shoot up temporarily. This can be extremely dangerous for people with blood pressure that is already high. However, strength-training is so good for your muscles, bones and joints that fitness experts are saying that even people with high blood pressure should consider lifting very light weights in addition to their aerobic exercise.

People in their 70s and older have built up their strength by doing biceps curls, military presses and other exercises starting with one-half to one pound weights.

For the biceps curl, stand against a wall and hold your weights with your arms fully lowered, palms facing forward. Without moving your back, bend your elbows to bring the weights to shoulder height. Lower and repeat.

Biceps curl

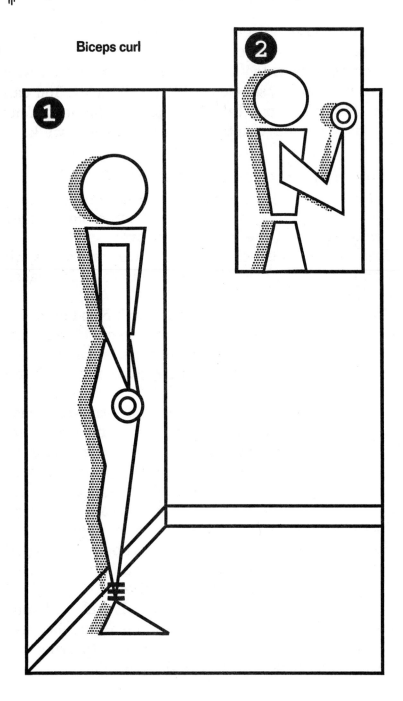

For the military press, sit on a straight-backed chair with your back straight against the backrest. Push weights from

Military press

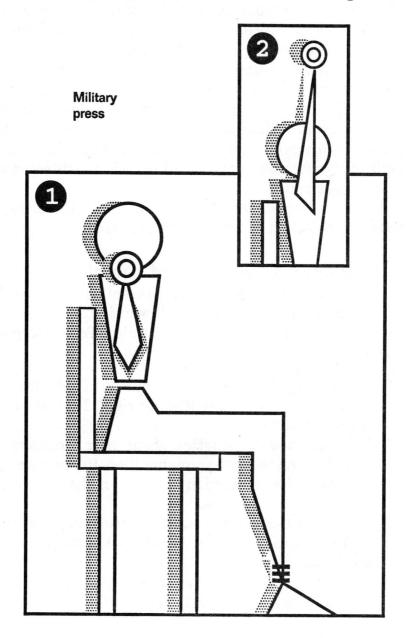

shoulder height to overhead until your elbows are straight. Lower the weights back to shoulder level, then repeat.

Only lift for 10 repetitions at the most, and then rest.

Check with your doctor before you begin lifting weights. You can make walking more challenging and give yourself an upper body workout by carrying hand weights when you walk.

Small hand weights, no more than five pounds per hand, will greatly increase your walking intensity. If you buy light-enough weights, you can do some simple arm exercises, such as shrugs (shrugging your shoulders as if you don't understand) and wrist curls (gently bending and straightening your wrists), while you walk.

Or, for a complete workout that includes the arms, try cross-country skiing or using a rowing machine.

End your exercise with a good stretch

A good stretch is like giving yourself a massage. You should treat your whole body to a few minutes of stretching after your walk or other aerobic activity. Try these gentle stretches:

- ☐ To stretch your neck, swivel your head left, then turn your neck until you are looking right. Return left and repeat 10 times.
- ☐ For your shoulder muscles, shrug your shoulders as if you're trying to touch your shoulders to your ears. Roll your shoulders forward in a circular motion, then backward. Repeat 10 times.
- ☐ To stretch arms and shoulders, interlace your fingers over your head, palms up. Then push upward and hold for 30 seconds.
- ☐ Stretch your fingers by spreading them out as far as you can, then make a fist. Repeat 10 times.

◻ Stretch your chest by clasping your hands behind your back, straightening your arms, lifting your chest and taking a deep breath.

Chest stretch

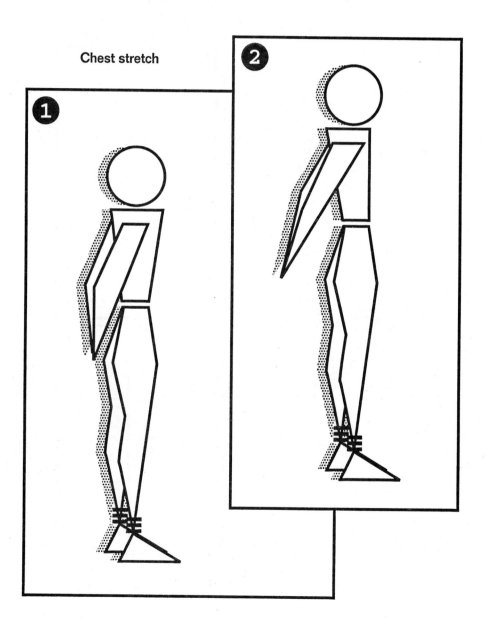

Thigh stretch

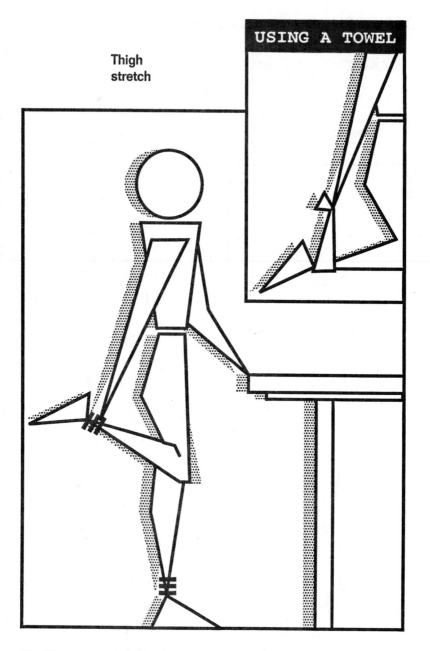

USING A TOWEL

☐ For your thighs, lean against a table or wall with your

left hand. Bend your right knee. With your right hand, grasp your ankle if you can. If you can't, loop a towel around your ankle and hold both ends in your right hand. Pull gently until you feel a mild stretch. Hold for 30 seconds, then switch legs and repeat.

❐ Stretching the hamstrings (shown on pages 118-119) at the back of your thigh is very important. Sit in a chair with your back straight. Place your right leg in another chair in front of you. Place your hands just above your knee, then, keeping your back straight, bend from your hips. Slide your hands down your leg until you feel a gentle pull. Hold for 30 seconds, then repeat for your left leg.

❐ To stretch your calves, or your lower leg muscles (as shown on page 120), face a wall and put both hands on the wall. Place your right foot farther from the wall than your left. Bend your left leg and keep your right leg straight with your heel on the floor. Move your hips toward the wall until you feel a gentle stretch in your right calf. Hold for 30 seconds, switch legs and repeat.

No age limit on exercise benefits

Even elderly people who are frail can improve their overall health and mobility with appropriate exercises, say researchers at the University of Michigan School of Medicine. Such exercises may even keep some older people out of nursing homes, says Tom Hickey, one of the researchers.

Seventy-five patients ranging in age from 65 to 98 tried a simple exercise program for six weeks. They tried gentle neck and shoulder rolls; spinal twists; side stretches; feet and arm extensions, flexes and circles; and slow, deep breathing.

Most of the patients were overweight and never exercised regularly. In addition, many of them suffered from arthritis,

Hamstring stretch

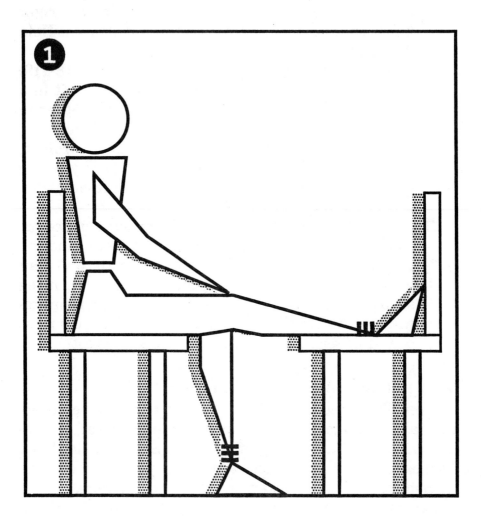

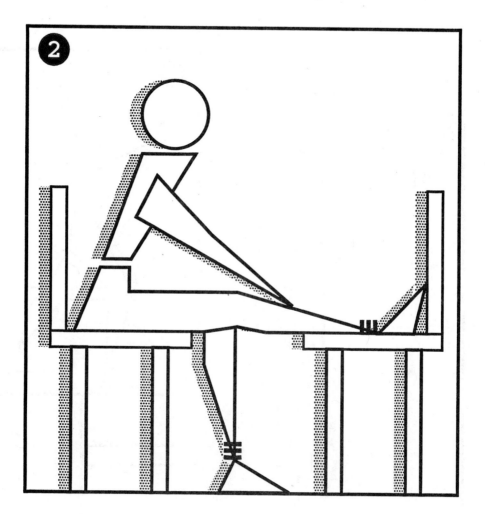

Calf stretch

high blood pressure, diabetes, heart disease or a combination of diseases.

They exercised twice a week in a program called SMILE, which stands for So Much Improvement with Little Exercise. After six weeks, most of them reported less stiffness in the joints and said they had more energy.

The researchers noted some drops in high blood pressure readings and in the time required to walk a certain distance.

Fitting exercise in your life, for good

➤ **Make the time.** You must choose an activity that you are willing to devote time to every day or every other day. Set aside a certain time and stick to it. Let everyone in your family know that during that time you are unavailable. It's your time to do something for yourself.

➤ **Find pleasure in your activity.** If you don't enjoy the type of exercise you are doing, you are less likely to make it a regular part of your life. Be willing to try several different activities. You may discover that a form of exercise you thought would be boring is perfectly suited to your needs and enjoyment.

Many people think walking every day sounds extremely boring. Here are a few suggestions for developing a lifelong habit:

❑ If quiet moments are hard to find at your house, use your walk as special time apart from the crowd.
❑ If you enjoy walking with others, choose a partner who shares your interest and will help you resist the temptation to cut your walk short occasionally.
❑ Choose a route that offers either the comfort of familiar surroundings or the challenge of a different view,

depending on your motivation.

❏ Use a miniature tape player to listen to music, learn a new language, or "read a book" from the many available selections on cassettes.

➤ **Variety is the spice of an exercise program.** Don't be afraid to choose a variety of activities that you enjoy. You may discover that aerobic classes during the week and a long walk or hike on the weekend are a perfect combination for you.

➤ **Stay positive.** Don't undermine your exercise by feeling guilty if you miss your planned activity. Look forward to your next time of exercise. Celebrate the successes you have enjoyed during your exercising. If you get discouraged, try doing the same routine or amount of exercise as your first time.

➤ **Get your spouse involved.** If you are married, having the support of your spouse can be very important. Finding an activity that you can do together can be great. Your spouse's support may make it easier for you to continue with regular exercise.

➤ **Find exercise partners.** Many people find that the support of a group makes regular exercise easier to continue. This doesn't mean you have to join an expensive fitness club or take a class. Just getting a small group of friends who are willing to meet and go for a walk on a regular basis can help. The companionship of the group, knowing you are not alone, and enjoying exercise as a social activity are very helpful.

➤ **Money motivates.** Some people find that a paid class is the best incentive for them to continue exercising. Even if you just have a little miser in you, you may feel the urge to attend all the classes because you don't want to waste the money. If this works for you, keep paying for classes in advance. However, for those on a tight budget, exercise doesn't have to cost a dime.

People can find all sorts of excuses why they can't exercise. They don't have time, they are too unfit, they are too tired or they are too old. No excuses.

Nobody is too old or unfit. Everyone can find 30 minutes sometime during the day. The National Exercise for Life Institute estimates that most Americans have 15 to 18 hours of free time every week.

As for the "I'm too tired" excuse, exercise gives you energy and makes you feel better. Do it for yourself and for your heart.

How to choose a workout time

The best time of day to work out is whatever time works best for you.

Morning workouts can help you feel ready to face daily stress. In general, morning workouts are better on your lungs, but your body might not be as flexible as in the evening. Some studies suggest that early-bird exercisers are most likely to stick with a workout program.

If you need to unwind and forget about the day's frustrations, evening workouts may be better for you.

According to Peter Raven, professor of physiology at the Texas College of Osteopathic Medicine, work out in the afternoon if you are trying to lose weight. That's when your body temperature and, subsequently, your metabolism rate go up.

Another consideration when choosing a workout time is mealtimes. Some people know that a pre-exercise meal will make their stomach hurt, while others like to scarf down a sandwich to boost their energy on the way to the gym.

But if your stomach doesn't tell you when to eat, let your health condition be your guide:

- ☐ Very overweight people who are exercising to burn calories would get the most benefits from eating first. Your body has to work harder to digest food when you exercise on a full stomach. You use more calories during and just after exercising on a full stomach than during and just after exercising on an empty stomach.

  On the other hand, don't despair if you prefer to exercise before you eat. Intense exercise will suppress your appetite for at least a half hour. Your body doesn't want to be faced with the task of digesting food when it's still cooling down from a workout.

- ☐ If you have heart disease, you should exercise before you eat. Aerobic exercise before a meal will get the blood flowing to your heart most effectively. Also, vigorous exercise after you eat a large meal can dangerously decrease the oxygen flow to your heart.

  Do take a short, brisk walk after your meal. The blood tends to form clots after you eat, so a walk will help prevent the clots from forming and lodging in an artery.

- ☐ Diabetics should exercise after they eat, within two hours of the meal. If you wait three or more hours after a meal or exercise in the morning, your blood sugar will be too low. Exercise can lower a diabetic person's blood sugar for eight hours.

  At least eat a snack before exercising and take a snack with you if you plan to exercise for over an hour.

If you don't have a special health condition, waiting until after exercising to eat has its advantages.

❑ You burn extra calories for at least an hour and some-times several hours after exercising. This is called "afterburn" or "excess postexercise oxygen consumption." (People who are obese don't get the same "afterburn" benefits as normal-weight people.)

❑ For about two hours after you exercise, your tired muscles need glycogen, their energy source. Carbohydrates and even candy bars eaten after exercising will be more easily converted to glycogen instead of being stored as fat.

❑ Exercising after a meal can cause a stomachache because your digestive system just doesn't get enough blood flow. Keep post-meal exercise moderate.

Your eating schedule should never keep you from exercising. Morning exercisers might like a light snack of cereal and milk before exercising and something more substantial afterward. Experiment to see what's best for you.

Exercising safely

Don't worry that you might not be able to get fit. Older bodies adapt to exercise in the same way that younger bodies do. You're never too old to reap the benefits of a healthy and safe exercise program.

But before you join a bench-aerobics class or even before you start walking, ask your doctor's advice about a program that's right for you.

Heart trouble, breathing problems like emphysema or chronic bronchitis, uncontrolled diabetes, seizures or arthritis prevent some people from starting or maintaining an exercise program. Certain medicines also can affect your ability to exercise.

When you're ready to begin exercising, here's how to stay safe:

❏ Wear a hat and gloves while exercising outdoors in cold weather to avoid losing body heat. But don't wear too many clothes! Layer your clothing so that you can adapt to varying temperatures. As soon as you start to sweat, shed a layer of clothes.

❏ Wear cotton sports socks and shoes that fit well. Your shoes should give your toes plenty of room and shouldn't slide on your heel. You may need to replace your shoes about every three months. Watch the midsole (the wide area between the toe and the heel) for wear. While the rest of the shoe may still look good, a worn midsole can cause shin splints and foot, ankle and knee troubles. To determine if your midsole is worn out, place your sneakers on a table and examine them from eye level. If either shoe doesn't sit evenly or looks lopsided, it's time for a new pair.

❏ Avoid accidents by exercising during daylight hours.

❏ Drink water before, during and after exercise to avoid dehydration. This is especially important for seniors because they have less total body water than younger people. This rule applies in cold weather as well as hot.

❏ Don't drink caffeine before you exercise if you have high blood pressure. It can place extra stress on your heart. Your heart rate may rise too high when you exercise if you drink caffeine first. Drinking caffeine before exercising has little effect on the heart rates of people with normal blood pressure.

❏ Always warm up if you'll be exercising vigorously, especially in cold weather. If you don't warm up first, you are more likely to be sore, and there is a greater risk that you will pull a muscle. Warming up also will allow your blood vessels to dilate, preventing your blood pressure from skyrocketing during strenuous exercise.

❏ Never stretch before you are warmed up. Stretching can pull or tear cold muscles.

❏ Exercise for at least 20 minutes, preferably 30 minutes. Anything less is not really going to help your heart.

❏ Slow down a little and take a few deep breaths if you get a cramp in your side.

❏ Cool down. Never stop any aerobic activity suddenly. Slow the jog down to a walk. Get off the stationary bike and walk around the room. Do anything, but keep your legs moving until your heart rate has gone back down to normal.

❏ Stop exercising and call your doctor immediately if you experience any of these symptoms:

> ➤ Chest pain
> ➤ Shortness of breath
> ➤ Pain in neck or jaw
> ➤ Faintness or dizziness
> ➤ Excessive fatigue
> ➤ Nausea or vomiting
> ➤ Heart racing
> ➤ Extreme muscle or joint pain

7 ||| Nutritional Guidelines

In the 1970s, Nathan Pritikin and his Pritikin program hit the news with a plan to stop high blood pressure and high cholesterol in their tracks.

The successful plan included a low-fat, low-calorie, low-salt diet and moderate daily exercise.

When a team of researchers from Loma Linda University studied the first 893 people to participate in the 26-day Pritikin Longevity Center program, they were amazed at the results:

✔ After the program, 83 percent of the people who were taking high blood pressure drugs were able to stop taking these drugs with their doctors' permission because their blood pressures had dropped to acceptable levels.

✔ Overweight participants lost an average of 13 pounds.

✔ Cholesterol levels dropped 25 percent. Many people who had been taking drugs to control their blood cholesterol were able to stop taking their cholesterol-reducing medicine.

✔ The level of other blood fats also dropped nearly 25

percent.

✔ Fifty percent of the diabetics were able, under medical supervision, to stop taking insulin.

✔ The study participants became more mentally alert and performed better on tests of mental ability.

✔ Many people lost their tiredness and required much less sleep.

The diet worked to help reduce high blood pressure in three ways. It was low in:

➤ calories so people could lose weight.

➤ sodium to help sodium-sensitive people.

➤ fat and cholesterol to help limit damage to the heart and arteries.

Since the '70s, tens of thousands of people have gotten good results with the Pritikin Program. It just goes to show that simple changes in your diet and your exercise habits can turn your health around.

New program actually reverses heart disease

The Pritikin findings have been confirmed by many studies over the past 20 years. In the late 1980s, Dr. Dean Ornish developed a program that helped people actually reverse heart disease and improve the blockages in their arteries. The coronary arteries literally began to look more clean and clear.

Author of *Dean Ornish's Program for Reversing Heart Disease*, Dr. Ornish is director of the Preventive Medicine Research Institute in Sausalito, California, and assistant professor of medicine at the University of California's School of Medicine.

Ornish's program focuses on stress management, diet and exercise as the keys to preventing and reversing heart disease. His healthy heart diet also works wonders for people who want to lose weight.

For people who have been diagnosed with heart disease, Ornish recommends a vegetarian diet that is less than 10 percent fat. This food plan, which Ornish calls The Reversal Diet, is a dieter's dream come true. You can eat whenever you feel hungry and still lose weight.

The diet includes fruits, vegetables, grains, legumes and soybean products. There are a few high-fat vegetarian choices Ornish says you should not eat such as avocados, olives, coconut, nuts, seeds and cocoa products.

You should also avoid all animal products with the exception of egg whites and 1 cup of nonfat yogurt or milk a day. Limit alcohol to 2 ounces per day or less and try to stay away from caffeine, which may worsen irregular heartbeats or provoke stress.

For people who want to prevent heart disease, Ornish recommends a diet that keeps your cholesterol levels at 150 mg or less. Many people can do this by simply limiting their daily intake of butter and oils, cheese, eggs, nuts and meats, especially red meat.

For many people, Ornish's program will mean many new changes, but the benefits are well worth the effort. And he believes that the closer you follow the program, the better you'll feel and the healthier you'll be.

In one of the recent programs Ornish conducted, 82 percent of the participants experienced a significant reversal in their coronary artery disease within the first year — all without drugs or surgery.

Your arteries can clean themselves!

If you are inspired by these study results, read on to learn about the basic components of a healthy diet.

The new Food Guide Pyramid

The Four Basic Food Groups is a concept most Americans

have heard since elementary school. And health-conscious mothers and fathers try hard to provide daily servings from those four famous food groups to keep their families healthy.

But did you know these groups have changed? The United States Department of Agriculture and the Department of Health and Human Services have rearranged the four equal food groups to form the new Food Guide Pyramid.

These new food guidelines emphasize a low-fat diet that includes a variety of foods. Following the Pyramid's guidelines will help you maintain a healthy weight and reduce your risk of high blood pressure.

Instead of the Four Basic Food Groups, the new Pyramid divides food into the six different groups listed below. We'll start at the top of the Pyramid and work our way down.

☐ Fats, oils and sweets. This group includes salad dressings, oils, cream, butter, margarine, sugars, soft drinks, candies and sweet desserts.
   The foods in this group provide lots of calories and/or fat, but they have little nutritional value. Use foods in this category sparingly.

☐ Milk, yogurt and cheese group. Eat two to three servings from this group each day. Teens, young adults up to age 24 and women who are pregnant or breast-feeding need three servings each day.

☐ Meat, poultry, fish, dry beans, eggs and nuts. Eat only two to three servings from this group daily. Total servings should equal five to seven ounces. These foods are especially important for providing dietary protein, calcium, iron and zinc.

☐ Vegetables. Eat three to five servings each day.

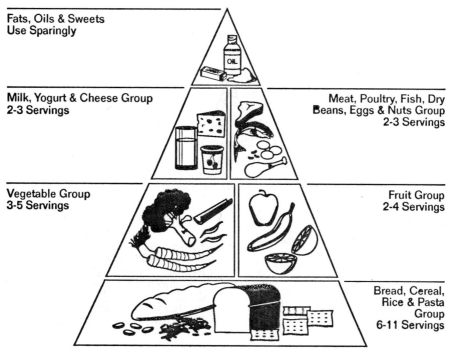

Fats, Oils & Sweets
Use Sparingly

Milk, Yogurt & Cheese Group
2-3 Servings

Meat, Poultry, Fish, Dry
Beans, Eggs & Nuts Group
2-3 Servings

Vegetable Group
3-5 Servings

Fruit Group
2-4 Servings

Bread, Cereal,
Rice & Pasta
Group
6-11 Servings

How many servings do you need each day?

	Women & some older adults	Children, teen girls, active women, most men	Teen boys & active men
Calorie level*	about 1,600	about 2,200	about 2,800
Bread group	6	9	11
Vegetable group	3	4	5
Fruit group	2	3	4
Milk group	**2-3	**2-3	**2-3
Meat group	2, for a total of 5 ounces	2, for a total of 6 ounces	3, for a total of 7 ounces

* If you choose low-fat, lean foods from the 5 major food groups and use foods from the fats, oils and sweets group sparingly, you will take in the calories you need for your sex, age and activity level.
**Women who are pregnant or breast-feeding, teen-agers and young adults to age 24 need 3 servings.

What is a serving size?

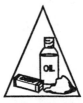

Fats, Oils and Sweets
Limit calories from these,
especially if you need to lose weight

Milk, Yogurt and Cheese
1 cup of milk or yogurt
1 1/2 ounces of natural cheese
2 ounces of processed cheese

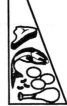

Meat, Poultry, Fish, Dry Beans, Eggs and Nuts
2 to 3 ounces of cooked lean meat, poultry or fish
Count 1 egg as 1 ounce of lean meat (about 1/3 serving)
1 1/2 cups of cooked beans

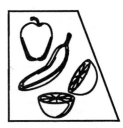

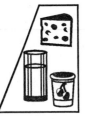

Vegetables
1/2 cup of chopped raw or cooked vegetables
1 cup of leafy raw vegetables

Fruits
1 medium piece of fruit
3/4 cup of juice
1/2 cup of canned or chopped fruit
1/4 cup of dried fruit

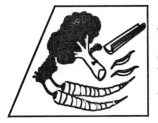

Breads, Cereals, Rice and Pasta
1 slice of bread
1/2 cup of cooked rice, pasta or cereal
1/2 cup of cooked cereal
1 ounce of ready-to-eat cereal

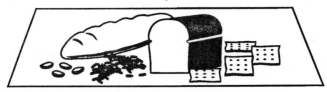

❏ Fruits. Eat two to four servings of fruit every day. Most people need to eat more fruits and vegetables than they do now. An apple a day will no longer do the trick. It appears that you'll need at least five (three vegetables and two fruits) a day to keep the doctor away.

❏ Bread, cereal, rice and pasta. Eat six to 11 servings daily.

Measuring serving sizes

The actual number of servings you need from each food group depends on how many calories your body needs each day.

How many calories you need depends on your age, sex, size and level of physical activity. Find your daily calorie count using the chart in Chapter 5, "Benefits of Weight Loss."

Many people think eating the recommended number of servings per day would mean tons of extra food. However, serving sizes are smaller than you think.

Listed below are some examples of typical serving sizes:

❏ Bread, cereal, rice and pasta group: One serving equals one slice of bread; one ounce of ready-to-eat cereal; or one-half cup of cooked rice, cereal or pasta.
❏ Fruit group: One serving equals one medium apple or banana; one-half cup of chopped, cooked or canned fruit; or three-fourths cup of fruit juice.
❏ Vegetable group: One serving equals one cup of raw, leafy vegetables; one-half cup of other types of raw or cooked vegetables; or three-fourths cup of vegetable juice.
❏ Milk, yogurt and cheese group: One serving equals one cup of milk or yogurt, 1 1/2 ounces of natural cheese or two ounces of processed cheese.

❐ Meat, poultry, fish, dry beans, eggs and nuts group: One serving equals two to three ounces of cooked, lean meat, poultry or fish; 1 1/2 cups of cooked, dry beans; or three eggs.

Even the six to 11 servings of bread, cereal, rice or pasta add up quickly. Consider your meals and snacks for a typical day.

For breakfast, you have a small bowl of cereal and one slice of toast. That's two servings already.

For lunch, you have a sandwich. You've quickly moved up to four servings. Your afternoon snack of three or four small crackers quickly raises your daily grains total to five. A half cup of rice or pasta at dinner brings your total up to the recommended six servings.

Although serving sizes are based on actual measurements of food amounts, you don't need to measure food at every meal. Serving sizes simply provide guidelines to help you estimate how much food you should eat without gaining or losing weight.

However, if you are interested in losing weight, exercise regularly and cut back on fats and sugars. Continue to eat the recommended number of servings from each food group. Otherwise, you may not get all the nutrients you need to keep your body strong and healthy.

Eating vegetarian to lower blood pressure

Even though the new food pyramid includes meat, becoming a vegetarian also can be a healthy choice.

Meat-eaters claim the only way to get enough protein and other nutrients is to eat meat. Sorry, meat-eaters, but doctors are siding with vegetarians in the debate over healthy diets.

Vegetarians tend to have fewer weight problems, lower

blood pressure and overall better health than meat-eaters. Plant sources provide all the proteins you need as long as you eat a variety of grains, nuts, seeds and legumes every day. In fact, doctors say that it would be very difficult to actually plan a vegetarian diet that didn't provide enough protein.

If you eat enough calories to maintain your ideal body weight, you're probably getting plenty of protein.

Plus, in most cases, a well-balanced, meat-free diet provides more iron, calcium, zinc and vitamin D than a nonvegetarian diet.

There are different types of vegetarian diets, and they are grouped into three categories:

➤ Semivegetarians avoid red meat, but they eat fish and poultry.
➤ Lacto-ovo vegetarians don't eat any meat or fish, but they do eat dairy products such as cheese, milk and eggs.
➤ Total vegetarians, or vegans, avoid animal products of any kind.

Vegetarian diets typically have two main advantages over regular diets. They're usually much lower in cholesterol and saturated fats than meat-eater's diets, and they're rich in complex carbohydrates, fiber, vitamins and minerals. Vegetarian diets typically have two to three times more fiber than traditional diets.

Since 60 to 70 percent of a vegetarian's diet comes from carbohydrate-rich vegetables, fruits, beans and grains, it's a perfect choice for athletes or anyone who wants an extra burst of energy.

As for variety, taste and cost, how does a vegetarian diet stack up? Very well, actually. Think about it. There are only a few different types of meats, most of which are relatively expensive.

But there are literally dozens of delicious vegetables, fruits, legumes and cereals, allowing for an almost endless variety of inexpensive dishes.

If you're thinking of going meatless, or if you already are, there are a couple of things you need to keep in mind. Total vegans (who eat absolutely no meat or dairy products) probably need to consider either eating vitamin B12 fortified foods or taking B12 supplements, since this vitamin comes mainly from meat.

Also, make sure your diet is low in fat. Choose low-fat cheeses, milk and other products, and watch out for the high-fat content of many types of nuts.

As with any type of eating style, proper meal planning is the key to good nutrition. The American Dietetic Association offers a consumer education pamphlet, *Eating Well — The Vegetarian Way*, for people interested in learning to plan well-balanced vegetarian diets.

To receive your free copy, call the American Dietetic Association at (312) 899-0040 or write to them at 216 West Jackson Blvd., Suite 800, Chicago, IL 60606-6995.

Healthy grocery shopping

Eating healthy starts at the grocery store. But with so many different products claiming to be low-fat and low-salt, how do you know which ones are really healthy?

In January 1993, the Food and Drug Administration issued new guidelines for food labels. Since most people now risk dietary excess rather than dietary deficiency, the new labels emphasize fat, sodium, carbohydrates and protein. Vitamins and minerals are listed, but they are not given the emphasis they had on past labels.

The label also has a new term, Daily Value (DV), to tell you how much of each nutrient you need. Beside the listed nutrients, Daily Value tells you what percentage of each nutrient one serving provides. Amounts of nutrients are listed in grams or milligrams. The recommended Daily Value is based on a 2,000 calorie diet.

Even if you don't eat exactly 2,000 calories a day, it's still easy to calculate how a certain food fits into your overall food intake. The Daily Values for sodium and cholesterol stay the same no matter how many calories you eat.

A chart appears at the bottom of each label listing the nutrients needed for a 2,000-calorie diet and a 2,500-calorie diet, making calculations easier. The 2,500-calories-a-day diet would only apply to younger men, teen-age boys and very active people.

At the very bottom of the label is the reminder that one gram of fat contains nine calories, one gram of carbohydrate contains four calories and one gram of protein contains four calories.

All the new labels follow the same basic format.

> ➤ **SERVING SIZE** — This appears at the top of the label. Serving sizes will now be the same for similar foods. That will make it easier to compare nutrient values of different brands. The new regulations prevent companies from making serving sizes smaller to make the amount of fat or other ingredients appear smaller.

> ➤ **FAT** — The label lists total fat as well as saturated fat and the number of calories in the product that come from fat. Meat labels may list stearic acid, a type of saturated fat, separately from other fats. It is rumored that stearic acid has possible health benefits, but re-

searchers aren't definite. For now, simply consider stearic acid as a saturated fat.

On food labels for children under age 2, information concerning calories and fat may not be provided. Fat is necessary during the first few years of life to ensure adequate growth and development.

The FDA reasoned that including this data on labels of children's food might make parents think that fat intake for young children needs to be restricted, which is not the case.

➤ **CHOLESTEROL** — 300 milligrams is the maximum daily allowance.

➤ **SODIUM** — 2,400 milligrams is the maximum daily allowance.

➤ **CARBOHYDRATES** — The total number of carbohydrates one serving contains is listed. Total carbohydrates should supply at least 60 percent of daily calories. On a 2,000 calorie diet, carbohydrates should provide at least 1,200 calories.

➤ **FIBER** — At least 20 grams of fiber or 11.5 grams per 1,000 calories daily is probably necessary to stay "regular" and help reduce the risk of cancer and other diseases.

➤ **SUGAR** — This category includes sugars that occur naturally in food as well as added sugars. The FDA has not decided on a set amount of sugar to recommend. Some nutrition experts recommend 50 grams or less per day.

➤ **PROTEIN** — A Daily Value for protein is not required

although some companies may choose to include it. Protein should provide 10 percent of a 2,000 calorie diet. That would mean about 200 of your calories would come from protein.

Companies can now make claims about foods they distribute that might reduce risks of certain illnesses. Any product that promotes a health benefit must meet strict FDA guidelines.

Grain products, fruits and vegetables that contain at least .6 grams of soluble fiber per serving and are low in fat and cholesterol may reduce the risk of heart disease and cancer.

Adequate intake of calcium may help reduce risk of osteoporosis. Reduced sodium consumption may lower blood pressure and possibly decrease risk of stroke and heart failure.

If you have allergic reactions to food colorings, this FDA guideline may brighten your day. Any color additive now has to be referred to by name instead of just by the word color.

Also, any flavorings or other ingredients that contain protein hydrolysates, many of which are high in sodium, have to be identified. These disclosures will be helpful for people on sodium-restricted diets.

With the new FDA label guidelines, claims such as low calorie, low fat, low sodium and low cholesterol are much more trustworthy than they have been in the past. Here are some of the claims you can expect to see.

Some of the labels may still have loopholes, but if you know what to look for, you won't be confused.

LOW CALORIE — A low-calorie product has 40 calories or less per serving. A low-calorie meal or main dish, such as frozen dinners and entrees, contains 120 calories or less per 100 grams, about 3.5 ounces.

LOW FAT — A low-fat food must have three grams or less of fat per serving. On individual foods, low-fat claims are trustworthy. However, on meals and main dishes that claim to be low-fat, make sure that there are no more than two grams of fat per 100 calories. Lobbyists for the dairy industry managed to bypass the regulation standard and get the low-fat label put on 2-percent milk, which actually has five grams of fat per serving. Only skim or 1-percent milk has three grams or less of fat.

LOW IN SATURATED FAT — Saturated fat should make up no more than one gram of all the fat contained in a single serving. In meals or main dishes, less than 10 percent of the calories should come from saturated fat.

LOW CHOLESTEROL — A single serving of a low cholesterol product must contain 20 milligrams (mg) or less of cholesterol. Saturated fat must not exceed two grams. A low-cholesterol meal or main dish should contain no more than 20 mg of cholesterol for every 100 grams of food. A 10-ounce meal should contain about 60 mg of cholesterol.

LOW SODIUM — A low-sodium food contains 140 mg or less of sodium per serving. Prepackaged meals should contain no more than 140 mg of sodium per 100 gram serving. A 10-ounce meal would contain about 400 mg of sodium. A 16-ounce meal should not exceed 600 mg of sodium.

VERY LOW SODIUM — There should be only 35 mg or less of sodium per serving.

LIGHT or LITE — These words have several possible meanings.

For foods that get half or more of their calories from fat, like cheese and hot dogs, a light version of these foods contains no more than half the fat of the original product.

Less fatty foods can be called light if the fat content has been cut by half or the calories by a third. The label must tell you which has been done.

A main dish can be called light if it meets FDA regulations for being low fat or low calorie.

Light may mean the product has half its usual sodium content, but the label must say light in sodium.

If the food is already light or low calorie, then light can be used to mean the product contains half the normal amount of sodium. In this case, the word sodium does not have to be mentioned.

Light may be used to describe a product's color or texture, but the label must make this clear.

On foods like brown sugar, cream or molasses, the word light can be used without explanation if it has traditionally been part of the name.

LESS or FEWER — Foods that contain 25 percent less of some nutrient than a similar food can be labeled less or fewer.

REDUCED — A reduced product has been altered by the manufacturer and contains 25 percent less of a nutrient or calories than the regular product.

FREE — A serving contains none or only very small amounts of fat, cholesterol, sodium, sugar and/or calories.

PERCENT FAT FREE — This phrase tells what part of a food's weight is fat free. However, this label claim can be very tricky to interpret correctly. Percent fat free refers to the fat that makes up a food's weight, not how many calories fat contributes to a food's overall calorie total. For example, a food serving that weighs 100 grams can have two of those grams come from fat and legitimately claim on the label that the food is 98 percent fat free. If you figure the number of calories the fat grams contribute to total calories, the fat percentage is startlingly different. If one serving of this same food contains 75 calories, those two grams of fat make up 18 of the total calories. (Each fat gram contains 9 calories). Eighteen fat calories of a 75 calorie total means that in one serving of food, 24 percent of your calories will be coming from fat, not 2 percent as the label may seem to imply.

GOOD SOURCE OF — A product that claims to be a good source of certain vitamins, minerals, calcium, fiber or other nutrients must contain 10 to 19 percent of the recommended Daily Value of that item. A good source food contains at least 10 percent. A high source food contains at least 20 percent. A product can make a good or high source claim if it contains any food that meets these definitions.

If a label makes a claim that the product is a good source of calcium or other nutrients yet the item exceeds Daily Value recommendations for fat, saturated fat, sodium or cholesterol, the FDA requires a disclosure on the front of the product that says *See back panel for more information about saturated fat and other nutrients.* The disclosure is required when 30 percent of the Daily Value for these nutrients is contained in a main dish or 40 percent in a meal.

LOW — Product contains 5 percent or less of the recommended Daily Value of a nutrient.

MORE — A serving of a food labeled "more" contains 10 percent more of the recommended Daily Value of a nutrient than the regular product. Food serving sizes of less than two tablespoons have to meet tighter guidelines to be labeled low in sodium, fat, calories or other nutrients. Most low foods can be eaten frequently without exceeding dietary guidelines.

The new regulations do not require companies to label fresh meat, poultry or seafood. However, for manufacturers who choose to label these products, the Department of Agriculture has created several new terms to help consumers choose healthier cuts of meat.

Few cuts of meat can be labeled low fat, but there will be categories of lean and extra lean. Keep in mind that manufacturers can take the fat and sodium counts from either fresh or cooked meat, depending on which makes the numbers lowest.

LEAN — Lean meat contains less than 10 grams of fat, four grams of saturated fat and 95 milligrams (mg) of cholesterol per serving.

EXTRA LEAN — Extra lean meat contains less than five grams of fat, two grams of saturated fat and 95 mg of cholesterol per serving.

These new guidelines may not turn you into a label lover, but they can at least give you the reassurance that most label claims are reliable.

The USDA's Human Nutrition Information Service offers additional information on healthy eating habits. For more information, write:

U.S. Department of Agriculture
Human Nutrition Information Service
6505 Belcrest Road
Hyattsville, MD 20782

You also can contact your local county extension office, public health nutritionist or dietician (at the local health department or hospital) for more information on healthier eating.

In this chapter, we've covered the basics of a healthy eating plan that will get your blood pressure under control. The following chapters will provide you with more details on fighting fat, getting your fill of fiber and other dietary measures to lower your blood pressure naturally.

8 Fighting Fat in Your Diet

Good nutrition and blood pressure control mean you're going to have to do battle with fat. But you can fight fat without feeding the fat phobia that seems to be popular in some circles these days. You don't have to avoid fat completely. In fact, your body needs a certain amount of fat to function properly.

Fat provides the energy you need to exercise, protects your internal organs against jarring or repetitive actions such as exercise or motorcycle riding, helps control your body temperature and aids in several other body processes as well.

Plus, your body has become accustomed to fats. Cooks have traditionally used fats to bring out the flavor and aroma of foods.

Fats help give foods a creamy, flaky or tender texture. A meal that contains fats also makes you feel fuller than a meal that doesn't. So, controlling your fat cravings is difficult.

Your goal should be to limit fat to 30 percent of your daily calories. That's the level recommended by both the U.S. Department of Health and Human Services and the American Heart Association.

To make life simple, just make sure that all of the foods you eat meet this 30-percent guideline. No food that you eat should have more than 3 grams of fat for every 100 calories. If you decide to splurge on a favorite high-fat food, compensate by limiting your fat calories for the rest of the day or week.

If you feel up to counting fat grams every day, here are more detailed guidelines:

To determine how much fat will make up 30 percent of your diet, simply multiply your total day's calories by .30, then divide that number by 9 (each gram of fat has 9 calories). Your final figure is the number of grams of fat you can include in your diet each day.

> For example: 1,600 calories x .30 = 480 (calories from fat)
> Then, 480 / 9 = 53 grams of fat per day.

A 1,600-calorie diet should contain no more than 53 grams of fat, a 2,200-calorie diet gets 73 grams of fat and a 2,800-calorie diet allows 93 grams of fat.

The chart on the following page lists the calories, fat grams and percent of calories from fat in different favorite foods from some of the more popular fast food eating places. You may be surprised at the results.

Some fats are worse than others

The kind of fat you eat is as important as how much you eat. Fats are made up of a combination of saturated, polyun-

Fast Food Danger			
Fast Food Item	Fat Grams	Calories	Percent of Calories From Fat
Apple Turnover	14	255	49%
Baked Potato with Broccoli & Cheese	18	376	43%
Burger King Cheeseburger	15	317	43%
Chicken Club Sandwich	25	479	47%
Chocolate Shake (medium)	12	320	34%
Danish	18	400	41%
Enchilada	21	396	48%
Fish Sandwich	27	469	52%
Kentucky Fried Chicken Breast (extra crispy)	21	353	54%
McDonalds Big Mac	35	570	55%
McDonalds French Fries (regular)	12	220	49%
Onion Rings (fried)	16	285	51%
Pepperoni Pizza (1 slice)	12	306	35%
Sausage Biscuit	31	467	60%
Taco	10	187	48%
Wendy's Breakfast Sandwich	19	370	46%
Wendy's Frosty (medium)	18	520	31%

saturated and monounsaturated fats.

Stay away from saturated fats as much as possible. They raise blood cholesterol and triglyceride levels. They are primarily found in animal and dairy products, such as meat, egg yolks, milk, butter, cheese, cream and a few vegetable fats, such as coconut oil, palm oil and hydrogenated vegetable shortenings.

Saturated fats are generally hard or solid at room temperature. Less than 10 percent of your calories should come from saturated fats.

Unsaturated fats can be called either polyunsaturated fats or monounsaturated fats. Studies show that foods high in polyunsaturated fats can reduce cholesterol levels but also may reduce your levels of HDL cholesterol (the "good" kind).

Foods high in monounsaturated fats (such as canola, olive and peanut oils and oatmeal) also reduce cholesterol levels. Plus, they don't lower your HDL levels, according to some experts.

New research comes out every day regarding ways to lower your cholesterol levels.

In fact, some authorities are now questioning whether monounsaturated fats are indeed better for you than polyunsaturated fats.

Experts definitely agree, however, that lowering your overall saturated fat intake will give you more energy and help your arteries remain clear.

Listed below are some tips to help you avoid saturated fats:

❏ Eliminate or drastically reduce consumption of egg yolks, organ meats and most cheeses. Don't want to give up your favorite high-fat cheese? Make a low-fat version by zapping it in the microwave for a minute or two. Any oil you can pour off will significantly reduce the cheese's fat content. This method works well for fajitas, cheese sandwiches or cheese toppings on casseroles.

❏ Reduce your consumption of butter, bacon, beef, whole milk, cream, chocolate and almost any food of animal origin.

❏ Never eat beef, lamb or pork more than three times per week. Choose lean cuts of meat and cut off all visible fat before cooking.

❏ When preparing chicken or turkey, be sure to cut off the skin before cooking because much of the fat is in the skin. Eat the light meat because it contains less fat than the dark meat.

❏ Eat smaller portions of meat by using dishes that combine meat with vegetables (especially legumes like beans), pasta or grains.

❏ Avoid duck, goose, gravies, sauces, casseroles, pot pies, bacon bits, croissants, fried foods, prepackaged cake mixes, biscuit mixes, pancake mixes, ice cream, whole milk, evaporated milk, artificial or nondairy creamers and sweetened condensed milk.

Some oils are better than others

Many people grew up eating foods cooked with butter, shortening and even lard — full of saturated fat. Today we know there are other ways to prepare food without adding all that extra fat to our diets.

Canola, sunflower, corn and olive oils are all fairly low in saturated fat.

Sesame oil and peanut oil are a little higher, but butter, cocoa butter (used in making chocolate) and coconut oil are the worst possible choices for people trying to lower their cholesterol levels.

Although all of the oils (except butter) listed in the chart on the following page contain no measurable amounts of dietary cholesterol, you must use oils low in saturated fat to lower your cholesterol level.

Canola oil (7% saturated fat) is one of the best available cooking oils. Olive oil (14% saturated fat) also is good to use.

Product	Saturated fat	Cholesterol	Poly-unsaturated fat	Mono-unsaturated fat
Canola oil	7%	0 mg	35%	58%
Safflower oil	9%	0 mg	78%	12%
Sunflower oil	11%	0 mg	42%	47%
Corn oil	13%	0 mg	62%	25%
Olive oil	14%	0 mg	12%	74%
Hydrogenated sunflower oil	14%	0 mg	40%	48%
Sesame oil	15%	0 mg	44%	42%
Soybean oil	15%	0 mg	60%	24%
Margarine, bottled	17%	0 mg	47%	36%
Margarine, tub	17%	0 mg	37%	46%
Peanut oil	18%	0 mg	33%	49%
Margarine, stick	19%	0 mg	33%	47%
Cocoa butter	62%	0 mg	3%	35%
Butter	66%	31 mg	4%	30%
Palm kernel oil	87%	0 mg	2%	11%
Coconut oil	92%	0 mg	2%	6%

This chart is deceptive in one respect. Any fat that is hard at room temperature, such as stick margarine, is not good for your cholesterol. Margarine has been hydrogenated, or hardened, and that process adds trans fatty acids. Trans fatty acids are almost as bad for you as saturated fat, so stick margarine is about the same as butter as far as your cholesterol is concerned. Diet margarines and soft margarines are better choices.

Satisfy your fat tooth with fat substitutions

The latest stand-in for butter or margarine is prune puree. Cooks from all over are creating culinary magic with this versatile fat buster.

Just mix up your favorite brownie, cake, cookie or bread recipe and substitute prune puree for the exact amount of butter, shortening or oil the recipe recommends.

Consider that 1 cup of prune puree has 407 calories and 1 gram of fat, while 1 cup of butter has 1,600 calories and 182 grams of fat and 1 cup of oil has 1,944 calories and 218 grams of fat. Now you can begin to understand why bakers are so excited about prunes.

Prunes contain large amounts of pectin which helps hold in the air bubbles that make baked goods rise. Prunes also contain fairly large amounts of sorbitol, a sugar alcohol, which helps keep baked goods moist and gives them the flaky, tender taste of shortening or butter.

To make enough prune puree for several recipes, mix one pound of dried, pitted prunes with 1 cup of hot tap water. Keep your prune puree in a covered jar in the refrigerator.

For more information on cooking with prunes, send a stamped, self-addressed envelope to Prune the Fat, P.O. Box 10157, Pleasanton, CA 94588-0157.

Applesauce and apricot purees also are good substitutes for butter and margarine in baked goods recipes. In some cases, you may only be able to replace three-quarters of the butter or margarine. Experiment to see which substitution works best for you. The only drawback to using applesauce and apricots as fat substitutes is that these baked goods tend to become soggy and moldy within a day or two.

When baking with fat substitutes, use cake flour instead of all-purpose flour. This will help keep your baked goods tender. Also, be careful not to overbake fat-reduced recipes, which dry out more quickly than traditional variations that call for butter or oil.

Some researchers even believe that as you reduce the amount of fats you eat, your cravings for them will decline. Researchers at the Fred Hutchinson Cancer Research Center in Seattle found that people who switch from high-fat to low-fat foods soon develop a taste for lower-fat foods.

High-fat foods take longer to leave the stomach than lower-fat foods and may contribute to indigestion and a bloated feeling.

You don't need to make all these changes overnight. Slowly, gradually begin putting the guidelines into practice. Introduce healthy foods as you slowly eliminate some of the unhealthier foods. Remember that even slow, gradual changes in your eating habits are better than no changes at all.

Learning to control your fat cravings is just like learning any new habit — a little tough at first, but easier every day you do it.

9 ‖ The Importance of Fiber

Here's one solid piece of nutritional advice: Eat more fiber.

One hundred years ago, the typical American diet contained an adequate amount of natural food fiber. Most bread was made with whole wheat flour which contained bran, the outer fibrous part of the wheat kernel.

High blood pressure and coronary heart disease were rare, and few people were troubled with appendicitis, diverticulosis, cancer of the large bowel, constipation, hemorrhoids, diabetes or obesity.

Then, in the last quarter of the 19th century, American industry made two discoveries which were hailed as breakthroughs. The first invention was the development of high-speed steel roller mills for flour milling.

Food companies could produce a fine white flour that tasted better than most whole wheat flour and was less likely to spoil.

The second development was the growth of the canning industry. The canning process greatly reduced food fiber content.

These two changes took place over several years, and no one noticed that anything was wrong. But in the 20th century, scientists became puzzled at the persistent rise in certain death rates and obesity.

In the 1940s and 50s, Dr. Denis Burkitt, a British surgeon, noticed that he never found a case of diverticular disease or cancer of the colon in the thousands of rural tribesmen of East Africa that were autopsied.

Further research showed that obesity, appendicitis, heart attacks, constipation and hemorrhoids also were extremely rare. Dr. Burkitt thought that the amount of fiber in the diet was the key. He and other doctors investigated what happened to tribes who moved to African cities and adopted a low-fiber diet.

The results confirmed the hypothesis: On a diet that had been depleted of bran and other fiber, many Africans became obese and developed all the other ills of Western civilization. Dr. Burkitt also linked high blood pressure with a lack of fiber in the diet.

More recently, scientists have found that a high-fiber diet can dramatically reduce your risk of developing high blood pressure. Of great significance is a scientific study that involved more than 30,000 men.

These men participated in the study to determine how dietary fiber affects blood pressure levels. The results of the study indicated that people who eat less than 12 grams of fiber a day have a 60 percent greater risk of developing high blood pressure compared with people who eat 12 grams or more of fiber daily.

This study and many others demonstrate the huge importance of adding fiber to your family's diet.

Two types of fiber

While most of us generally lump all fiber into one big category, researchers are a little more specific. They divide what we refer to as plain old fiber into two categories: soluble and insoluble fiber.

Both are made up of the parts of plants — beans, grains, vegetables and fruits — that your body can't digest because enzymes in your intestinal tract can't break it down. (You don't find fiber in animal foods.) Some foods have both kinds of fiber, but most foods are higher in one than the other. It's important to eat both kinds.

Insoluble fibers are fibers that don't dissolve in water. They help prevent constipation. Too much can make diarrhea symptoms worse. Insoluble fiber passes through your digestive system pretty much unchanged from the way it went into your mouth.

When the insoluble fiber gets into the intestines, it dramatically reduces the amount of time food spends in the digestive tract.

This reduces the possible harmful effects of wastes staying in the intestines longer than necessary. That's one reason researchers believe insoluble fiber helps prevent colon cancer.

Soluble fibers are fibers that can dissolve in water. They help lower fat and cholesterol in your blood. When soluble fiber gets to the intestines, it actually swells as it rapidly soaks up water.

Soluble dietary fibers have been shown to attach to and remove bile acids in the digestive tract. Bile acids are produced by the liver to aid in digestion.

The removal of these acids helps slow the development of

micelles, which are necessary for the absorption of cholesterol and other lipids.

Fewer micelles mean less cholesterol and even less digested sugar can get into the bloodstream.

Soluble fiber contributes to good health by lowering the total amount of cholesterol circulating in the bloodstream, especially LDL cholesterol. This helps reduce the risk of developing high blood pressure, atherosclerosis, heart disease and strokes.

It also helps diabetics regulate their blood glucose levels, leading to a reduction in the amount of insulin needed.

In one study, a group of 20 men with cholesterol levels over 260 were given diets containing 17 grams of soluble fiber each day. This fiber was added to the men's diets from oat products and beans.

This is equivalent to one serving of hot oat bran cereal and five oat bran muffins per day or several servings of cooked beans and bean soups. After only three weeks on this high soluble fiber diet, the men averaged a 24 percent drop in LDL cholesterol.

Beyond the general description of the work of soluble fiber on bile acids, researchers are not entirely clear about just how soluble fiber produces all its benefits.

This is because so many different studies have been done, using different methods and different ways to examine the fiber.

However, many researchers agree that the benefits you will get from soluble fiber is related to the amount you eat. When a moderate amount of soluble fiber is eaten each day, a 10 to 20 percent reduction in cholesterol may be reasonably expected.

Some natural sources of soluble and insoluble fiber are listed on the following page.

Natural Sources of Fiber

Insoluble fiber	Soluble fiber
Bananas	Apples
Broccoli	Apricots
Brown rice	Barley
Brussels sprouts	Berries
Cauliflower	Cabbage
Corn	Carrots
Lentils	Celery
Pasta	Chickpeas, split peas
Potatoes	Grapefruit
Spinach	Nectarines
Wheat bran cereal	Oat bran, oatmeal
Wheat germ	Okra
Whole-wheat bread	Oranges
Whole-wheat crackers	Peaches
	Peas
	Pinto, kidney, navy, lima beans
	Sweet potatoes
	Tangerines
	Turnips
	Zucchini

For more information about the fiber and fat content of many foods, see Chapter 26 in the back of this book.

Feeling your oats

Oat bran has soluble fiber to help reduce high cholesterol levels and insoluble fiber to help prevent many types of digestive problems and cancers.

Oat bran is good for you for a number of reasons. It is readily available in fairly unprocessed forms. The less processing, the better it is for you. That means it will retain proteins, carbohydrates and vitamins B and E.

Oat bran helps protect against high blood pressure, cancer, high cholesterol, heart disease, obesity and diabetes.

A new study suggests that two to three ounces of oat bran added to your diet every day for about six weeks could reduce your cholesterol levels by 7 to 10 percent. Funded by a grant from the Quaker Oats Company, a group of Chicago scientists tested the effects of oat bran on the cholesterol levels of 140 volunteers, all of whom had high cholesterol.

The volunteers were divided into seven groups. All groups started eating a low-fat diet. Group one, the control group, ate one ounce of a wheat cereal each day. Groups two, three and four added one, two and three ounces of oatmeal to their diet. And groups five, six and seven ate one, two and three ounces of oat bran daily.

At the end of six weeks, the volunteers tested their total cholesterol levels and their LDL cholesterol levels. Group one, the control group that ate wheat cereal, showed no drop in cholesterol levels.

In fact, the group experienced a slight rise in cholesterol. Wheat bran is an insoluble fiber only.

The group that ate two ounces of oatmeal daily experienced a drop of 2.7 percent in total cholesterol and a 3.5 percent drop in LDL cholesterol.

The group that ate two ounces of oat bran daily experienced a 9.5 percent drop in total cholesterol and a 15.9 percent drop in LDL cholesterol.

The oat bran was better at reducing cholesterol levels than the oatmeal because of the oat bran's higher concentration of a kind of fiber known as beta-glucan fiber. It requires three ounces of oatmeal to achieve the same cholesterol-lowering effects as two ounces of oat bran.

Other studies were conducted by Dr. James Anderson at the University of Kentucky. In 1984, he reported that his subjects' high cholesterol levels fell by 21 percent when they were given 3.5 ounces of oat bran per day for 21 days.

The same doctor also conducted a study at the Massachusetts Institute of Technology that compared oat bran versus wheat bran and their effects on cholesterol levels. Students who ate 1.5 ounces of oat bran a day saw their cholesterol levels drop by 9 percent. Wheat bran had no effect on blood cholesterol levels, Anderson reported.

Keep in mind that a 9 percent drop in cholesterol readings for healthy college students cuts the likelihood of an early heart attack by as much as 30 percent.

A special warning: Beware of high-fiber claims in foods that are commercially prepared. Many nationally known companies began marketing high-fiber products when wheat germ and oat bran became popular several years ago.

Many of these products either contain so little extra fiber or add so much fat that the good of the fiber is almost canceled out.

For example, you would probably say that a muffin would make a better snack than a cookie or that an oat bran waffle would make a better breakfast than a doughnut. But that's not always true. One company's oat bran muffin has more fat and more calories than a creme-filled doughnut.

Nutritionists at Tufts University set out to see what is good and bad in commercially prepared muffins. Some manufacturers were reluctant to say what's in their muffins. But through laboratory testing Tufts found:

☐ A simple raisin bran muffin sold through a national

doughnut chain had 418 calories, 13 grams of fat and 692 mg of sodium. (Keep in mind that it is usually necessary to eat several muffins to get the needed dietary fiber.)

❑ A nationally distributed grocery store oat bran muffin had 220 calories, 8 grams of fat and 380 mg of sodium.

❑ An apple and spice muffin from a doughnut shop had 327 calories, 11 grams of fat and 382 mg of sodium.

❑ Another doughnut shop offered a corn muffin. Its totals? It had 347 calories, 13 grams of fat and 577 mg of sodium.

These figures should cast some doubt in your mind about the "healthy" muffins now being sold. Your best bet may be to make your own oat and high-fiber products. That way, you know exactly what is going into them. Learn to read labels and ask questions.

An oat-bran fat substitute lowers cholesterol

Lower your blood cholesterol level by eating ice cream? The U.S. Department of Agriculture scientists say they have come up with a new process that extracts the fat-fighting part of oat bran and turns it into a creamy substance that could be used to replace many kinds of fats in foods, including ice cream.

Called Oatrim, the white, tasteless flour is loaded with beta-glucans, the part of oat bran that researchers believe lowers cholesterol levels. Researchers treat oat bran with enzymes to produce either a flour or a powder.

In animal tests, Oatrim slashed cholesterol by 18 percent. Even better, it hits hardest at LDL cholesterol, the bad kind, while it seems to slightly increase HDL or good cholesterol. Adding about an ounce of Oatrim to an instant breakfast drink gives you more cholesterol-lowering beta-glucans than three ounces of pure oat bran, researchers say.

Oatrim also is being used in breads, brownies, cakes, cookies and muffins.

You can buy Oatrim in its powdered form to use for cooking at home, including baking. You can find it at some health food stores.

Peas and beans add bulk to diet

Pinto, white, kidney and other cooked, dried beans and peas are excellent dietary sources of soluble fiber. When measured in raw weight, these legumes provide an average of 19.9 grams of total dietary fiber and 7.8 grams of soluble fiber per 100 grams.

Legumes make tasty additions to soups, stews and entrees and can significantly reduce your risk of atherosclerosis and high blood pressure by reducing cholesterol levels. Based on scientific studies, eating beans for three weeks, either cooked alone or in soups, can result in a 15 to 23 percent decrease in total serum cholesterol and a 13 to 24 percent decrease in LDL cholesterol.

Gummy food additives can be healthy

Gums are a form of dietary soluble fiber that are generally indigestible. They receive their name based on their ability to produce gel-like substances when they are in a liquid. A common example is the guar seed.

This seed is the Indian cluster bean cultivated in India for animal feed and in the United States for use as food and drug additives.

Recent research indicates that these food additives also can help reduce cholesterol levels. A scientific study showed a 16 percent reduction in cholesterol in seven healthy volunteers who were fed 36 grams of guar seed for two weeks in addition to their normal diet. An additional group of volunteers enjoyed an 11 percent drop in cholesterol after two weeks of eating 15 grams of guar per day.

Further studies also show that adding gums to the diet can produce a reduction in LDL cholesterol.

An apple a day ...

A French study has found that eating two apples a day can lower your cholesterol level by at least 10 percent and by as much as 30 percent. Apples and prunes have been considered healthy foods for a long time, but their beneficial effect on cholesterol levels has only recently been discovered.

Apples and prunes are two common food sources rich in pectin, a soluble fiber. Pectins change from an insoluble form in unripe fruit to a much more soluble form in ripened fruit.

Scientific studies reveal that consuming up to 15 grams of pectin per day for a few weeks can result in a 5 percent reduction in total serum cholesterol.

Because apples and prunes are high in pectin and have been shown to help lower cholesterol, they are excellent snacks and an important part of a healthy diet.

The #1 cholesterol-lowering fiber

If you've taken Metamucil, Fiberall or another natural bulk laxative to get relief from constipation, you've had psyllium, which some studies show works better to lower cholesterol than any other fiber.

Psyllium is the fiber part of seed husks from the common plant, English plantain. The fiber dissolves in water and forms a kind of gel in the digestive system.

Even though psyllium is all soluble fiber, the bacteria in your stomach don't break it down as quickly as other soluble fibers. That means it also works like an insoluble fiber to increase stool bulk and prevent constipation.

Psyllium seems to lower both total cholesterol levels and LDL cholesterol levels. The people who volunteered for a recent study took psyllium twice a day. They mixed three packets of instant Metamucil into a 12-ounce glass of water.

The volunteers each drank one glass of Metamucil before breakfast and one after dinner. They also drank a 12-ounce glass of water after each glass of Metamucil.

The volunteers also participated in the American Heart Association diet while they tested the psyllium. The combination of the AHA diet and the psyllium drinks resulted in a 17.3 percent decrease in total cholesterol in men and a 7.7 percent decrease in total cholesterol in women. The study also showed a 20 percent decrease in LDL cholesterol in men and an 11.6 decrease in LDL cholesterol in women.

Researchers suggest that psyllium is probably most effective in lowering cholesterol when it is combined with the American Heart Association diet. (You can contact the American Heart Association for a copy of this diet.)

In a different study, other researchers found that daily doses of just three teaspoons of psyllium can lower cholesterol levels in the blood by 5 percent and can slash levels of bad cholesterol by 10 percent or more.

For every percentage point you lower your total cholesterol level, your risk of heart attack drops by two percentage points. In addition, the fiber supplements can raise the proportion of good HDL cholesterol while they lower bad LDL cholesterol.

The researchers gave the psyllium to people who had mild to moderate cases of hypercholesterolemia, (too much cholesterol in the blood).

The 75 people had already been put on low fat diets to treat their condition. Most received some benefit from just that step alone.

In addition to the low fat diet, half of them took the extra psyllium daily for up to 16 weeks during the experiments. The people who took the fiber laxative had dramatic cuts in cholesterol levels.

They took each teaspoonful of psyllium with eight ounces of water. Besides the beneficial effects of lowering cholesterol, the psyllium supplements had no serious side effects.

About one out of six people reported minor discomforts, such as temporary feelings of fullness with some abdominal cramping. One in 12 had bloating and increased amounts of intestinal gas.

Only one experienced a significant laxative effect. These side effects were minor, and they did not require the treatment to be discontinued.

The psyllium fiber worked even better than oat bran. Overall, eight out of 10 people who took the psyllium (in the form of Metamucil) had lower LDL cholesterol and total cholesterol levels after eight weeks. The control group, which had been given a fake supplement, experienced almost no changes.

Easy ways to eat more fiber

Besides lowering your risk of high blood pressure, heart disease and stroke, fiber works as a natural laxative to help keep you regular.

It can be a real diet booster as well. Loading up on fruits and vegetables can help you feel full. You should aim for 20 to 35 grams of fiber a day.

Here are some easy ways to eat more fiber:

❑ Substitute whole wheat flour for white. Use whole-wheat or spinach pasta instead of regular. Replace white rice with brown.

❑ Eat vegetables with their skins. The skins contain high levels of fiber. Some vegetables high in fiber are winter squash at six grams a cup, and broccoli and spinach at four grams a cup each.

❑ Eat fruits with seeds, such as blackberries, raspberries, strawberries and figs, which are good sources of fiber. Here are some other high-fiber fruits:

High-fiber fruits	
Raisins	Kiwi
Blueberries	Dates
Apple	Pear

❑ Make a good supply of bran muffins and keep them on hand for breakfasts and snacks and to serve with dinner.

❑ Try to reduce the amount of time high-fiber foods are cooked. Cooking breaks down some types of fibers and may slightly reduce the fiber content of the food.

❑ Avoid mechanical food preparations which ruin fiber in food before it is cooked. This includes peeling, mashing and grating prior to cooking. Instead, leave the peels on often-peeled vegetables. The peels not only provide fiber when eaten, they also add important vitamins and minerals. Cut fruits and vegetables into chunks rather than grating them.

❑ When given a choice, always select whole grains over more processed foods. More whole-grain breads are available, and cookies are now sold with less sugar and more fiber.

❑ When preparing recipes, try substituting coarse whole wheat flour for one-fourth to one-half of the amount of regular flour called for. Remember, if you are using oat flour, do not substitute it for more than one-third of the regular flour. It may interfere with the way things bake. (Is your flour coarse enough? Most of it shouldn't be able to pass through your sifter.)

❑ Peas and beans are excellent sources of fiber and they are easy to store. They also are high in protein. They easily form the main dish at a nonmeat meal, and they come in many varieties:

Beans and peas	
Broad beans	Lentils
Black beans	Lima beans
Pinto beans	Baked beans
Kidney beans	Green peas
Chickpeas	Black-eyed peas

❑ Try mixing mashed legumes (peas or beans) into ground beef. This not only stretches the meat, it adds fiber and reduces the total amount of fat eaten. This mixture also makes a good base for Mexican-style dishes.

❑ Sprinkle oat bran and wheat bran on cereals, vegetables, desserts and even ice cream.

❑ Make sure you drink plenty of water as you increase

the amount of fiber you eat. If you don't, the fiber can make constipation worse. You may experience gas and bloating as you increase the amount of fiber in your diet. If you increase the fiber gradually, your system will adapt better.

Breakfast cereals easiest way to boost fiber intake

Your cholesterol levels throughout the day seem to be directly affected by the food you choose for breakfast, according to a five-year study. Adults who "break the fast" with ready-to-eat cereal "have significantly lower fat and cholesterol intakes than those who [eat] other foods at breakfast" or even those who skip breakfast altogether.

The National Health and Nutrition Examination analyzed the food intakes of 11,864 Americans. To determine whether breakfast really is the most important meal of the day, researchers divided respondents into one of these three categories:

➤ cereal eaters
➤ breakfast eaters (other than ready-to-eat cereal)
➤ breakfast skippers

The noncereal breakfast eaters had the highest fat intakes, followed by breakfast skippers.

Among men and women aged 50 to 74, the study indicates that serum cholesterol levels were lowest for those people eating breakfasts that include cereal and highest for those who skip breakfast altogether.

Having cereal for breakfast seems to help keep cholesterol levels under control, an important factor in controlling your heart disease risk. The breakfast skippers apparently ate higher cholesterol meals later in the day, the study indicates. In addition, they don't get the cholesterol lowering benefits of the high-fiber breakfast cereal.

Eating a high-fiber cereal for breakfast can result in weight loss, too. Men and women who eat high-fiber cereal for breakfast tend to feel less hungry throughout the day, compared with those who eat other breakfast foods or cereals with low amounts of fiber. Therefore, high-fiber cereal eaters tend to eat less food during breakfast and lunch.

Researchers asked men and women between the ages of 24 and 59 to eat a 7:30 a.m. breakfast of orange juice and cold cereal with milk. They ate either Post Toasties (lowest in fiber), Shredded Wheat, Bran Chex, All Bran or Fiber One (highest in fiber of the five).

Three and a half hours later, they ate a buffet lunch. The high-fiber eaters consumed about 100 fewer calories at breakfast and about 50 fewer calories at the lunch buffet than those who had eaten lower-fiber cereals, according to the report.

Saving 50 calories at lunch doesn't seem significant, but "theoretically could result in substantial weight loss if continued long-term," the researchers conclude. High-fiber hot cereals like oatmeal probably would give many of the same benefits.

The cereals listed below are high in fiber:

High-fiber cereals

Kellogg's Cracklin Bran	Kellogg's All-Bran
Kellogg's Bran Flakes	Kellogg's Bran Buds
Kellogg's Raisin Bran	Quaker Corn Bran
Ralston Purina Bran Chex	Post Bran Flakes
Ralston Purina Raisin Bran	Post Fruit and Fiber
General Mills Fiber One	Loma Linda 100% Bran

General Mills Bran Muffin Crisp

10 | The Shakedown on Salt

S alt itself isn't bad for your health. You may know that in the Bible Jesus says, "Ye are the salt of the earth," indicating that even thousands of years ago salt was a valuable commodity for preserving food and stimulating taste buds.

The word "salary" comes from the Latin word "sal," meaning salt. Roman soldiers were sometimes said to be "worth their salt" because they were often paid in salt rather than actual money. Salt, also known as sodium chloride, is made up of 40 percent sodium and 60 percent chloride. It is essential to life, and it is an important mineral in the body. Without it, we would die.

Salt maintains fluid levels between the cells and the blood system and acts as an electrolyte to help chemical and electrical reactions in the body.

Why, then, all the fuss about removing salt from your diet? What has happened is that we have simply overdosed on a good thing to the point that it has become a bad thing. Too much salt in your diet begins to have a negative effect on your health.

Our bodies are equipped to handle only so much salt. Normally, the kidneys handle any extra salt by allowing the salt to be flushed out in the urine.

Diets containing large amounts of salt over long periods of time tend to overwhelm the kidneys' ability to regulate salt. Over time, this can lead to high blood pressure.

The Greenland Eskimos and the Amazon Indians, who eat very little salt, have very little high blood pressure. But in the north of Japan, high blood pressure is common among the people whose diet contains large amounts of salt.

Of course, in such societies other factors may be at work, but the strong relationship between salt consumption and high blood pressure should not be underestimated.

Training your taste buds

A low-sodium diet is one of the basic, natural ways to lower high blood pressure, but many people are hesitant because they think that a salt-free diet is bland.

However, researchers at the University of Minnesota discovered that your desire for salt and your tastes change when you start a low-salt diet.

Many participants in earlier studies said that once they were on a low-salt diet, many foods they once enjoyed were now too salty.

Participants on a low-salt diet compared salted crackers at regular intervals. After a short time, the crackers with the most sodium were considered too salty.

By the sixth week, the participants experienced a change in taste, preferring less salt.

As you reduce the amount of salt in your diet, you will

experience new flavor sensations that were masked by the large amounts of salt you ate.

The true flavor of vegetables can be hidden by cooking with too much salt. In this sense, excessive salt can be a taste destroyer rather than a flavor enhancer.

One scientific study on salt consumption deals with twins. One twin was put on a low-salt diet. The other twin continued to consume a diet high in salt.

After a few weeks, the twin on the low-salt diet learned to consume less salt and preferred to eat less salt.

The other twin was still in the habit of consuming more salt and continued to prefer the high-salt diet.

Counting your salt grams

According to many scientists, some people are "salt-sensitive." These people react more quickly to smaller amounts of salt in their diets and develop high blood pressure much sooner than people who are not salt sensitive.

If you are wondering if you are one of those salt-sensitive people, try this three-step test:

1) Record blood pressure and salt intake under normal circumstances.

2) Restrict salt to 2 grams per day and record blood pressure.

3) Increase salt by one gram per day to determine threshold levels in those who responded to restriction.

According to Dr. Hugo Espinel of the Blood Pressure Center in Metropolitan Washington, this test can help you find the level of salt intake that is safe for your blood pressure.

In addition to salt-sensitive people, researchers have

found that African-Americans, elderly people and people who are already suffering from high blood pressure are more sensitive to changes in dietary salt intake than most people.

However, researchers have found that most people can benefit from lower blood pressure levels simply by cutting back on the amount of salt in their diets.

Getting salt down into the range of 500 milligrams (mg) per day (1/4 teaspoon of salt = 500 mg) seems to be the most effective. Since most Americans consume between 6,000 and 12,000 mg of salt each day, it shouldn't be too difficult to cut back some.

Recent studies indicate that some people need as little as 200 mg a day. A healthy amount for most people is from 500 mg up to no more than 1,000 mg of salt per day.

However, there are exceptions. Hard labor, profuse sweating, pregnancy and breast-feeding might increase the need for salt up to 2,000 mg per day.

You may find it hard to believe that you eat a lot of salt every day, but the processed foods that we eat are usually filled with salt.

This can account for up to 75 percent of salt intake. Any food that comes in a can, a frozen package or a box is likely to have salt added as a preservative or flavor enhancer.

Table salt and salty products can be easy to avoid, but it is this hidden salt that often has consumers stumped.

The Food and Drug Administration (FDA) requires soft-drink manufacturers to list the sodium content of their drinks on their bottles or cans.

Many products list their nutritional information, but be wary of their advertising and labeling. The higher up on the ingredients list salt appears, the higher the content. Check labels very carefully.

A slice of bread may contain over 200 mg of salt, a bowl of

cornflakes over 300 mg, a bowl of canned soup over 1,000 mg, a chicken dinner from a fast food restaurant over 2,000 mg and a large dill pickle over 1,000 mg.

The following chart shows how much sodium some popular foods from the different food groups contain:

Food	Portion	Sodium (mg)
American cheese	1 ounce	405
bacon	3 slices	420
bacon bits	1 Tbsp.	165
beef bouillon	1 cup	782
bologna	1 slice	289
Canadian bacon	2 slices	710
catsup	1 Tbsp.	178
cheese Danish	1 Danish	319
chicken breast	1 breast	770
chicken consomme	1 cup	635
chicken noodle soup	1 cup	1107
chili	1 cup	1061
chocolate ice cream	1 cup	100
cottage cheese	1/2 cup	425
cream cheese	1 ounce	85
croissant	1 roll	450
dill pickle	1 slice	430
fried chicken	2 pieces	800
fried onions rings	3 ounce	485
ham	1 slice	373
hamburger	1 patty	500
Hamburger Helper	1 cup	980
hot dog	1 hot dog	639
Italian bread	1 slice	175
Italian sausage	1 sausage	618

Food	Portion	Sodium (mg)
macaroni and cheese	1 cup	1086
manhattan clam chowder	1 cup	1808
minestrone	1 cup	1830
mixed nuts	1/4 cup	240
mustard	1 tsp.	65
olive	1 olive	19
Parmesan cheese	1/4 cup	466
peanuts	1/2 cup	594
pepperoni pizza	1/4 of 12 in. pie	1256
pickles, sweet	1/2 cup	645
pizza rolls	1 serving	380
pork sausage	1 patty	420
pretzels	1 cup	756
quarter-pound hamburger with cheese	1 sandwich	1225
relish	1 Tbsp.	122
sausage biscuit	1 biscuit	1210
smoked pork sausage	1 link	1020
soft pretzel with cheese	1 pretzel	1175
soy sauce	1 Tbsp.	1029
steak sauce	1 Tbsp.	265
teriyaki sauce	1 Tbsp.	690
tomato juice	6 ounces	660
tomato soup	1 cup	872
tortilla snack chips	15-18 chips	200
tuna salad	1 cup	434
vegetable beef soup	1 cup	957
wheat bread	1 slice	132

The many disguises of salt

Many people find it difficult to cut back on sodium in their diets because they don't recognize the sodium when they see it.

Listed below are some common sodium-containing compounds that you should look out for when you do your grocery shopping:

Compound	Commonly used as
Salt (sodium chloride)	Used in cooking or at the table; also used in canning and preserving.
Monosodium glutamate (also called MSG)	A seasoning used in home and restaurant cooking and in many packaged, canned and frozen foods.
Baking soda (sodium bicarbonate)	Used to leaven breads and cakes; added to vegetables in cooking; used as an alkalizer for indigestion.
Baking powder	Used to leaven quick breads and cakes.
Disodium phosphate	Present in some quick-cooking cereals and processed cheeses.
Sodium alginate	Used in many chocolate milks and ice creams to make a smooth texture.
Sodium benzoate	Used as a preservative in many condiments, such as relishes, sauces and salad dressings.

Compound	Commonly used as
Sodium hydroxide	Used in food processing to soften and loosen skins of ripe olives and certain fruits and vegetables.
Sodium nitrite	Used in cured meats and sausages.
Sodium propionate	Used in some pasteurized cheeses and in some breads and cakes to inhibit growth of molds.
Sodium sulfite	Used to bleach certain fruits, such as maraschino cherries and glazed or crystallized fruits that are to be artificially colored; also used as a preservative in some dried fruits such as prunes.

Easy ways to eat less salt

If you are concerned about giving up flavor in your cooking, a little creativity can help add spice to your food while lowering the salt content. You do not have to sacrifice flavor when you cut down on sodium if you follow these suggestions:

☐ Don't add salt to pasta or other starchy foods that will be topped with other foods. The toppings usually add enough flavor so that you don't even notice the missing salt.

☐ Balance your salt intake. If your breakfast is high in salt, eat low-salt meals for the rest of the day.

☐ Remove the salt shaker from your table.

❑ Use lemon juice on food instead of salt.

❑ Don't use onion salt or garlic salt as spices because they are just flavored salt. Use real onion or garlic for more flavor without the salt.

❑ Avoid store-bought mixes for biscuits, cakes, pancakes, muffins, cornbread, etc. If you prepare your own, you can control the ingredients.

❑ Read all labels to determine the sodium content and buy low-sodium products whenever possible. Remember to avoid any sodium-containing additives, too.

❑ Learn about the many natural herbs, spices and fruit peels that are available. You may decide to grow your own or experiment with store-bought herbs.

❑ Use one of several salt-free mixtures of herbs and spices that are available for seasonings.

❑ Don't use potassium chloride salt substitutes. They can increase potassium levels in your body and may even cause heart rhythm abnormalities.

❑ Enjoy Mexican, Cajun and Tex-Mex foods. The strong spices give flavor without adding salt. Beware of Oriental food. It can be high in MSG which is high in sodium.

❑ To spice chicken dishes, add fruits such as mandarin oranges or pineapples.

❑ Marinate chicken, fish, beef or poultry in orange juice or lemon juice. Add a honey glaze.

❑ Marinate meat in wine or add wine to sauces or soups. If you thoroughly cook the dish, most of the alcohol will evaporate, but the flavor will be enhanced.

❑ Use fresh vegetables whenever possible. However, if you must use canned vegetables, wash them in cool water before using. Rinsing will help remove some of the salt added when processing.

❑ Just a little green pepper, parsley, paprika or red pepper can add a lot of flavor to a meal.

❑ Be sure to keep your meals attractive and include a variety of colors and textures. Most people are more tempted to add salt when the meal appears bland.

❑ Drink water with your meals and avoid soft drinks. Soft drinks are high in sugar which dulls your taste buds and makes it more difficult to give up salt. Also, many carbonated drinks are high in sodium. Even some sugar-free soft drinks contain sodium as sodium saccharin, an artificial sweetener.

If you are eager to prepare meals without adding salt, try experimenting with the following seasonings:

Seasoning	**Used with these foods**
Allspice	Lean meats, stews, tomatoes, peaches, applesauce, cranberry sauce, gravies
Almond extract	Puddings and fruits
Basil	Fish, lean meats (especially lamb), stews, salads, soups, sauces, fish cocktails
Bay leaves	Lean meats, stews, poultry, soups, tomatoes
Caraway seeds	Lean meats, stews, soups, salads, breads, cabbage, asparagus, noodles
Chives	Salads, sauces, soups, lean meat dishes, vegetables
Cider vinegar	Salads, vegetables, sauces

<u>Seasoning</u>	<u>Used with these foods</u>
Cinnamon	Fruits (especially apples), breads, pie crust
Curry powder	Lean meats (especially lamb), veal, chicken, fish, tomatoes, tomato soup, mayonnaise
Dill	Fish sauces, soups, tomatoes, cabbages, carrots, cauliflower, green beans, cucumbers, potatoes, salads, macaroni, lean meats, fish
Garlic (not garlic salt)	Lean meats, fish, soups, salads, vegetables, tomatoes, potatoes
Ginger	Chicken, fruits
Lemon juice	Lean meats, fish, poultry, salads, vegetables
Mace	Hot breads, apples, fruit salads, carrots, cauliflower, squash, potatoes, veal, lamb
Mustard (dry)	Lean meats, chicken, fish, salads, asparagus, broccoli, brussels sprouts, cabbage, mayonnaise, sauces
Nutmeg	Fruits, pie crust, lemonade, potatoes, chicken, fish, lean meat loaf, toast, veal, pudding
Onion (not onion salt)	Lean meats, stews, vegetables, salads, soups

<u>Seasoning</u>	<u>Used with these foods</u>
Paprika	Lean meats, fish, soups, salads, sauces, vegetables
Parsley	Lean meats, fish, soups, salads, sauces, vegetables
Peppermint extract	Puddings, fruit
Pimiento	Salads, vegetables, casserole dishes
Rosemary	Lean meats, sauces, stuffings, potatoes, peas, lima beans
Sage	Lean meats, stews, biscuits, tomatoes, green beans, fish, lima beans, onions,
Savory	Salads, lean meats, soups, green beans, squash, tomatoes, lima beans, peas
Thyme	Lean meats (especially veal and pork), sauces, soups, onions, peas, tomatoes, salads
Turmeric	Lean meats, fish sauces and rice

Dining out

If you eat out often, take a look at these tips for eating less salt at restaurants:

- ❏ Don't add salt to your food. Try freshly ground pepper.
- ❏ Be familiar with low-sodium foods that you prepare at home and order similar items.

❏ Avoid menu items that you normally avoid cooking because of the high-sodium content.
❏ When you order, be very specific about what you want and how you want it cooked. Request that your food be prepared without any salt or sodium-containing seasonings, such as MSG.

Some medicines contain salt

One final tip about how to cut down on your sodium intake: Beware of medications. Many popular over-the-counter medications contain sodium. Be sure to always read labels carefully. Listed below are a few medications that are sodium-free.

Bayer Aspirin	Vanquish
Bufferin	Sudafed
CoTylenol	Tylenol
Comtrex	Sine-Aid
Coricidin	Ecotrin
Pepto-Bismol	Contac
Phillips' Milk of Magnesia	Nytol
Robitussin-DM	Sine-Off
Triaminic Syrup	Sominex
Triaminic Expectorant	Excedrin

Could a low-salt diet send your blood pressure soaring?

A few, very rare people are salt-resistant.

Dr. Brent M. Egan, a blood pressure specialist, told the audience at a recent annual American Heart Association meeting that a low-salt diet may actually be harmful for some people.

He and his colleagues studied 27 men who were put on a very low-salt diet for one week. They then ate their regular diet for two weeks and then repeated the low-salt diet once more.

Some of the men with normal blood pressure were "salt-resistant," says Dr. Egan, meaning that their blood pressure did not automatically fall when their salt intake was reduced.

In fact, blood pressure actually increased by as much as five points in some men who reduced salt intake, he reports.

Studies have shown that insulin, a hormone produced by the pancreas, in some cases contributes to hardening of the arteries by helping the body produce excessive cholesterol.

Insulin also encourages the body to retain salt in the kidneys, the report says.

Many men in the study had higher levels of insulin, and Dr. Egan suggests that the body may "adapt" to a low-salt diet by producing more insulin.

If your blood pressure doesn't fall after two months on a low-salt diet, talk with your doctor. Dr. Egan says, the diet "apparently is not helping."

11 ‖ The Protective Role of Potassium

$\mathbf{E}$at your bananas and you'll lower your blood pressure. Bananas are rich in potassium, and scientific studies suggest that a diet high in potassium can help protect against high blood pressure.

Potassium appears to work by stimulating the body to get rid of excess sodium, which directly lowers blood pressure. Unfortunately, societies which have high levels of salt consumption also have low levels of potassium consumption and vice versa.

Potassium also may affect the release of certain hormones and chemicals into the blood that can influence blood pressure.

Take a look at these potassium/blood pressure studies:

❏ A recent study at Duke University showed a significant drop in blood pressure in just two months when participants were given potassium supplements. Researchers also suggest that increasing the amount of potassium in your diet may lower cholesterol and decrease your risk of stroke. According to the researchers, people who ate the most fruits and vegetables (which are rich in potassium) had 25 to 40 percent fewer fatal strokes than groups with lower potassium intakes. And women seem to benefit more from a high potassium diet than men.

❏ In another study at the Temple University School of Medicine, 10 men were put on either low potassium or normal potassium diets, then given a saline (containing salt) infusion. The blood pressure levels of the men on low potassium diets increased significantly while on the diet and increased more after the saline infusion. The men on the normal potassium diets experienced no rise in blood pressure, even after the saline injection.

❏ To further prove that potassium lowers blood pressure, a separate team of Italian researchers tested the effects of increased potassium on a group of people who were already taking medicine for high blood pressure. The test group increased the amount of potassium-rich foods they ate by more than 60 percent for a year. They consumed about 4,460 mg of potassium daily by including three to six servings of peas, beans, fruits and vegetables in their meals every day. They also cut back slightly on fats. As a result, these people were able to cut by more than half the amount of medicine they took for high blood pressure.

❏ A 12-year California study indicated that men in the lower third of the population in potassium consumption are more than 2 1/2 times more likely to have a stroke than men who consume more of this valuable mineral.

In addition to its blood pressure lowering abilities, potassium appears to protect blood vessels from developing atherosclerosis, the hardening and thickening of blood vessel walls. Based on a study conducted at the University of Mississippi Medical Center, potassium works like this:

☐ It slows down your body's production of free radicals. These free radicals react with cholesterol in the blood and make it more attracted to blood vessel walls to form plaques.

☐ It keeps muscle cells within the vessel wall from growing and thickening too much.

☐ It blocks the action of platelets, the part of the blood responsible for clotting.

The dangers of too much potassium

In spite of all the good news about potassium, don't run out and buy potassium supplements. Too much potassium in the blood (called hyperkalemia) is much more serious and life-threatening than low potassium (called hypokalemia).

People with renal insufficiency (kidney failure) can't get rid of excess potassium in their urine. This results in a large amount of potassium in their blood after a potassium-rich meal or after taking a potassium supplement.

People who have diabetes mellitus have a defect in the kidney's ability to regulate potassium levels.

In addition to those health conditions, there are several medications that can interfere with potassium metabolism and cause a buildup of excess potassium in the blood. Some of those medications include: potassium-sparing diuretics, ACE inhibitors, beta-blockers, heparin and nonsteroidal anti-inflammatory agents (NSAIDs), such as aspirin and ibuprofen.

People using these medications or people with diabetes or kidney disease should use extreme caution in eating large amounts of potassium-rich foods or taking potassium supplements.

Potassium do's and don'ts

The recommended dietary allowance for potassium is from 1,600 to 2,000 mg.

But you might need to raise your potassium intake to about 3,500 mg a day for it to help lower high blood pressure. For the best results, follow these potassium do's and don'ts:

Do's:
✔ Steam or microwave vegetables to preserve potassium.
✔ Do try to eat a diet that includes more fresh fruits and vegetables, rather than canned or processed. You will automatically raise your potassium intake and lower your sodium intake.
✔ Check the list on the following page of high potassium foods for a wide range of tasty suggestions.

Don'ts:
✗ Don't rely on meat, poultry or fish for your potassium. Although they are good sources of potassium, they are higher in calories and fat than vegetables, fruits, peas and beans.
✗ Don't take large doses of a potassium supplement unless prescribed by a doctor because high levels of potassium might cause a heart attack. Some diuretic

drugs reduce natural potassium. If you are taking one of these drugs, your doctor will give you a prescription for potassium supplements.

Best natural sources of potassium

Vegetables	asparagus, artichoke, broccoli, carrots, cauliflower, eggplant, romaine lettuce, mushrooms, peppers, baked potato, spinach, turnips
Peas and beans	pinto beans, kidney beans, chickpeas, broad beans, lentils, string beans, peas
Fruits	apples, apricots, bananas, cherries, grapefruit, grapes, oranges, peaches, pears, plums

12 ‖ The Calcium Advantage

alcium is best known for its bone-building abilities,
but it also plays an important behind-the-scenes role
in beating high blood pressure.

Scientists are still searching for the exact way in which
calcium helps to lower blood pressure, but they suspect that,
much like potassium, it has something to do with the muscle
cells throughout your body. Not getting enough calcium in
your diet destroys the balance of calcium inside and outside
your cells. The cell membrane gets "leaky," and both sodium
and calcium leak into the cells. Too much calcium gets into
the cells and that causes the muscle cells in the artery walls
to constrict, or tighten.

When those muscle cells begin to tighten up, the blood
vessels get narrower, and blood pressure goes up. Calcium
also affects the levels of certain hormones in the blood which
tend to influence blood pressure levels.

In one study conducted by James H. Dwyer, Ph.D., from

the University of Southern California School of Medicine, calcium seemed to be one of nature's best protectors against high blood pressure. The study involved over 6,600 men and women and indicated that each gram (one gram equals 1,000 mg) of calcium consumed a day lowered the risk of high blood pressure about 12 percent.

Another team of researchers studied more than 1,900 Japanese men and found that high calcium intakes, especially from dairy products, helped lower systolic blood pressure.

Scientists from Harvard Medical School found that the risk of high blood pressure can be reduced by 22 percent in women who take in at least 800 mg of calcium each day compared with women who take in only 400 mg a day. Another study indicates that people with high blood pressure consume 20 to 25 percent less calcium than people who don't have high blood pressure.

To sum up the benefits of calcium in the diet, a group of researchers recently analyzed many of the scientific studies performed over the past decade.

They found that when people with high blood pressure increase their daily calcium intake, systolic blood pressure falls an average of 5 to 7 mm Hg and diastolic blood pressure falls an average of 3 to 4 mm Hg.

Scientists also have found that some people may be more calcium sensitive than others. These people may experience blood pressure drops as great as 20 to 30 mm Hg systolic and 10 to 15 mm Hg diastolic in response to increased calcium.

As many as 30 to 45 percent of people suffering from high blood pressure may fall into this calcium sensitive group.

People who have high blood pressure caused by eating too much salt seem to get the most benefits from calcium. In other words, calcium seems to dull some of the negative effects of a high-salt diet. The more salt seems to affect someone's blood pressure, the more calcium supplements seem to improve their blood pressure, Dr. Lawrence Resnick at the New York Hospital-Cornell Medical Center reports.

Plus, sodium seems to compete with calcium for absorption by your bones. Getting more sodium than calcium in your diet can speed bone loss and deterioration.

Eating a high-calcium diet while you're expecting a child may help cut down on pregnancy-related high blood pressure, too. Although blood pressure usually rises in the last three months of pregnancy, scientific studies showed that blood pressure levels remained constant in women who received 1,500 mg of calcium per day.

High blood pressure in pregnancy can sometimes be dangerous for the growing baby. Pregnant and nursing women need more calcium to provide for the developing baby and to produce breast milk.

Are you meeting your calcium requirements?

The Recommended Daily Allowance (RDA) of calcium is 800 mg per day for most people, and 1,200 mg per day for pregnant women and nursing mothers.

Most people don't get this much. The National Institutes of Health wants to raise the RDA to encourage Americans to eat more calcium-rich foods.

They say that people ages 11 through 24, when bones grow most rapidly, need 1,200 to 1,500 mg of calcium per day.

Women ages 25 to 50 and men 25 and older need 1,000 mg a day. Women who have gone through menopause need between 1,000 to 1,500 mg to prevent bone fractures.

If you're a woman 65 or older, shoot for at least 1,500 mg per day to make up for bone loss due to aging. From 1,000 to 1,500 mg may sound like a lot, but you can be halfway there before dinner if you eat properly. An 8-ounce glass of milk with breakfast and a cup of yogurt with lunch gives you nearly 600 mg. Have two cups of greens or broccoli plus a little low-fat cheese with dinner, and you've given your body the daily calcium it needs.

Remember, when you select high-calcium dairy products, select low-fat dairy products, like skim milk, cottage cheese and yogurt.

What if you can't digest milk?

Milk and dairy products remain the best sources of calcium, but if you have lactose intolerance that doesn't do you much good.

To make up for that, eat extra helpings of vegetables like kale, turnip greens, collard greens and mustard greens during dinner.

Consider other excellent calcium sources like clams, oysters and shrimp, or try snacking on canned sardines or salmon, including the bones.

Calcium supplements are available at most grocery stores and come in liquid, tablet or chewable forms. While these may help if you can't have dairy products, avoid them if you can get calcium naturally. Some of these supplements contain lead.

To equal the calcium in one cup of milk (291 mg), you'd need to eat:

> 2 cups of broccoli
> 1 cup of greens (collards, turnip, kale or mustard)
> 2 cups of cottage cheese
> 1 ounce of Swiss cheese
> 4 ounces of salmon, with bones and oil
> 5 cups of green beans

Don't overdose on calcium. If your diet is healthy, you probably don't need calcium supplements. More than 2,000 mg a day is too much. Going over that once in a while is OK, but too much calcium may cause other problems, like kidney stones, over a long period.

Making the most of your calcium intake

You may be taking in plenty of calcium, but is it doing your body any good? Counting milligrams toward your daily allowance means little if your body isn't absorbing the calcium you eat and drink.

Getting your body to absorb more calcium is a function of two old reliables — eating right and exercising regularly.

> ➤ **Get more calcium by eating less protein.** Many Americans don't get enough calcium because they eat a diet high in protein. Too much protein interferes with your body's ability to use calcium.
> High-protein foods dump fatty acids into the blood. Since your body produces acid naturally, this extra acid increases blood toxicity and puts a strain on your kidneys. Your body's first instinct is to correct this by "robbing" the skeleton of calcium, which is then lost through your urine.
> Eating less protein reverses this trend, and helps your body keep the calcium you take in.

> ➤ **Fortified foods enhance calcium absorption.** Certain calcium sources are more easily absorbed by your body than others. Fortified orange juice and yogurt are excellent sources that your body absorbs better than calcium supplements or antacids.
> In other words, a supplement or an antacid tablet may

provide the same amount of calcium that a glass of orange juice provides. But your body doesn't absorb all the calcium in the supplement or antacid. You get more calcium benefits from the orange juice or yogurt.

➤ **Get your calcium at mealtime.** Researchers learned in a recent study that your body absorbs more calcium when you take it in at mealtime than when you take it without other food.

Getting your calcium with meals is not only smart, it's easy to do. The best calcium sources are dairy products; fortified orange juice; and green, leafy vegetables, foods we ought to eat at breakfast and dinner anyway. If you must take calcium supplements, it's best to do so with meals. That seems to increase their effectiveness.

➤ **Remember your potassium and vitamin D.** Potassium and vitamin D both work to regulate acid levels in your blood.

This affects how much calcium your body soaks up and uses to help build strong bones. Potassium, vitamin D and calcium work together, so make sure you get plenty of each. Having an 8-ounce glass of orange juice provides about two percent of the daily requirement of calcium and gives you 430 mg of potassium.

➤ **Don't forget to exercise.** Getting all your nutrients may not help if you don't exercise regularly. The way your body uses calcium is affected by the amount of exercise you get. Regular exercise helps your body absorb calcium better and guards against bone disease and high blood pressure.

13 ‖ Magnesium — The Miracle Mineral

Magnesium plays an important role in virtually every system of your body. In fact, the more researchers learn about its powers, the more magnesium sounds like a miracle mineral — able to lower blood pressure, reduce high cholesterol, help prevent cancer and diabetes, keep your heart and lungs healthy, soothe PMS symptoms, zap headaches, relieve stress and even build stronger muscles.

Doctors even give magnesium injections to heart attack victims, more than doubling their chances of survival.

Evidence is mounting that magnesium can lower blood pressure safely. Studies have shown that people who don't get enough magnesium through their diets tend to have higher blood pressure than folks who eat magnesium-rich foods.

So researchers looked to see if taking magnesium supplements would lower blood pressure in a group of women with high blood pressure who were not taking any medication for their condition.

Half the women received a dose of magnesium equal to about twice what most of us get in our meals; the other half received an inactive pill known as a placebo.

The blood pressure of the women taking the magnesium supplements dropped significantly. In fact, the systolic blood pressure fell by almost three points. The diastolic blood pressure was reduced an average of almost three and a half points.

Just how does magnesium work its blood pressure reducing magic? Researchers aren't sure but suspect part of the reason is that magnesium helps neutralize stress-induced hormones that are known to hike blood pressure.

Other studies show that higher levels of dietary magnesium play a definite role in fighting the bad effects of high blood pressure and high fat diets.

For example, in animal tests, results showed that high blood pressure caused by too much salt in the diet was actually prevented by adding magnesium to the drinking water at four to eight times the recommended dietary allowance.

In another test, this time with rabbits on normal cholesterol diets, the researchers showed that increasing magnesium levels to about five times the recommended dietary allowances resulted in 30 to 40 percent reductions in blood levels of cholesterol and other blood fats when compared with low magnesium diets.

Equally significant, rabbits on high cholesterol diets got megadoses of magnesium and cut their blood fat levels by more than half, the test showed.

There also is evidence to support the theory that magnesium helps prevent alcohol induced high blood pressure. Rats given ethanol and magnesium supplements had significantly lower blood pressure levels than rats given ethanol alone.

Experts believe more than eight of every 10 people don't get enough magnesium. Most people consume only about 40 percent of the daily amount of magnesium they need.

At the highest risk are alcoholics and those taking water pills (diuretics), digitalis and other heart drugs, and some antibiotics and anti-cancer drugs.

These substances bind with magnesium and prevent its absorption into the body. If you are at risk for a magnesium deficiency, ask your doctor if you should be taking supplements.

Soft drink fans also may cut down their magnesium absorption to harmful levels because of the binding effect of the phosphates in the drink. For example, a regular 12-ounce soft drink may bind up to 30 mg of magnesium and flush it out of the body before it can do its good work.

The RDA for magnesium is 350 mg for males over 18 and 280 mg for females. The RDA for pregnant women and lactating (milk producing) mothers is even higher, up to 355 mg. Three or four soft drinks a day could cause significant deficiencies in magnesium absorption, even in those few people who get enough of the mineral every day.

People living in hard water areas often get lots of magnesium because magnesium is present in hard water. They seem to have low rates of heart attacks and lower blood pressure. But people living where drinking water is soft could have severe deficiencies because the water contains very little magnesium.

Some experts believe that it's difficult to get enough magnesium in the diet just by eating the right foods. One researcher said magnesium would be the one supplement he would recommend for everyone.

You should take magnesium with calcium, researchers recommend. Dolomite is a good, inexpensive supplement that contains both minerals.

However, remember to take it between meals because

magnesium neutralizes stomach acid and acts like an antacid.

Although several studies have not shown any serious side effects when magnesium is taken in doses larger than the RDA, one study suggested large doses of magnesium could be linked to low blood pressure and depressed breathing in some people. Check with your doctor before taking large doses of magnesium.

Magnesium-rich foods

Nuts	Whole-grain cereals
Figs	Peas and beans
Corn	Bananas
Lemons	Seafood
Apples	Grapefruit
Leafy, dark-green vegetables	

14 | The Strengthening Power of Vitamin C

Vitamin C should get at least a B for its role in regulating blood pressure. Two studies have shown that people with high levels of vitamin C in their blood tend to have low blood pressure.

Researchers at the Medical College of Georgia checked 67 healthy men and women ages 20 to 69 and found that those with high levels of vitamin C in their blood averaged a blood pressure reading of 104/65. Others with one-fifth those blood levels of vitamin C, but still within acceptable, healthy levels, averaged blood pressure readings of 111/73.

Researchers at Tufts University checked 241 elderly Chinese-Americans and found the same result: The lower the blood levels of vitamin C, the higher the blood pressure.

In two very small studies, people who took 1,000 mg of vitamin C a day reduced their systolic blood pressure by four to eight points over four weeks. In another study, people took 400 mg of vitamin C a day for four weeks, but they weren't able to reduce their blood pressures.

The jury is definitely not in on vitamin C, but chances are good that it may help lower blood pressure slightly. Scientists think that vitamin C might protect against high blood pressure because it helps maintain healthy connective tissue, known as collagen, within the blood vessel walls.

Vitamin C helps keep the collagen healthy, which strengthens and supports the blood vessel walls and makes them more resistant to high blood pressure. The current RDA for vitamin C is 60 mg per day, although some scientists think that number should be higher. Some natural sources of vitamin C are citrus fruits and dark-green vegetables like broccoli.

Check the following chart for fruits and vegetables high in vitamin C:

Foods	Serving	Vitamin C (mg)
Kiwi fruit	(2)	145
Orange juice	(1 cup)	105
Papaya	(1 cup)	87
Strawberries	(1 cup)	83
Orange	(1)	82
Broccoli, raw	(1 cup)	79
Grapefruit juice	(1 cup)	76
Green or red pepper	(1/2)	76
Cantaloupe	(1/4)	57
Brussels sprouts, cooked	(1/2 cup)	53
Grapefruit	(1/2)	53
Tangerines	(2)	52
Snow peas	(1/2 cup)	51
Cauliflower, cooked	(2/3 cup)	47
Cabbage, shredded	(1 cup)	40
Raspberries	(1 cup)	35
Honeydew	(1/10)	33
Watermelon	(2 cups)	27
Spinach, raw	(1 1/2 cups)	24

15 ‖ The Caffeine Controversy

Caffeine's effect on blood pressure is grounds for a hot debate in the scientific world. Some researchers say cutting caffeine out of your diet is a sure way to bring your blood pressure down.

Other experts say drinking caffeine just sends your blood pressure up temporarily, and only does that when you're not used to the jolt. They say that once you've adjusted to a certain level of caffeine, your blood pressure won't be affected at all.

If you're trying to decide whether to kick the caffeine habit, here are some points for you to consider:

☐ Caffeine definitely causes a temporary increase in blood pressure unless you've built up a tolerance to it. Scientific studies have found that systolic and diastolic blood pressure levels were raised an average of nine points after drinking two cups of coffee.

☐ Everyone is different. Cutting back on coffee may help

you lower your blood pressure considerably. In one study, 34 male volunteers were given grapefruit juice containing caffeine. Half the men were characterized as being at high risk for high blood pressure, because they had a parent with high blood pressure or consumed a high-fat, high-sodium diet.

Fifteen minutes after drinking the caffeinated juice, the men in the high-risk group had higher blood pressure levels than the low-risk group. People with risk factors for developing high blood pressure seem to react more to caffeine than people without those risk factors.

❏ Never drink caffeine before you exercise when you have high blood pressure. That can cause your blood pressure to skyrocket.

❏ Caffeine may affect your blood pressure more if you are under stress. A group of researchers from the University of Oklahoma say that if you have a high-stress job, more than five cups of coffee a day can send your blood pressure soaring. Don't drink caffeinated drinks before going into a stressful situation.

❏ In addition to raising blood pressure, excess caffeine can provoke arrhythmia, an irregular heartbeat, which can be very dangerous for some people. In fact, in one scientific study, patients with existing heart rhythm problems got worse after taking the equivalent of three to five cups of caffeinated coffee each day.

❏ Caffeine can intensify the effect of some stimulants, common cold remedies and hormones. It can cause extremely high blood pressure when combined with certain antidepressants. So, make sure your doctor or pharmacist knows how much caffeine you drink.

❏ Caffeine can affect cholesterol levels slightly, but recent research has suggested that any rise in LDL ("bad") cholesterol that it causes is offset by an equal rise in HDL ("good") cholesterol.

Almost every person in America takes in caffeine in one form or another daily. Most coffee lovers drink about three and a half cups a day. A five-ounce cup of automatic drip coffee contains between 80 and 150 mg of caffeine. (That's cup, not mug. Mugs hold 10 ounces, or up to a whopping 300 mg of caffeine.) Most experts recommend you get no more than 250 to 500 mg of caffeine per day, depending on your weight, age and general health.

Someone who is used to a lot of caffeine can find quitting, or even cutting back, pretty rough going. Flu-like symptoms, insomnia, jangling nerves and a nasty headache are frequent consequences. Withdrawal symptoms usually start within 18 to 24 hours, but can begin earlier.

In fact, the "lift" your morning cup of coffee gives you may be simple relief from early withdrawal symptoms. If you need to cut down, do it gradually.

Since it is possible to develop a tolerance for caffeine, it's best to stick to a maximum intake. Be aware that caffeine "hides" in unexpected places, and you may be consuming much more than you know. Read labels and check this chart and the chart on the following page.

Beverages	Milligrams caffeine
Coffee, automatic drip (5 oz. cup)	80 - 150
Coffee, perked (5 oz. cup)	64 - 124
Coffee, instant (5 oz. cup)	40 - 108
Coffee, decaf (5 oz. cup)	2 - 5
Cocoa, hot (5 oz. cup)	4 - 6
Tea, brewed, 3 min. (5 oz. cup)	36 - 40
Tea, brewed, iced (12 oz. glass)	36 - 40
Cola drinks (12 oz. can)	36 - 46

Beverages	Milligrams Caffeine
"Specialty" Coffees	
Espresso, 1.5 oz. (demitasse cup)	15 - 30
Cappuccino (3 oz. espresso, 3 oz. milk)	30 - 60
Foods	
Chocolate bar, average size	15 - 30
Baking chocolate, unsweetened, 1 oz.	25
Chocolate cake, slice	20 - 30
Drugs (adult dose)	
No-Doz	200
Aqua-Ban	200
Excedrin	130
Fiorinal	80
Anacin, Empirin, Midol	64
Darvon Compound	60
Norgesic	60

Drug/caffeine interactions

Many common medications interact with the caffeine you take in and can cause harmful side effects.

Some drugs slow the body's disposal of caffeine. These can result in insomnia, irritability, nervousness or heart palpitations when combined with caffeine:

➤ Birth-control pills
➤ Verapamil (Calan, Verelan) — prescribed for heart problems
➤ Cimetidine (Tagamet) — prescribed for ulcers

Drugs that stimulate the nervous system also can cause insomnia, anxiety or palpitations when combined with caffeine. These include:

> ➤ Appetite suppressants
> ➤ Theophylline (Slo-Phyllin, TheoDur) — prescribed for asthma
> ➤ Amantadine (Symadine, Propagest) — prevents flu
> ➤ Oral decongestants (Sudafed, Propagest)
> ➤ Thyroid hormone (Synthroid, Levothroid)

Caffeine can interfere with the sedative effects of the benzodiazepine tranquilizers (Halcion, Valium, Xanax).

And, perhaps worst of all, combined with the antidepressant monoamine oxidase (MAO) inhibitors (Marplan, Nardil, Parnate), caffeine can cause severe high blood pressure or abnormal heart rhythms.

16 | The Final Word on Fish Oil

Fish oil does work to lower blood pressure, but don't get too excited about it. A little rush of adrenaline may undo all the good your weeks of popping fish oil supplements have done.

Recently, three researchers decided to get to the bottom of all the confusing reports about fish oil. They pooled together the results of the fish oil studies that met their scientific standards, and they came up with one large study of 1,356 people.

The researchers found that fish oil can lower blood pressure, but the effects aren't nearly as breathtaking as some scientists have claimed. Whether or not fish oil benefits you at all depends on your health.

☐ If you're healthy with normal blood pressure (less than 140/90 mm Hg), fish oil supplements will do nothing for you. Don't take them in an attempt to keep from developing high blood pressure later. You won't get anything out of it except, possibly, an upset stomach.

☐ If you have high blood pressure but don't have heart disease, fish oil supplements may or may not help you lower your blood pressure. You have to take a lot of fish oil to get any effect at all. On average, people with high blood pressure can lower their systolic blood pressure (the upper number) by 4 mm Hg and their diastolic blood pressure (the lower number) by 3 mm Hg by taking 7.7 grams of omega-3 fatty acids a day. That's about 15 fish oil capsules every day.

☐ If you have hardening of the arteries because of heart disease or high cholesterol, you may really benefit from fish oil. Three of the four studies on the effect of fish oil on blood pressure in people with heart disease showed systolic decreases of 10 to 17 mm Hg and diastolic decreases of 3 to 10 mm Hg. Those results are pretty good, but only four small studies have been done, so you may not want to put too much stock in the findings yet.

The higher your cholesterol levels and the worse your heart disease, the better fish oil works. People with heart disease and high cholesterol levels have high levels of thromboxane in their bodies. Thromboxane is a vasoconstrictor, which means it raises blood pressure by narrowing your blood vessels.

Fish oil contains the omega-3 fatty acid eicosapentaenoic acid (EPA), which seems to lower blood pressure by stopping your body from making thromboxane.

EPA also seems to help lower your blood pressure by stimulating your body to make a certain type of vasodilator, which causes the blood vessels to relax and dilate.

If you have high blood pressure and you're ready to try fish oil, don't let us discourage you. One thing is certain: Fish oil works better for some people than for others. It may be your miracle cure.

Instead of taking fish oil supplements, eat cold water fish that contains omega-3 fatty acids, such as cod, tuna, salmon, halibut, shark and mackerel, three times a week. You'll get the fish oil benefits without the unpleasant side effects, such as diarrhea, gas, burping, a bad aftertaste and an upset stomach.

Dietary sources of fish oil

The highest levels of the two kinds of beneficial fish oil ingredients (EPA and DHA fatty acids) are found in fresh or frozen fish that normally live in deep, cold waters.

Eating canned fish is not recommended, since the canning process destroys most of the omega-3 oil. Best of the saltwater breeds are mackerel (Atlantic, king and chub), Pacific and Atlantic herring, European anchovies, Chinook salmon, sablefish, sturgeon, tuna and mullet.

Cod is a cold water fish, but it has relatively little omega-3 oil in its flesh. Instead, the cod stores omega-3 in its liver. But many doctors advise against a regular supplement of cod liver oil, since too much can cause overdoses of vitamins A, D and E.

Among freshwater fish, highest omega-3 levels are found in lake trout and whitefish. Shellfish like lobster, crab and shrimp have smaller amount of omega-3, as do mollusks like scallops and clams.

Don't like fish that much? You can still get some omega-3 through plant sources, but most plants generally are lower in omega-3 than the same amounts of fish. However, there are exceptions. For example, oat germ is a good source of omega-3, better than all but 15 kinds of oil-rich fish. Three and one-half ounces of oat germ have more omega-3 than the same amount of sockeye salmon or mullet.

Common dry beans have more omega-3 than ocean perch, Pacific halibut, red snapper and many other kinds of fish.

The lettuce-like purslane, used in soups and salads in Mediterranean countries, is high in EPA. Also good are tofu, walnuts, wheat germ oil, several kinds of beans, soybean products and rapeseed (canola) oil.

Margarine also is a rich source of omega-3, largely because it's made from soybeans. Unfortunately, it also has more saturated fats than fish or other plant sources of omega-3.

Based on an uncooked serving size of 100 grams (approximately three and one-half ounces), the following fish are highest in total omega-3 fatty acids.

Food	Total fat in grams	Omega-3 in grams	Omega-3 % of fat
Albacore tuna	4.9	1.5	31
Round herring	4.4	1.3	30
European anchovy	4.8	1.4	29
Atlantic salmon	5.4	1.4	26
Atlantic sturgeon	6.0	1.5	25
Lake whitefish	6.0	1.5	25
Mullet	4.4	1.1	25
Bluefin tuna	6.6	1.6	24
Lake trout	9.7	2.0	20
Mackerel	11	2.2	20
Atlantic herring	9.0	1.7	19
Bluefish	6.5	1.2	19
Pacific herring	13.9	1.8	13

The following are plant sources high in omega-3 fatty acids. The comparisons are based on a serving size of 100 grams (approximately three and one-half ounces).

Food	Total fat in grams	Omega-3 in grams	Omega-3 % of fat
Soybeans, sprouted, cooked	4.5	2.1	47
Common dry beans	1.5	0.6	40
Navy beans	0.8	0.3	38
Leeks, raw	2.1	0.7	34
Pinto beans	0.9	0.3	33
Kale, raw	0.7	0.2	29
Spinach, raw	0.4	0.1	25
Strawberries, raw	0.4	0.1	25
Rapeseed (canola) oil	100.0	11.1	11
English walnuts	61.9	6.8	11
Walnut oil	100.0	10.4	10
Dry soybeans	21.3	1.6	8
Wheat germ oil	100.0	6.9	7
Soybean oil	100.0	6.8	7
Black walnuts	56.6	3.3	6
Oat germ	30.7	1.4	5
Wheat germ	10.9	0.7	6

17 ‖ Licorice Alert

Those who like to snack on licorice candy every day may be left with a bad taste in their mouths after hearing this news: Real (not artificially flavored) licorice can raise your blood pressure. Adults who eat large quantities of licorice every day run a higher than normal risk of developing high blood pressure and heart disease.

Apparently, licorice or licorice extract causes your body to retain sodium and fluids and lose potassium, which raises blood pressure and puts a strain on your heart.

Researchers recommend that licorice lovers with high blood pressure cut way back on their treat and eat it only on special occasions.

Of course, most licorice that is sold in the United States is now made with artificial flavoring, usually anise oil, so it's safe for you to eat. The ingredient you want to avoid is glycyrrhizic acid. This ingredient is highly concentrated in some licorice candies and in some laxatives and tobacco products.

Side effects of eating too much licorice besides high blood pressure are headache, a puffy face, swollen ankles, weakness and extreme fatigue.

Many herbalists are great believers in the healing powers of real licorice. They will argue that licorice is a remedy for coughs, colds, ulcers and arthritis. Licorice does have healing properties, especially for coughs.

But one popular herbal cough remedy contains an ounce of licorice root in one quart of water. You are supposed to drink one-half pint at bedtime. That dose of glycyrrhizic acid could be toxic for a person with high blood pressure.

It's best to avoid all but the smallest amounts of licorice if you have high blood pressure, especially if you are taking diuretics. Licorice can increase the side effects of diuretic drugs.

See Chapter 29 for a chart of more herbs that can positively or negatively affect your blood pressure.

18 || What You Need to Know About Cholesterol

Cholesterol is a fatty, waxy substance found only in animal products. Most of the cholesterol found in the body is produced in the liver, but 20 to 30 percent comes from the food we eat.

A high level of cholesterol in your blood is a significant risk factor for the development of high blood pressure. But despite its bad reputation, cholesterol is essential for life. Here's why.

Cholesterol is a building block of the outer membrane of cells in the body; it's a principle ingredient in bile, a fluid that helps us digest our food; it's present in the fatty sheath that insulates nerves; and it helps with the production of many hormones in the body.

Scientists believe that the ideal blood cholesterol level is below 200 mg. Average levels for Americans are between 200 and 240 mg. Levels above 240 are considered to be high.

Medical researchers have discovered that cholesterol and

other fats are carried in the bloodstream in protein-fat combinations called lipoproteins. The two major types of lipoproteins are high density lipoproteins (HDLs) and low density lipoproteins (LDLs).

HDL is known as good cholesterol because it helps remove cholesterol from the blood. This cholesterol is carried to the liver for storage or removal, thus reducing the risk of high blood pressure and heart disease.

On the other hand, LDL, also known as bad cholesterol, circulates in the blood, depositing fat and cholesterol in the tissues and on artery walls. LDL molecules carry more cholesterol than HDLs and are less soluble (able to be dissolved) in the blood. Therefore, their cholesterol can be easily deposited in the inner linings of arteries. This directly increases the risk of high blood pressure and heart disease.

Studies show that the higher the LDLs, the greater the risk of heart disease. However, the higher the HDLs, the lower the risk of heart disease.

Arteriosclerosis, or hardening of the arteries, is the result of too much cholesterol in the blood. The cholesterol plaques build up inside the artery walls, eventually narrowing the arteries and hardening the arterial walls. Both of these processes contribute to the development of high blood pressure.

A heart attack occurs when a portion of a cholesterol plaque breaks off and gets lodged in one of the narrowed vessels of the heart and prevents blood flow. When this happens to a blood vessel in the brain, it is called a stroke.

As early as 1913, Russian pathologist Nikolai Anitschkow showed that he could produce cholesterol deposits, or plaques, in the arteries of rabbits just by feeding them a cholesterol-rich diet.

In 1947, a study of seven nations showed a direct relationship between a country's incidence of heart disease, the level of cholesterol in the blood, and the amount of animal fat in the national diet.

The Finns, who eat a high-fat diet, had the highest cholesterol levels and the highest rate of heart disease. Americans had the second highest cholesterol levels and second highest heart disease rate. But in Japan, where diets are low in fat, cholesterol levels were the lowest and heart disease risk was low.

Although most people think of hardening of the arteries as something that afflicts elderly people, the process of atherosclerosis can begin in youth. A study revealed that 77 percent of American soldiers killed in the Korean War were found in autopsies to have some degree of hardening of the arteries.

The average age of the soldiers was 22 years. The arteries of the opposing young Korean soldiers of comparable age, who ate mostly rice and vegetables, showed no atherosclerosis.

Most Americans consume about 40 percent of their total calories from fat. High-fat diets can cause hardening of the arteries which leads to higher and higher blood pressure over the years. Low-fat diets are associated with low blood pressure. Cutting fat intake levels in half can have a dramatic effect in reducing the number of cases of high blood pressure.

The American Heart Association recommends that fats make up only 30 percent of total calorie intake; others suggest even lower levels of only 10 to 15 percent. These levels are substantially lower than the levels found in typical American diets.

Dietary cholesterol means the cholesterol you eat. The American Heart Association recommends no more than 300 mg per day. Most food labels list cholesterol.

Serum cholesterol, blood cholesterol, and total cholesterol all mean the same thing — the cholesterol in your body. This is what is measured when you have a cholesterol test.

The cholesterol test: What your numbers mean

One of the first steps in reducing your risk of high blood pressure and heart disease is to find out what your cholesterol level is.

Simple screening tests, done without fasting, measure only your total cholesterol and your HDL cholesterol, the good kind. These tests can give inaccurate results.

Even the complete cholesterol test, called the lipid profile, can vary each time you are tested. These measure total cholesterol, HDL cholesterol, LDL cholesterol (the bad cholesterol) and triglycerides.

For accurate numbers, you should not eat or drink anything except water for 12 hours before the test, and you shouldn't exercise for 24 hours.

Also, if you're taking any medication, such as blood pressure pills or birth control pills, make sure the person testing you knows. These will affect the results.

Relax when blood is being drawn and sit still. Say something if the tourniquet stays on your arm more than a minute. This can affect the results. Finally, get tested more than once, especially if readings are not normal. Studies show that cholesterol levels may vary by season, so try again in a month or so.

Total cholesterol = HDL cholesterol + LDL cholesterol + (Triglycerides ÷ 5)

The value of triglycerides in predicting heart disease is

not clear, but scientists know a lot about LDL (low-density lipoprotein) and HDL (high-density lipoprotein). These numbers are very important. You want to have a low LDL and a high HDL.

Don't worry as much about your HDL levels as about your LDL levels. Studies show that not all people with low HDLs are at high risk for a heart attack. If you have a simple cholesterol screening, you may only get your total cholesterol and your HDL cholesterol. That's because HDL levels are easier to test (you don't have to fast beforehand).

The following chart shows the accepted standard for total cholesterol levels and the new standards for LDL and HDL cholesterol levels:

	Cholesterol Level	Guidelines
TOTAL	less than 200 mg/dl 200 to 239 mg/dl 240 mg/dl and over	desirable borderline high high
LDL	less than 130 mg/dl 130 to 159 mg/dl 160 mg/dl and over	desirable borderline high high
HDL	less than 35 mg/dl	too low

15-step plan lowers high cholesterol naturally

If you're thinking you don't have to worry about cholesterol because you don't have heart trouble, you may want to think again. About 25 percent of American adults over age 20 have blood cholesterol levels that are considered high. More than half of all Americans have levels that are borderline-high.

Eating the typical American diet of fatty meats, processed cold cuts, dairy products, fried foods, eggs and commercially baked breads, cakes and cookies can lead just about anyone down the high-cholesterol path.

Only a small fraction of the population can eat high-fat diets and have low cholesterol.

You don't need to eat any cholesterol. Your body makes all it needs. Any extra you get is either eliminated from your body or is deposited in your arteries. That's when problems begin.

Of course, even if your cholesterol is a little high, it doesn't mean you'll have a heart attack, but elevated cholesterol is one of the main risk factors. And if your cholesterol isn't high, you may want to take steps to keep it that way.

Fortunately, that's fairly easy to do. Most people can lower or maintain their cholesterol just by making a few additions and subtractions to their diets. Here are several ideas:

➤ **Don't chew the fat.** Strangely enough, eating cholesterol doesn't raise blood cholesterol as much as eating a type of fat called saturated fat. Like cholesterol, saturated fat is found mainly in animal products, like cheese, butter, cream, whole milk, ice cream, lard and marbled meats. Some vegetable oils — palm oil, palm kernel oil, coconut oil and cocoa butter — also are high in saturated fat.

These oils are used in commercially baked goods, coffee creamers and nondairy whipped toppings, so read the labels. Since eating cholesterol also can raise blood cholesterol levels, go easy on egg yolks, which contain 213 mg of cholesterol, and on organ meats, such as liver.

Unsaturated fats, both polyunsaturated and monounsaturated, have been shown to reduce blood cholesterol levels. Polyunsaturated fats come from plant and vegetable sources, such as cottonseed, soybean, corn and safflower. Sunflower and sesame seeds, walnuts and pecans also are high in polyunsaturates. Polyunsaturated fats are usually soft or liquid at room temperature.

Monounsaturated fats, like olive oil, have been found to lower high blood pressure also. Increasing your monounsaturated fats while decreasing your saturated fats should help lower your blood pressure naturally.

➤ **Forgo frying.** Trim all fat off meat before cooking. Remove fatty skin from chicken and turkey. Don't fry foods. Roast, bake, broil or poach them instead. Use fat-free basting or marinating liquids, such as wine, tomato juice or lemon juice. If you use oil for sautéing or baking, use olive or canola, both very low in saturated fat. Use margarine that lists a liquid oil as the first ingredient. Watch out for the term "hydrogenated," which means some of the fat has been made saturated.

➤ **Eat your vegetables and complex carbohydrates.** The lowest-fat foods of all are vegetables, fruits, grains (rice, barley and pasta), beans and peas. Substitute these for meat and high-fat dairy products. Don't douse your pasta in butter or your baked potato in sour cream. Use tomato-based sauces instead of cream-based. Use lemon juice, low-sodium soy sauce or herbs to season vegetables. Make chili with extra beans and seasonings, and leave out the meat.

➤ **Lose weight.** People who are overweight usually have high cholesterol levels. Most people can lower their levels and raise their HDL levels by dropping a few pounds. Follow the guidelines for eating less fatty foods and more fruits, vegetables, grains and beans, and you will slowly but surely lose weight.

➤ **Include the family.** Children older than age 2 can join in the low-fat lifestyle. Eating habits carry into adulthood, so teach your kids to make healthy choices. Don't, however, start before age 2. Babies need extra fat calories to grow properly.

➤ **Snack to your heart's content.** Don't be afraid to snack several times a day on low-fat foods, such as yogurt, fruit, vegetables, bagels and whole-grain breads and cereals. As a matter of fact, evidence points to lower cholesterol levels in people who eat small meals several times a day. Eating often keeps hormones like insulin from rising and signaling your body to make cholesterol. Just make sure your total intake of calories doesn't go up when you eat more often.

➤ **Go a little nutty.** If you like nuts, especially walnuts, sprinkle a few on your cereal, bake them into muffins or pancakes, or add them to casseroles or stir-fries. In one study, walnuts were shown to decrease blood cholesterol levels by 10 percent more than an already low-fat, low-cholesterol diet. While walnuts are high in fat, it is mostly polyunsaturated fat, the kind that lowers cholesterol.

Walnuts also are an excellent source of an important dietary fatty acid (n-3 linolenic acid). Scientists think hazelnuts and almonds may have the same cholesterol-lowering effect. Be sure to decrease other sources of fat to allow for the calories in the nuts.

➤ **Even some chocolate is OK.** Studies indicate that

the primary type of saturated fat in chocolate, stearic acid, has no effect on cholesterol levels. When a chocolate bar was substituted for a high-carbohydrate snack on a low-fat, low-cholesterol diet, the chocolate did not increase LDL cholesterol, and even seemed to raise HDL cholesterol, according to one study. But chocolate is high in fat and calories, so take it easy.

➤ **Note the color of your wine.** If you enjoy a glass of wine with dinner occasionally, there is no need to stop, especially if it's red wine. A low rate of heart disease in some areas of France, despite a high-fat diet, led researchers to investigate the wine. It seems that some of the nonalcoholic ingredients in red wine keep your body from producing LDL cholesterol and will raise your HDL levels.

One 5-ounce glass a day for women and two for men is considered moderate. But if you don't drink, there's no need to start. Alcohol consumption can have several bad side effects, too. At least one study has shown purple grape juice to have the same good effects as red wine.

➤ **Eat the "stinking rose."** The cholesterol-lowering effects of garlic have been repeatedly demonstrated in people with normal and high cholesterol. Garlic may raise HDL levels, too. Garlic also works against heart disease by dilating the blood vessels, lowering blood pressure and making the blood less sticky and less likely to clot. If the odor bothers you, try it in tablets. These have been shown to be just as effective as the cooked or raw cloves.

➤ **Niacin works, but be careful.** Niacin, one of the B vitamins, is proven to lower total cholesterol and raise HDLs. It is one of the cheapest and most effective cholesterol-lowering drugs. But without a doctor's supervision, it may not be safe. Doses high enough to lower cholesterol have been shown to cause very high blood sugar or liver damage. In one study, liver problems developed at 1,500 mg a day. If you have very high cholesterol, check with your doctor about this treatment.

➤ **Vitamin E looks promising.** Study after study has documented the good effects vitamin E has on cholesterol, even on HDL levels, and on your risk of heart attack. Doses of up to 800 international units (IUs) appear to be safe, but 100 IUs seems to be enough for a beneficial effect. This is more than you can get in your diet alone. Many scientists say large, long-term studies are still needed to prove that it's safe to take large doses of vitamin E.

➤ **Calcium can help.** In one study, when 56 people took a calcium carbonate supplement, their total cholesterol went down 4 percent and their HDL cholesterol went up 4 percent. They took 400 mg of calcium three times a day. No side effects were reported.

➤ **Fill up on fiber.** Oat bran caught the national fancy a few years ago when some studies showed that it drastically lowered cholesterol levels. Later studies showed inconsistent results, but scientists generally believe that soluble fiber, the kind found in oat bran, helps lower LDL cholesterol. Other sources of soluble fiber are barley, beans and many fruits and vegetables. These are also low-fat foods. Psyllium, a type of soluble fiber, may even raise your HDL cholesterol.

➤ **Keep moving.** Evidence shows that exercise can lower LDL cholesterol and boost HDL cholesterol. But exercise alone can't perform this magic. People who exercise and still eat high-fat diets or who are overweight may not reap the cholesterol-lowering benefits. Both aerobic exercise (walking, jogging, swimming, bicycling and cross-country skiing) and strength training (lifting weights or using weight machines) work to improve cholesterol levels. An analysis of 11 studies on weight training showed that this exercise lowered LDL cholesterol by 13 percent and raised HDL cholesterol by 5 percent. If you lift weights, use light weights (even one pound will do) and do many repetitions.

➤ **Try vitamin C.** Vitamin C deficiencies have been linked to low HDL levels. Boosting your vitamin C intake may improve your HDL levels.

19 || Diabetes and Insulin Resistance

Insulin is a natural hormone produced by the pancreas. It's needed to help process dietary sugars and carbohydrates for your body to use as energy. When you eat, your body absorbs sugar and nutrients from the food, causing your blood sugar to rise.

This elevated blood sugar level triggers, or stimulates, the release of insulin from the pancreas into the bloodstream. Insulin enables the cells in the body to take in the glucose and either use it immediately for energy or store it as glycogen, and your blood sugar levels go back to normal.

Insulin is such a vital hormone that humans cannot survive without it. In fact, people who suffer from Type-I diabetes mellitus do not produce insulin, so they must give themselves daily shots of insulin in order to survive.

People with Type-II diabetes mellitus have some insulin, but their bodies often require more insulin than they can produce. They frequently require insulin injections, too.

Scientists are now finding that too much insulin can be a significant factor in high blood pressure. Recently, a group of researchers analyzed the results of 11 different studies on the effects of insulin on blood pressure conducted between 1983 and 1991.

They found a definite link between insulin and high blood pressure, although it has not been proven to be a direct cause of high blood pressure.

In addition to controlling blood sugar levels, insulin also causes the kidneys to retain sodium. Scientists think this might be part of the reason why insulin has a bad effect on blood pressure levels.

Many scientists also believe that high levels of insulin in the blood may be a silent heart disease risk factor for 25 percent of the trim and otherwise healthy people in the United States.

This was confirmed recently by a report presented to the American Diabetes Association by Dr. Annick Fontbonne, a researcher at the French National Institute of Health and Medical Research.

Scientists believe that a long-term excess of insulin in the bloodstream damages the cardiovascular system, although how remains a mystery. Some scientists think that high insulin levels damage the artery walls.

This could lead to a buildup of fat that narrows the blood vessels. This narrowing of blood vessels directly contributes to high blood pressure, a known risk factor for cardiovascular disease.

Many overweight people have a problem called insulin resistance. This occurs when the pancreas produces the correct amount of insulin, but the cells aren't able to use the insulin properly to take in the sugar they need. As a result, blood sugar levels rise, and the pancreas then churns out even more insulin to meet the body's demand.

Type-II diabetes (also called noninsulin-dependent diabetes) results from high blood sugar levels due to the body's inappropriate response to insulin.

It affects 10 million Americans, usually overweight people over age 40. People with type-II diabetes are two to four times as likely as nondiabetics to develop heart disease, scientists report.

However, not all insulin-resistant people are diabetic. They have too much insulin in their bodies, but their blood sugar levels are OK. Dr. Gerald M. Reaven of Stanford University School of Medicine has researched insulin resistance for more than 20 years. He has identified what he calls "syndrome X," the heart disease risk factors that insulin-resistant, but otherwise healthy, people have. The risk factors are:

- ❏ high blood pressure
- ❏ high triglycerides (a form of fat in the bloodstream)
- ❏ low levels of high-density-lipoprotein (HDL) cholesterol

Although Type-I (insulin-dependent) diabetics have a definite heart disease risk, Dr. Reaven is having a difficult time convincing diabetes specialists that people who are insulin-resistant, whether they are diabetic or not, are at risk as well. The syndrome X theory is controversial. Yet, it may explain why people in countries such as India and Pakistan have lower cholesterol levels but a greater incidence of heart disease than people in other countries.

Many researchers believe syndrome X is hereditary, but further research will try to determine if other factors, such as obesity, trigger it.

Other studies have identified insulin levels as a heart

disease risk factor for men. In a report recently presented to the American Diabetes Association, Israeli researcher Michaela Modan said that tests for insulin resistance could predict coronary heart disease risk sooner than cholesterol and blood lipid tests.

Dr. Modan suggests that finding a simple test for insulin resistance might pave the way for mass screening of people for this important indicator of heart disease.

The technique Dr. Modan used was an oral glucose tolerance test. The test involved taking repeated blood samples over a two-hour period. This method is effective, but it is not simple enough for mass screenings, she says.

20 ‖ The Effects of Stress on Your Body

If you've ever suspected that your high-pressure job is bad for your health, you could be right. Stressful jobs certainly have the ability to make people feel overly tense, and now several scientific studies have shown that middle-aged men in stressful jobs tend to have a higher risk of developing high blood pressure.

According to one study, men who have jobs with high demands over which they have little or no control are three times more likely to suffer from high blood pressure than men who don't.

These workers also are more likely to suffer from physical changes to the heart that could lead to heart disease over time. The researchers report that the risk of job-related hypertension increases with age, and they suggest that anxiety, frustration and anger may aggravate high blood pressure.

Another team of researchers, along with Dr. Thomas G.

Pickering, professor of medicine at New York Hospital — Cornell Medical College's Cardiovascular and Hypertension Center, used 24-hour ambulatory blood pressure monitors to measure how high-stress jobs affect blood pressure. The researchers gathered 264 men between the ages of 30 and 60 to participate in the study.

All of the volunteers were employed at one of the following eight work sites: a newspaper typography department, a federal health agency, a stock brokerage firm, a liquor marketer, a hospital, a sanitation vehicle repair facility, a department store warehouse and the headquarters for a large insurance company.

Twenty percent of the volunteers in the study were classified as having high-stress jobs, which were defined as jobs that were very demanding with little decision-making.

The researchers provided each of the 264 men with ambulatory blood pressure monitors, which took measurements every 15 minutes over a 24-hour period, including on the job, at home and during sleep. After gathering the blood pressure recordings and analyzing the information, the researchers came up with some alarming news.

Apparently, the high-stress jobs resulted in higher blood pressure readings compared with the low-stress jobs. The alarming news, however, is that the job stress raises blood pressure at work, at home and even during sleep.

The researchers found that job stress was associated with a 7 mm Hg increase in systolic blood pressure (the top number) and a 3 mm Hg increase in diastolic blood pressure (the bottom number). These increases in blood pressure were noted throughout the 24-hour period, including time spent sleeping, as if the job stress had more or less reset the entire blood pressure system.

And if stress weren't enough, job happiness and job security are two more factors that seem to influence your blood pressure. Researchers at the University of Pittsburgh discovered that being unhappy at work can raise your blood pressure.

In a study of 288 men who had blue-collar jobs, the researchers found that the more dissatisfied the worker was with his job, the higher his risk of having high blood pressure.

If the man felt insecure about his job, had little opportunity for promotion, didn't feel part of the decision-making process or worked with employees who were not supportive, he was more likely to have high blood pressure.

Although scientists continue to study how jobs affect blood pressure, they suspect that the increased blood pressure is one of the body's natural reaction mechanisms to stressful situations. With so-called "reactive" high blood pressure, the body reacts to stressful or threatening situations by releasing a hormone called renin from the kidneys.

This prepares your body for "fight or flight," pumping adrenaline and speeding up the heart, sending more blood to the brain and muscles. It also causes sodium retention and elevates blood pressure. Some people naturally produce too much renin.

These people usually have a "Type A" personality. Often, they are stereotyped as competitive, aggressive, tense, impatient and easily irritated. They also usually have high blood pressure. Some aggressive men don't have enough of an enzyme that normally regulates your body's chemical reaction to stress.

However, blood-pressure-raising stress doesn't just come from the workplace, and it doesn't just affect adults. Craig Ewart, a psychologist at the School of Public Health at Johns Hopkins University, believes that many teen-agers experience enough stress to more than double their risk of early-onset high blood pressure.

Issues that tend to evoke that kind of stress among teen-age girls include social rivalries and struggles for dominance.

Teen-age boys, on the other hand, experienced stress as a result of feeling unsupported in their daily struggles. The frustration associated with typical teen issues seems to be at the center of stress that causes high blood pressure among teens.

Many studies suggest that the way a person handles stress, frustration or anger, whether he holds it in or takes it out on others, for example, does not seem to be a factor in the development of high blood pressure.

Talking may be hazardous to your health

Talking too much may irritate your friends, but did you know it could also be a health hazard? Studies by Dr. James Lynch of the University of Maryland Medical School show that listening, rather than talking, lowers blood pressure. According to reports, 98 percent of the 178 people studied had their blood pressures surge when they started talking.

The highs and lows of blood pressure levels won't hurt people with normal blood pressure, Dr. Lynch explains, but in someone with high blood pressure, the highs can be dangerous.

Dr. Lynch used an automatic blood pressure monitor and recorded continuous blood pressure readings during conversations with patients. In people with high blood pressure, talking about intimate problems raised their blood pressures to dangerous levels, according to Dr. Lynch.

Many people with high blood pressure do not speak calmly, which causes their blood pressures to rise even further. Dr. Lynch claims that the louder and faster a person talks, the higher his blood pressure. People who emphasize their words, talk "breathlessly," use hand motions, interrupt or talk over someone else seem to experience the highest rise in blood pressure.

Dr. Lynch believes that slower speaking, combined with breathing more deeply and regularly during speech, helps to lower blood pressure. Anyone with speech-induced blood pressure problems can learn to speak more slowly, he says.

Learning to listen and focusing on what the other person is saying might lower stress and reduce the load on the heart. Most people with chronic high blood pressure do not really "listen" to a conversation, Lynch explains.

These people are so worried about how they will reply that they are defensive even when they are listening, and their blood pressure doesn't drop as much as it does in a person who truly listens.

In a University of Pennsylvania study, Drs. Katcher and Beck compared blood pressure levels during three different situations: while the participants just sat and did nothing, while they watched fish in a small tank and while they talked.

The highest level was during speech, but the lowest level was while watching the fish. Being quiet isn't the key to lowering your blood pressure. You need to relax and focus on something or someone else.

Dr. Lynch believes that the most important thing his studies have shown is that you can lower your blood pressure by learning to listen to others.

The next time you visit your friends or family, listen to what they have to say. Your blood pressure will thank you for it.

The benefits of positive thinking

In addition to contributing to lower blood pressure, some scientists think that happiness, contentment and good social vibes can increase your resistance to disease. Take a look at these encouraging studies:

☐ People with cancer who are relaxed and optimistic about their chances of survival live longer than anxious people trying to cope with cancer on their own, say researchers at the University of California at Los Angeles.
Thirty-four people with a deadly skin cancer went through a six-week program of relaxation techniques, coping strategies and cancer education. Another group the same age, sex and with the same seriousness of cancer didn't receive counseling. Ten of the 34 people in the uncounseled group died within six years, but only three of the group that received counseling died.

☐ Your chances of surviving a heart attack are better if you have emotional support. In one study of heart attack victims, those with supporting companions and family members had better survival rates and less severe heart problems than people without support.

☐ A group of 110 people aged 60 to 70 gave their immune systems a boost by living in a resort facility for 11 days and learning about exercise, diet, stress management and changing their lifestyle. Blood samples were taken before and after the program. The people who reported feeling less stress after the program had increased levels of disease-fighting white blood cells in their bodies.

Is laughter really the best medicine?

Laughter seems to help people keep positive attitudes in sometimes bleak surroundings, and it also helps keep your body healthy. Laughter is a complex and coordinated arrangement of 15 separate facial muscles and is accompanied by changes in the normal breathing pattern.

Laughter causes an increase in your pulse rate and breathing rate, which increases the amount of oxygen in your blood.

The muscles involved in laughter undergo a light physical workout during the laughter, which helps to improve and maintain muscle tone. And, during hearty, boisterous laughter, a larger group of muscles undergoes a stronger workout. This is especially helpful for people who are bedridden.

Following bouts of laughter, the involved muscles begin to relax. This helps to ease muscle tension that builds during the day and helps to break the spasm-pain cycle that is often seen in many nerve problems and in rheumatism.

People who suffer from lung problems like emphysema also benefit from laughter. Doctors refer to this laughter therapy as "humor respiration." The laughing, chuckling and chortling involved in humor respiration help to increase air exchange in the lungs, increase blood oxygen levels, and clear mucous plugs out of the airways. And laughter just seems to make people feel better.

Laughter also causes a temporary increase in heart rate and blood pressure, which serves to exercise the heart muscle and increase circulation of blood, oxygen and nutrients from the heart to the whole body.

Increased blood circulation helps promote the movement of important immune system elements throughout the body, helping the body to fight infection and illness. Increased circulation also reduces the risk of blood clots forming in vessels and, therefore, reduces the risk of some types of heart attacks and strokes.

Although scientists are still conducting studies on the effects of laughter on the nervous system and the brain, they suspect that laughter has beneficial effects on mental functions such as alertness and memory.

As scientists learn more about the benefits of laughter and mirth, they hope to use it as a complement to the natural healing process and possibly add "laughter therapy" to many medical treatment routines.

Feelings and attitudes have always seemed to play an important role in achieving and maintaining good health. Scientists are just trying to figure out why.

Man's best friend — a natural remedy for stress?

Dogs might offer more than the morning newspaper and your evening slippers. Sometimes a dog can be nature's best remedy for stress or illness.

The presence of a dog can act as a "natural drug" for its owner by helping to lower blood pressure and other bodily responses to stress. The dogs seem to help reduce the effects of stress because they provide unconditional love and support without criticizing the owner's actions.

Researchers studied 96 people with heart disease after they were released from a heart unit in a hospital. They found that the people who owned pets had a higher survival rate one year after release from the hospital than the people who did not have pets, even after accounting for individual differences in the extent of heart damage and other medical problems.

In fact, owning a pet seemed to be a better indicator of a successful recovery than the presence of a spouse or extensive family support.

In another study, 345 elderly pet owners reported fewer doctor visits per person over one year than did 593 elderly people without pets. Some study evidence indicates that touching, stroking and cuddling pets reduce a person's heart rate and blood pressure.

Scientists say, however, that these benefits probably do not extend to people who are afraid of animals or are uncomfortable around animals. But for those who enjoy the company of a pet, the faithful companions might help you enjoy a longer, more stress-free life.

Follow these tips to help relieve stress

❐ Take care of your body and you'll take life in stride. Exercise, a proper diet and adequate rest can make all the difference in your ability to handle stress. A balanced diet of vegetables, fruits, grains, dairy products and small amounts of meat will help keep your immune system strong. Avoid caffeine because it is a stimulant and can worsen anxiety. Don't smoke, either. Exercise will relax you, help you rest better and help you feel good about yourself. However, high-intensity exercise on the level of a marathon runner can cause your body to put out too much of the stress hormones and depress your immune system. Too little exercise is a more common problem than too much.

❐ Practice good breathing. Lie flat on your back on a carpeted floor. Prop up your head and put a cushion under your knees so you are completely comfortable and relaxed. Breathe in slowly (to the count of 10), hold for two seconds, then breathe out slowly (another count of 10). Many people feel that they are practicing good breathing just by breathing in slowly, but slow exhaling is just as important. By doing these deep breathing exercises for only three to five minutes each day, you will feel relaxed and might lower your blood pressure and pulse rate.

☐ Be nice. Bolster your immune system and your marriage. A stressful argument with your spouse can instantly cause a drop in your white blood cell count and make you more susceptible to disease. Reduce your stress by discussing issues with your spouse calmly.

☐ Resist drinking alcohol. The numbing effect of alcohol may seem to decrease stress in the short term, but the social stigma of drinking, your own feelings of worry and guilt, and the harm it does to your body will actually increase your stress over the long haul.

☐ Get some of that old-time religion. Religion is a wonderful stress reliever because God and your church give you social networks and personal support to help you cope. Religious people also tend to avoid self-destructive behaviors like drinking and drugs. But, you have to attend church regularly for it to help.

☐ Seek out humor. Laughter really is the best medicine. It releases "feel-good" chemicals in your brain and enhances blood flow. Laughter increases your heart rate, blood pressure and muscle tension. When you stop laughing, these levels temporarily drop below normal, leaving you feeling very relaxed.
Find movies, comedians and books that make you laugh, put cartoons on your refrigerator and office bulletin board, and don't take yourself so seriously all the time.

☐ Make your home smell nice with flowers, spices, perfumes or fragrant sprays. Pleasant smells may trigger brain chemicals that work against stress. Your nose quickly adapts to your own body fragrance, so simply wearing your favorite perfume won't help.

❑ Control your time so it doesn't control you. A day with too much or too little to do can make you stressed and anxious. Plan to help others a few times a week. Your own worries will look smaller when you get involved with others.

❑ Avoid disastrous thinking. If you describe situations as awful, horrifying and terrible, you may not be seeing things realistically. How you perceive a threat to your happiness or well-being will determine your body's response. Overstating threats will only create unnecessary stress.

❑ Focus on a relaxing scene. Imagine yourself lying on a beach and feel the sun making you warmer and warmer, melting your stress away.

❑ Accept your own personal limitations. Accept the limitations of money. You will always want more than you have, and you may have to sacrifice some things to get what is important to you.

❑ Accept the limitations of your situation. If your plane is delayed or if you are stuck in a traffic jam, worrying and getting angry will not make the situation better.

❑ Your approach to life has a lot to do with how much stress you create for yourself. For example, if you are a perfectionist about your own work and expect others to adhere to your high standards, you are setting yourself up for plenty of stress-filled days. Learning to accept things that are less than perfect could be important for your health. Even if you accept a few less-than-perfect projects, you will lower your stress.

☐ Also, remember your strengths and weaknesses. No one can do all things well. Try to improve your strengths and your weaknesses. Don't be too hard on yourself when you discover that you cannot excel at everything.

☐ Cool your competitive edge. Rather than constantly comparing yourself to others, set your own goals based on your own performance. Don't be constantly trying to get the best parking space or get ahead of "that" car in traffic. Many times these minor competitions contribute to unnecessary stress in our lives.

☐ Acknowledge your successes. Celebrate the things you accomplish, no matter how small. If you have a job that is repetitive and it's difficult to see any progress, create and celebrate your own accomplishments.

☐ Reach out to others. Doing something for someone else may help to put your problems into better perspective. You will become less self-centered as you appreciate the people around you.

☐ Make time for yourself every day. Do something that you enjoy.

☐ Don't try to bear other people's stress. Learn to recognize that their problems are not your fault. You can be supportive and loving without carrying their stress.

☐ Get help if you need it. Asking for help is not a sign of weakness but rather a sign that you know your own limitations.

❏ Don't be afraid to cry. Research has shown that crying is a natural and healthy way to deal with stress. Crying helps focus your emotions and provides a needed release.

❏ Music is now being recognized and used by professional therapists to help relieve and treat stress. Music can change your breathing rate, your heart rate and the level of stress you are experiencing. Music that causes you to relax will be most helpful. Songs from your past that you associate with good times can bring back those good feelings. Therapists prefer music without lyrics so you don't get caught up in listening to the words. After having a stressful experience, just lying down with your eyes closed and listening to relaxing music should alleviate some of the symptoms of stress.
Music also can help prepare a person for a stressful situation. For example, if you dread going to the dentist or you have an important business meeting, play your calming music on the way there. The right music can help you approach stressful events in a calm and peaceful manner.

❏ Avoid bringing stress from your job home. Taking your frustrations out on your family and friends may add to their stress. There is a place for discussing your problems with your family, and your family should be able to support you. But learn the difference between having their support and making them share the burden of your stress.

❏ Share your concerns, your fears, your dreams and your anxieties with your closest friend or spouse. Talking helps put your problems into correct perspective.

❒ Supplement your diet with vitamins. Stress may increase the need for niacin (vitamin B3) and thiamine (vitamin B1). Researchers in France and Dr. Burton M. Altura of Brooklyn, New York, have discovered that low magnesium levels make it more difficult to deal with stress.

❒ The best way to prepare your body to cope with stress is to get plenty of rest (seven to eight hours of sleep each night) and to avoid eating high-fat or high-salt foods.

Take five: 5-minute stress relievers

These exercises are perfect for relieving stress during a hectic day at the office. After a tense meeting with the company president, a run-in with a co-worker or a rush to meet a deadline, take five.

Stress reliever No. 1:

➤ Sit in a comfortable position and close your eyes (unless it makes you nervous to close your eyes at work).

➤ Point your toes back toward your face and tighten your shins. Hold for five to 10 seconds. Release and relax for 20 to 30 seconds.

➤ Point your toes downward and tighten your calves, thighs and buttocks. Hold for five to 10 seconds, then release and relax for 20 to 30 seconds.

➤ Take a deep breath, arch your back slightly and push your stomach out. Hold for five to 10 seconds, then relax for 20 to 30 seconds.

➤ Hunch your shoulders forward and up to your ears. Wrinkle your face up like an old, dried apple. Hold for five to 10 seconds, then relax.

After each step, note the difference between body tension and relaxation. You should feel your muscles relaxing in waves throughout your body.

Stress reliever No. 2:
➤ Raise your right arm out to your side while breathing in. Breathe out. Breathe in and stretch your right arm up to the ceiling. Breathe out.
➤ Repeat with left arm.
➤ Let your arms come down slowly while you breathe out. Continue to breathe deeply for about 20 seconds.
➤ Place your feet shoulder-width apart. Slowly let your head hang forward until your chin touches your chest.
➤ Start to curl forward and bend over very slowly. Breathe deeply. Let your arms dangle and hang down as far as you can comfortably. Don't strain or bounce. Sway gently from side to side.
➤ Now, on each inhale, raise back up a little. On each exhale, relax. In this way, slowly roll your body up until your spine and head are straight.

Your body should feel looser and more relaxed.

21 ‖ Smoking and Your Health

Cigarette smoking is dangerous, especially if you have high blood pressure. Smoking is a major risk factor for cardiovascular disease.

Secondary cigarette smoke poisons the environment with many toxic substances and increases the risk of disease among the friends and family members of smokers.

Cigarette smoke contains more than 4,000 chemicals that can possibly harm your body. Each year smoking is blamed for countless cases of lung cancer, heart attacks and other serious health problems. Breaking the cigarette habit greatly reduces the risk of serious illnesses.

Nicotine is very addictive. To stop smoking, you must unlearn your smoking behavior and break the nicotine addiction.

But before we get to some guidelines that should help you along your path to becoming smoke-free, here's another really good reason to consider kicking the habit.

A night on the town turns deadly

Ever heard of someone walking out of a smoky bar and dropping dead on the spot? This strange and all-too-common incident may not be just a coincidence. Smoking and drinking alcohol seem to increase your risk of a life-threatening form of stroke.

Both smoking cigarettes and drinking alcohol can temporarily send your blood pressure skyrocketing, causing a sudden increase in the flow of blood to your brain. The blood vessels in the brain burst because they can't handle the extra blood flow.

Finnish researchers studied the smoking and drinking habits of people 15 to 60 years old who suffered an aneurysmal subarachnoid hemorrhage (SAH). SAH is a type of stroke caused by a damaged blood vessel on the surface of the brain ballooning out and bleeding into the space between the brain and skull. About a third of the people in the study died from the bleeding.

The risk of stroke went up more than fourfold for men who had drunk more than 120 grams of alcohol (that's about six mixed drinks or nine 12-ounce beers) within 24 hours of the stroke.

Women who had drunk more than 40 grams of alcohol (that's about two mixed drinks or four glasses of wine) on the day of the stroke were more than six times as likely to have an SAH as women who had not been drinking alcohol.

Most of these alcohol-related strokes occurred during the hangover period. Your blood pressure can be dangerously high when you're withdrawing from alcohol.

Men who smoked at least 20 cigarettes a day were seven times more likely to have the brain hemorrhage than men who had never smoked. Women who were smokers, no matter how many cigarettes they smoked, doubled their risk of

SAH.

Smoking is probably at the root of almost half of all SAHs. Over the long term, smoking weakens the walls of the blood vessels in the brain, leaving you at risk for stroke. Even smoking just one cigarette may have the short-term effect of increasing your blood pressure for two to three hours.

Thousands of Americans die of stroke every year, making it the third largest cause of death in the United States. Reduce the chances of it happening to you. Don't drink heavily and don't smoke.

Quitters are winners

"Better late than never." This time-tested cliché has never been more true than it is with smoking. It's better to stop smoking late in the game than never at all. Unfortunately, many people who have smoked cigarettes for 20 years or more think that stopping smoking after that much time is really pointless. "The damage is done now ... stopping won't help anything," is their common excuse.

The good news is that it will help. The lungs start healing almost immediately after you quit smoking. Researchers conducted a five-year study on 7,181 elderly men to test the effects of smoking cessation after many years of smoking, and the results were encouraging.

Men who were current smokers experienced twice the rate of dying from smoking-related illnesses, such as heart attack, strokes and cancer, compared with people who had never smoked.

However, former smokers (those who quit smoking) experienced the same low rate of dying from heart problems as people who had never smoked.

And those results were true for people who stopped smoking 20 years ago, or for those who stopped smoking two days before the study began. No matter how old you are or how long you have smoked, you can still cut your risk of dying from heart disease or cancer if you quit smoking.

Kicking the habit may be easier if you're black

If you are trying to kick the smoking habit, your chances of success are better if you are African-American. Black smokers find it easier to quit smoking than white smokers because they are generally less addicted to nicotine than their white smoking counterparts.

A recent study indicates that an incredible 98 percent of black former smokers were able to quit smoking without any outside help or intervention. However, only 85 percent of white former smokers were able to quit on their own.

Apparently, black smokers found it easier to refrain from smoking in nonsmoking areas or situations than the white smokers in the study. Black smokers also reported smoking fewer cigarettes each day compared with white smokers, and they waited longer in the mornings before having their first daily cigarette.

These results indicate that African-American smokers usually have a lower level of nicotine dependence than white smokers, which makes it easier for them to quit smoking.

Tips for kicking the cigarette habit

The American Cancer Society, the American Lung Association, Merrell Dow Pharmaceuticals and many other organizations have compiled these guidelines to help you quit smoking:

❑ Decide you want to quit. Be positive about your decision. Then choose a day to quit and stick to it. If you are a heavy smoker while at work, you may want to quit on a Friday afternoon. By Monday morning, you'll have two smoke-free days behind you and should be better prepared for the stress of your first smoke-free workday.

❏ Examine your reasons for wanting to quit. Besides the physical damage of smoking, you may be helping your family and friends, as well as saving time and money. Write down at least 10 reasons for quitting. Review these reasons daily and keep adding to the list.

❏ Identify the times and feelings you associate with smoking. Do you smoke after meals or while you are under stress? When possible, avoid situations that you associate with smoking.
If you feel the desire to smoke every time you have a cup of coffee or an alcoholic drink, cut out the coffee and alcohol as well. You may have to limit your social life until you feel secure about not smoking. Learning when you smoke and relearning those activities without smoking can be the most difficult part of kicking the habit.

❏ Organize pleasant and busy activities for the day you will quit. Plan to do things with other people, preferably nonsmokers. Keeping an active schedule may help you get over the first few days. You may want to have some kind of treat or celebration to start your non-smoking campaign.

❏ If you are quitting "cold turkey," try to remove all temptations before you start. Throw away all cigarettes. Remove your ashtrays, lighters and matches.

❏ Keep your mouth clean. Brush and floss your teeth

often so your mouth will taste clean. You may want to visit a dental hygienist and have your teeth cleaned within the first few days after you quit smoking. If you schedule the appointment beforehand, this appointment could be your first goal as a nonsmoker.

☐ Chew sugar-free gum when you have the urge to pick up a cigarette. Gum helps keep your mouth occupied.

☐ If you miss having something in your hand to play with, try substituting a pen or pencil.

☐ If you feel the urge to smoke, go for a walk or take a bath or shower. Try doing more things with your hands, like crafts, sewing, woodworking, housework, gardening or writing letters.

☐ Keep a diary of how many cigarettes you smoke and how much money you spend on cigarettes each day. Document each day that you smoke fewer than the day before. Don't get discouraged and give up if you "slip" sometimes. Just do better the next day.

☐ Maintain or improve your physical health. Start exercising regularly. Eat healthy meals, including lots of fruits and vegetables. Drink more fluids, including fruit juices and water. You should drink at least eight glasses of water each day. Get lots of rest and relaxation. By getting your body in good condition, you will be better able to tolerate the physical symptoms of withdrawal from nicotine. Physical exercise will improve your breathing and blood flow, as well as provide a smoke-free activity.

☐ Get support. If your spouse smokes, try quitting together. You will be able to support and encourage each other. If not, involve someone else who will support you. This will improve your chances of becoming and staying a nonsmoker. Join a local support group. The American Lung Association, the American Cancer Society and the American Heart Association can give you names and addresses of groups meeting in your area.

☐ Remember that smoking is not just a bad habit. Smoking is an addiction to the drug nicotine and you will probably experience withdrawal symptoms. According to the Department of Health and Human Services, mood changes, irritability, aggressiveness, anxiety, difficulty in sleeping, drowsiness, weight gain, lower blood pressure, headaches, upset stomach and a decrease in heart rate are common physical reactions to nicotine withdrawal.

Usually, the withdrawal symptoms subside within a few days or a few weeks. Talk to your doctor about a nicotine replacement program, such as nicotine gum or nicotine skin patches. Nicotine gum is just like regular chewing gum except that it contains nicotine, the addictive substance in cigarettes that makes the smoking habit so hard to break.

The skin patch is an adhesive patch that contains nicotine. It delivers nicotine to the blood through the skin. Nicotine gum and nicotine skin patches replace the nicotine while you cut down on cigarettes. You can gradually lower the dose of the nicotine from the gum or patch and you'll soon be free of nicotine and cigarettes.

☐ Withdrawal from nicotine also may be eased by taking 1/2 teaspoon of baking soda in a glass of water two or three times a day. Apparently, the baking soda helps hold nicotine in the system and reduces withdrawal symptoms by giving the body more time to adapt to withdrawal.

☐ While trying to quit smoking, Earl Mindell's Vitamin Bible recommends a variety of supplements to help overcome the withdrawal from nicotine. A good multi-vitamin, 100 mg of a vitamin B complex, 100 mg of cysteine and 300 mg of vitamin C will help keep your body healthy during the time you are withdrawing from nicotine, says Mindell.

☐ Don't try to have just one cigarette. Just like a re-formed alcoholic, one cigarette can begin the smoking cycle again. Even in times of personal crisis, don't smoke.

☐ If you don't quit the first time you try, don't give up. Don't be too hard on yourself. There is a definite physical addiction to nicotine and it may not be easy to quit. You might need to try two or three times before you are successful.

☐ Don't be discouraged if you gain a few pounds as you quit smoking. Starting a regular exercise program, such as walking, will help you burn calories and keep your mind off smoking.

☐ Accept the fact that not everyone can quit "cold turkey." Although this method may work for some people, it does not work for everyone. If you feel that the cold-turkey method is not for you, try cutting back on the number of cigarettes you smoke each day. Count the number of cigarettes you smoke in an average day, then smoke one less each day. You may need to count them every morning. Keep a chart and leave out only the number of cigarettes that you can have that day.

☐ If you find you cannot quit at this point, switch to a low-tar, low-nicotine brand of cigarette. But do not increase the number of cigarettes you smoke each day.

☐ Congratulate yourself with each step you take toward being smoke-free. Giving up smoking is hard. Be proud of yourself each time you give up one cigarette.

☐ Reward your achievements. Celebrate your anniversaries of nonsmoking. Treat yourself after the first week, the first month and maybe every month after that. You deserve to celebrate.

22 ||| The Alcohol Question

Drinking alcoholic beverages can increase your risk of developing high blood pressure. According to recent scientific studies, alcohol consumption might be responsible for as many as 5 to 7 percent of all cases of high blood pressure and up to 25 percent of the cases referred to as essential hypertension, high blood pressure with no known, specific cause.

Scientists estimate that alcohol is probably responsible for as many as 11 percent of the cases of high blood pressure in men alone, making alcohol a significant risk factor.

The relationship between high blood pressure and alcohol is well-documented. Although scientists are still studying the effects of alcohol on blood pressure, many researchers believe that alcohol raises blood pressure by directly causing a constriction (or narrowing) of blood vessels, which makes it harder for the blood to squeeze through.

Alcohol also seems to increase the blood vessels' sensitivity to certain chemicals in the blood that can cause vessel constriction, leading to higher blood pressure.

Alcohol stimulates the sympathetic nervous system, the part of the central nervous system responsible for the fight-or-flight reaction. Stimulation of this part of the nervous system results in higher blood pressure.

Alcohol also seems to trigger the release of certain hormones (known as adrenocorticoid hormones) from the adrenal glands that can cause higher blood pressure. And, finally, alcohol makes blood pressure skyrocket because it damages the liver and kidneys and causes fluid buildup.

According to one study, one or two drinks a day didn't affect blood pressure, but excessive drinking caused blood pressure to rise dramatically.

Alcohol studies have varied in size from less than 100 to more than 80,000 volunteers, and almost all of the studies have shown that blood pressure rises when you drink alcohol (at least when you have three drinks or more per day).

The results of one clinical study on 16 men with high blood pressure levels who were heavy drinkers (six to seven drinks per day) showed that blood pressure levels went down significantly after the men stopped drinking alcohol.

The study also demonstrated that the men experienced a prompt rise in blood pressure after resuming their alcoholic habits.

Another study conducted on 46 men with normal blood pressure levels tested the effects of alcohol on blood pressure by substituting the men's regular beer with low-alcohol-content beer for six weeks.

Researchers found that a 350-milliliter reduction in the intake of alcohol (approximately three drinks) per week would result in lower systolic and diastolic blood pressure levels.

Researchers at Harvard Medical School confirmed that

blood pressure in women also is affected by heavy drinking. Women who drink two mixed drinks or three glasses of wine every day increase their risk of developing high blood pressure by 40 percent. The risk jumps to 90 percent in women who drink more alcohol than that each day.

A major new heart study agrees with the two-a-day limit. More than that amount of alcohol daily may drain a vital nutrient, calcium, from your body, says a report by the American Heart Association.

That harmful effect shows up even if you take extra calcium supplements, the study indicates. According to Dr. Michael H. Criqui, co-author of the study, blood pressure goes up and calcium is lost at more than two drinks per day for the average person.

Dr. Criqui and his co-workers recruited 7,011 men of Japanese descent to participate in the study. The results from the study warn that people who average more than two alcoholic drinks a day suffer at least two bad effects: The alcohol seems to raise their blood pressures, and the drinking seems to prevent the blood-pressure-lowering effects of calcium.

Previous studies show that drinking alcohol apparently leads to poor absorption of calcium in the intestines. In addition, a heavier drinker passes a lot of calcium through the kidneys in urine, draining the body's stores.

Heavy drinkers sometimes have bones that appear to be washed out in X-rays, because they lack calcium. That's added bad news for people at risk from osteoporosis, a bone-loss disease that strikes many women and some men over the age of 50.

You can't get around the bad effects of alcohol simply by taking more calcium every day, Dr. Criqui says. Alcohol seemed to influence blood pressure more than calcium or potassium.

The researcher recommends that you eliminate alcohol from your diet. For people who absolutely will not stop drinking completely, he recommends no more than two alcoholic drinks a day.

And because a diet rich in potassium and calcium may help reduce blood pressure, he suggests eating several servings every day of fruits and vegetables (containing potassium) and nonfat or low-fat dairy products (containing calcium).

Another study found that older men and women were more likely to have their blood pressures increased by heavy drinking. The researchers were not sure if the increase was caused by a different reaction to alcohol in older people or if alcohol has a cumulative effect after many years of heavy drinking.

Studies also reveal that drinking just two alcoholic drinks per day can undo all the blood-pressure-lowering effects of exercise.

Although alcohol can produce dangerously high blood pressure, the good news is this: High blood pressure that is caused solely by high alcohol consumption usually disappears within a few weeks of giving up alcohol.

Cutting back on alcoholic intake is effective in lowering blood pressure in people with high blood pressure and in people with normal blood pressure. Drinking less alcohol also can help prevent the development of high blood pressure.

With these facts in mind, habitual intake of alcohol should not exceed one or two drinks per day. Researchers recommend the following daily limits: one ounce of alcohol, which is equal to two ounces of 100-proof whiskey, eight ounces of wine or 24 ounces of beer per day.

23 ‖ Drugs That Can Raise Your Blood Pressure

Pop pain relievers regularly? Careful! Your doctor may not tell you that you could be sending your blood pressure right through the roof.

Massachusetts researchers recently found that people older than 65 who used nonsteroidal anti-inflammatory drugs (NSAIDs) were about one-and-a-half times more likely to need treatment for high blood pressure than people who weren't using NSAIDs.

NSAIDs are used to relieve just about every ache under the sun, from menstrual cramps to joint swelling. Over-the counter aspirin, ibuprofen (sold as Advil and Motrin) and naproxen (sold as Aleve), as well as dozens of prescription drugs, fall into the NSAID category. At this point you may be confused because you've heard that aspirin is good for your heart. This is still true. NSAIDs do make your blood less sticky.

People who have had heart attacks or strokes often take a low dose of aspirin every day to help prevent blood clots.

But some NSAIDs are much stronger than plain aspirin and have other undesirable side effects. They raise blood pressure by decreasing the amount of prostaglandins in your body.

Prostaglandins help to keep your blood pressure lower naturally by controlling the fluid level in your cells and dilating blood vessels.

The researchers studied nearly 10,000 Medicaid participants who recently had begun treatment for high blood pressure.

Those most likely to have started treatment were older people who had taken high doses of prescription NSAIDs for 30 to 90 days prior to the beginning of the study.

Researchers found that nearly one in 10 of those study participants being treated for high blood pressure had recently used NSAIDs.

If you're at high risk for developing high blood pressure and you are taking NSAIDs, you may want to consider changing to another form of treatment.

There are other effective pain relievers that aren't associated with raising blood pressure, such as acetaminophen, sold as Tylenol.

You also might want to try analgesic creams, which can be good options for some kinds of pain. Mild exercise is a great natural alternative for managing arthritis pain. Losing weight can help too, by lowering stress on your joints and heart.

Even with the possibility of raising your blood pressure, you may decide you get the best pain relief from the NSAIDs.

If you choose to continue using NSAIDs, use the lowest effective dose for the shortest possible period of time. Make blood pressure checks part of your routine, especially if you are at high risk for developing high blood pressure.

What other drugs are you taking?

Ask your pharmacist or your doctor if any prescription drugs you are taking can raise blood pressure. Birth control pills were first linked to high blood pressure in 1967 by Dr. John Laragh.

Over the years, several other studies have verified the suspicions. The longer "the pill" is used and the older you are when you take it, the higher your chances of developing high blood pressure.

Women taking birth control pills should have their blood pressure checked once every two months during the first year. If it is elevated, a different form of birth control should be used.

Once you stop taking birth control pills, blood pressure should return to a normal level within four months.

There are hundreds of drugs, including over-the-counter diet pills and decongestants, which list high blood pressure as a side effect. Even sodium-containing antacids could raise blood pressure in the salt-sensitive person. Be sure to read the warnings listed on any nonprescription or prescription drugs you may buy. Don't stop taking any medication without your doctor's approval.

24 || If Drugs are Prescribed

Drug treatment for mild to moderate high blood pressure has been extremely controversial within the medical profession because doctors are not sure when blood pressure levels are high enough to begin using prescription drugs.

A study in Sweden found that reducing blood pressure levels to lower than 150/85 in middle-aged men had no effect on their risk of heart or artery disease. The study at the University of Goteberg was conducted over 12 years.

However, another new study has shown that early drug treatment can save lives. People with mild high blood pressure who took drugs had 40 percent fewer fatal strokes and 38 percent fewer nonfatal strokes.

Therefore, treating mild or moderate high blood pressure with drugs might save lives.

Most people with high blood pressure need drug treatment, according to a study by the Joint National Committee on Detection, Evaluation and Treatment of High Blood Pressure.

Prescription drugs are the most common treatment for high blood pressure because they are easy to prescribe and easy for the patient to take. But they are often overprescribed because many doctors are hesitant to offer alternatives to drugs to their patients.

It is difficult for a doctor to make sure that his patient takes the prescribed medicine. It would be impossible for him to ensure that a diet and exercise plan was being followed. Most people want "a pill" from the doctor that will magically make them better.

If high blood pressure is diagnosed, your doctor should review your family history and administer some tests to make sure that it hasn't affected any of your vital organs. Your doctor also should test for rare causes of high blood pressure, like kidney problems, Cushing's disease or brain tumors.

A new procedure, involving resting for half an hour, taking the drug captopril and then having a special blood test will help doctors determine if narrow kidney arteries are causing your high blood pressure.

Narrow arteries leading to one or both kidneys cause high blood pressure in just 1 to 5 percent of all high blood pressure cases. If narrow kidney arteries are discovered, your doctor might decide you need angioplasty, a technique used to widen narrowed arteries using a balloon catheter.

Blood pressure was reduced in 90 percent of over 200 patients who had narrow kidney arteries and were treated by angioplasty, Dr. Heinrich Ingrisch reported from the Bogenhausen Clinic in Munich.

The success continued as 75 percent had normal blood pressure six months after the angioplasty, and of those, 77 percent maintained normal levels five years after surgery.

Yet, if high blood pressure from kidney-artery malfunctions goes undiagnosed, a person may be needlessly treated for high blood pressure.

Your eyes, stomach, blood vessels in the legs, kidney function, heart and nervous system should be checked. A complete blood count including thyroid hormone and renin levels, urinalysis (an analysis of the urine), a chest X-ray, and an electrocardiogram (ECG) may be needed to determine the damage, if any, to your heart, arteries and kidneys. Insulin levels also should be checked.

High levels of thyroid hormone in the blood may show that an overactive thyroid is causing or aggravating your high blood pressure. High or low levels of renin, a substance produced by the kidneys, also can affect the preferred treatment.

All of these factors will help determine whether or not your doctor will prescribe blood pressure medicine and, if needed, what kind of drug will be best for you.

Drug treatment is quite complex because many people have more than one ailment and need several different drugs. The interaction of those drugs and the actions that the drugs have on the body must be considered for each person. For example, some people with high blood pressure may have heart problems or high cholesterol levels which will need to be considered when deciding on the correct medication.

The disadvantages of blood pressure medications

Long-term treatment with blood-pressure-reducing drugs may increase the chance of developing diabetes in middle-aged men, a scientific study suggests.

But the risk seems to be greater in men who are "predisposed" to diabetes, according to Dr. Einar T. Skarfos, who led the Swedish study. The study does not prove that blood pressure drugs cause some cases of diabetes, but it suggests that continued use may trigger the disease in some cases.

Blood pressure drugs can cause side effects like headaches, poor appetite, upset stomach, dry mouth, diarrhea, stuffy nose, tingling or numbness in the hands or feet, dizziness, cramps, depression, rashes, chills, fever, constipation, aching joints, difficult urination or low sex drive.

In fact, a recent study involving 3,844 patients with high blood pressure found that 9.3 percent of them stopped drug treatment because of "definite" or "probable" side effects, and an additional 23.4 percent stopped drug treatment because of "possible" side effects.

Drug treatment is only effective when the drugs are taken as prescribed. Since high blood pressure may not have symptoms, many people stop taking their medication because they feel better. Other people forget to take their medication.

This can lead to dangerously high blood pressure levels. Never stop taking or change anything about your prescribed medication without your doctor's knowledge and consent.

Remember that high blood pressure is not cured, but it can be controlled. Learning to control your blood pressure is a lifelong commitment. If you and your doctor choose nondrug methods, they must be continued for the rest of your life, just as prescription drugs would be.

Choosing just one area, like reducing salt intake, may or may not help lower your blood pressure. But it is the effective combination of natural methods that will give you the best results.

In a study by Dr. James Mitchell, people lowered their diastolic pressure about 10 points by dieting or exercising. But when they combined diet and exercise, they lowered their blood pressure an additional four points.

The first step you should take to lower your blood pressure naturally is to talk with your doctor about the methods we've described. Have your doctor monitor your blood pressure levels as you gradually make changes in your diet and lifestyle. Your doctor will probably be as excited as you are when your body gradually needs less and less of the medication.

Drugs of first choice

Since many factors enter into blood pressure control, many different drugs are used for treatment. Usually doctors try the most widely accepted drugs first — drugs that usually work best for most people.

However, if these drugs don't control your blood pressure, other drugs that are stronger, more expensive or have more serious side effects are tried.

Diuretic drugs are usually prescribed first because they are effective and are relatively inexpensive. ACE inhibitors and calcium channel blockers also can be used as the first step in drug treatment, but these drugs are much more expensive.

Of an estimated 50 to 60 million Americans with high blood pressure, about 19 million are currently being treated with medications. If they only take one kind (and many people need combinations), twice a day, that comes to 38 million tablets swallowed daily. Medication alone costs billions of dollars each year.

Getting the most benefits from your medication

Take your medication as directed by your doctor and follow these healthful hints:

❏ Get your blood pressure checked regularly. It only takes a minute or two.

❏ Continue to take your medication even if you feel better. Your high blood pressure is not cured. Regular doses are necessary to keep it under control.

❏ Don't stop taking your prescribed medicine if your blood pressure is normal when you have it checked. The medication is probably why it's normal.

❏ Don't change the dose yourself. You might get too much or too little medicine. Either way it could be harmful. If you take less of your medicine than your doctor prescribes, you may increase the risk of complications such as stroke or heart attack. If you take more of your medication than you're supposed to, you increase the risk of having side effects from the drug.

❏ Don't stop taking a drug on your own, even if you feel light-headed, dizzy, tired, depressed or have trouble sleeping. Your drug can be controlling your blood pressure, but it might be giving you these or other side effects. Notify your doctor immediately when bothersome side effects occur. Many times your doctor will be able to give you a different drug. Your doctor needs to know how medication is affecting you in order to treat your condition properly.

❏ If you have questions about your high blood pressure or your prescription, don't ask a friend or relative. Their information or advice may be well-intended but wrong for you. Ask your doctor or pharmacist. They are the people qualified to answer your questions.

❏ Tell your doctor about all prescription drugs, daily vitamin or mineral supplements, and nonprescription drugs (aspirin, cold medicines, laxatives) that you take regularly. Many drugs interact with each other and lose or gain potency or cause serious side effects when taken together.

☐ Have all your prescriptions filled at the same pharmacy. This will help the pharmacist keep track of the drugs you are taking, which may protect you from dangerous drug interactions.

☐ Record any side effects you may experience while taking prescription drugs, and report them to your doctor.

☐ Follow label instructions. If there is a difference between your doctor's verbal instructions and the label instructions, contact your doctor immediately. If you don't follow the doctor's specific instructions, your medicine may be ineffective or harmful to you.

☐ Refill your prescription in advance so you won't ever have to miss taking your medication.

☐ Carry a day's supply with you at all times, and always remember to carry your medication with you (not in your luggage!) when you travel.

☐ Never take drugs prescribed for someone else. Drugs are prescribed after considering other drugs being taken, your age, weight, health history and other important factors. Exchanging medicine is dangerous. Don't do it!

☐ Ask questions about the drugs your doctor prescribes. If you are well-informed about your treatment and condition, you will know if something unusual occurs, and you will know when to contact your doctor for help. Do not be afraid to write down your doctor's answers to these questions so you can refer to them later.

   ➤ What is the name of the drug?

   ➤ What is it supposed to do?

   ➤ How long will it take before it is effective?

   ➤ How am I supposed to take it? How many pills and how many times a day?

➤ When am I supposed to take it? Should I take it at mealtimes, before meals, at bedtime?

➤ Are there any foods, drinks, other drugs or activities that I should avoid while taking this drug?

➤ What are the drug's side effects?

➤ What should I do if the side effects happen to me?

➤ Is written information available on this drug that I could have?

➤ How can I get this written information?

❐ Keep a list of all your current prescriptions in your wallet or purse. Include the name of the drug and what dose you are taking. When you visit your doctor, have him check your list and keep it up-to-date. The list will remind him of your current prescriptions, and keeping it with you could help avoid dangerous drug interactions. During an emergency, the list will provide valuable information for the attending doctor.

❐ Even if you're taking high blood pressure medication, you should still try to eat foods low in salt, improve your diet, get regular exercise and do all the things you can to help lower your blood pressure naturally. These changes will enable your doctor to prescribe the least amount of medication possible. In one study at the Indiana University School of Medicine, one-third of people who cut back on sodium were able to reduce their blood pressure and their medication.

❐ Always keep your doctor's appointments to have your blood pressure checked and your prescriptions refilled.

Types of blood pressure medications

When your doctor prescribes a drug, it belongs to a general category of drugs. All the drugs in the group act in a similar way to solve a problem.

Here are some brief descriptions of the major drug groups used to treat high blood pressure. The drugs are listed with the generic (or chemical name) first, followed by the brand names. Remember that many of the drugs can be purchased in generic form as well as by their brand names.

ACE inhibitors

ACE is an abbreviation of **A**ngiotensin **C**onverting **E**nzyme. ACE inhibitors work by interfering with a pathway in the body known as the renin-angiotensin-aldosterone system, which is involved in the regulation of blood volume flow and blood pressure.

The central chemical in this system is the substance called renin. Renin is released from special cells in the kidneys in response to lowered blood pressure, low blood volume or low sodium in the blood.

Once released into the bloodstream, renin stimulates the release of the next chemical known as angiotensin I, which is then converted to angiotensin II. Angiotensin II is known as a vasoconstrictor, which means that it causes blood vessels to constrict.

When angiotensin II is released into the blood, the blood vessels constrict and the blood pressure goes up. Angiotensin II then stimulates the release of a hormone known as aldosterone.

This hormone works on the kidneys and causes the kidneys to absorb excess salt, which also causes the blood pressure to rise.

The enzyme that converts angiotensin I to angiotensin II is called the Angiotensin Converting Enzyme (ACE). ACE inhibitors act by preventing this conversion. When angiotensin II is not available, the blood vessels do not constrict, so blood pressure is maintained at a regular level.

Also, without angiotensin II, no aldosterone is released, so extra salt is flushed out of the kidneys into the urine, which prevents blood pressure from rising. It is estimated that ACE inhibitors can produce a 15 to 25 percent reduction in blood pressure. This class of drugs was introduced in the 1980s.

New research suggests that ACE inhibitors can help your heart just when it needs it the most. In a recent three-and-a-half-year study of 2,231 heart attack victims, captopril (an ACE inhibitor) reduced the risk of a second attack by 25 percent, and cut the risk of developing heart failure by 22 percent. In addition, the risk of death was reduced by 19 percent.

A second study involving 4,228 people revealed a 29-percent reduction in the development of heart failure in patients being treated with enalapril (another ACE inhibitor). In the people who did develop heart failure, the onset was delayed by 14 months in the group taking enalapril.

The drug also reduced hospitalizations by 20 percent. All participants had some damage to the left ventricle, which reduces the heart's pumping efficiency.

A third study, which involved administering enalapril within 24 hours after a heart attack, was stopped after six months because there didn't seem to be any increase in survival rates. The benefits seem to be greater when drugs are given three to 16 days after a heart attack, as in the first study.

Heart attack victims have an increased risk of a second attack because of the damage to the left ventricle. They also are at risk for enlargement of the heart and heart failure, which are major predictors of death.

These studies indicate that for some people who already have damaged hearts, ACE inhibitors could be the latest weapons in the fight against heart failure.

ACE inhibitors should be used with caution by people with poor kidney function, people with autoimmune diseases (like rheumatoid arthritis or lupus), or people on drugs affecting white blood cells or immune response. They should not be used during pregnancy because they can cause injury or even death to the fetus.

While on ACE inhibitor treatment, excessive perspiration; dehydration; vomiting; mouth sores; fever; sore throat; swelling of the hands, feet or tongue; irregular heartbeat; chest pains; water retention; skin rash; changes in taste; difficulty in breathing; diarrhea; or any signs of infection should be reported to the doctor immediately.

ACE inhibitors caused cough in 7 to 25 percent of the people in a recent study. This figure is much higher than previously thought, and researchers suggest doctors try prescribing smaller doses.

Dizziness, headache and fatigue are the other most commonly reported side effects associated with ACE inhibitors.

Rash has been reported in about 4 to 7 percent of patients taking some of the ACE inhibitors. Loss of taste might occur with the use of captopril.

All of the ACE inhibitors can cause an excess of potassium in the body. This side effect is even more pronounced in people with poorly functioning kidneys and in those who are taking other medications that can increase potassium.

Since excess potassium can be dangerous for the heart, be sure to have your doctor check your potassium levels from time to time.

The incidence of decreased sex drive and impotence is usually less than 1 percent with ACE inhibitors.

Over-the-counter cough, cold or allergy medications should be avoided. Aspirin or indomethacin decreases the effectiveness of captopril and should be avoided. People also taking diuretics may experience a severe drop in blood pressure during the first three hours after receiving the first dose of an ACE inhibitor.

ACE inhibitors most frequently prescribed are:

> benazepril (Lotensin)
> captopril (Capoten)
> enalapril (Vasotec)
> fosinopril (Monopril)
> lisinopril (Prinivil, Zestril)
> quinapril (Accupril)
> ramipril (Altace)

ACE inhibitors are equally effective in younger and older people with high blood pressure.

Beta blockers

Your body has a type of built-in alarm system that switches on whenever you face an emergency or any sort of stressful situation. This system causes you to put forth your best efforts to deal with stressful situations.

If your blood pressure is normal, your alarm system is probably functioning as it is meant to — now and then raising your energy level, your "get up and go," and making you a capable, productive person.

If your blood pressure is high, however, your alarm system may be turned on too much of the time. You may not feel tense, but your nervous system could be too active. This could be an inherited condition, or it could result from your life situation.

Beta-adrenergic blocking agents, known as beta blockers,

work to keep your emergency nervous system blocked so that your heart will beat more slowly and your blood pressure will fall. They block the action of naturally occurring substances, like epinephrine (adrenaline), that stimulate the heart.

These stimulating substances, which are released into the circulation in response to physical exertion or other stress, cause an increase in heart rate and in the force with which the heart pumps blood.

By decreasing the rate and force of the heart contraction, beta blockers reduce blood pressure levels.

They also are used to treat angina (chest pain) and abnormal heart rhythms and can be used in the treatment of atrial fibrillation (dangerously rapid, nonrhythmic heartbeats).

Some beta blockers are used to treat heart attack victims because they seem to be beneficial in lowering the rate of having a second heart attack in certain patients.

Unfortunately, these drugs also may cause depression and dull your energy levels, leaving you drowsy or feeling lethargic most of the time.

You may begin to feel as if you don't care much about life anymore and chalk it up to just getting older. Beta blockers are often used to treat high blood pressure in older people.

Often these feelings come on so gradually that you may not realize that it is the drug that is causing you to feel this way.

Beta-blockers can also lower HDL cholesterol levels to such a degree that the risk of coronary heart disease may not be decreased even though your blood pressure is lowered.

But there is evidence that chromium, a trace element, helps counteract beta blockers' bad effects on cholesterol.

In a recent study, researchers found that 600 micrograms of chromium per day significantly raised HDL, and reduced the risk of coronary heart disease by 12 to 17 percent in men who took beta blockers three times a day.

Beta blockers should not be used (or should be used with great caution) by people with asthma, hay fever or a history of congestive heart failure or by pregnant women. Beta blockers may interfere with heart activity during major surgery and with the treatment of overactive thyroid, low blood sugar, diabetes, kidney disease or liver disease.

Beta blockers may change the effectiveness of insulin, anti-inflammatory drugs, antihistamines and antidiabetic drugs.

Avoid alcohol when taking beta blockers. Alcohol can cause dangerously low blood pressure when combined with a beta blocker. Smoking may reduce the effectiveness of the beta blocker propranolol.

If you have been taking a beta blocker and suddenly stop, your body may react by raising your blood pressure to dangerously high rates.

If you want to stop taking the medication, you must do it gradually and under the watchful care and consent of your doctor.

Beta blockers most frequently prescribed include:

acebutolol (Sectral)
atenolol (Tenormin)
betaxolol (Kerlone)
carteolol (Cartrol)
labetalol (Normodyne, Trandate)
metoprolol (Lopressor)
nadolol (Corgard)
penbutolol (Levatol)
pindolol (Visken)
propranolol (Inderal, Inderal LA)
timolol (Blocadren)

Vasodilators

These drugs act on the muscles of the blood vessels causing them to dilate and so lowering blood pressure. Side effects can include headache, flushing, stuffy nose, stomach upsets and rapid heart rate.

The vasodilator hydralazine may produce symptoms of rheumatoid arthritis or acute lupus erythematosus (like rheumatoid arthritis with skin rashes) when used over a long period of time, or when used by people who are slow to break down the drug

Minoxidil is usually used in more severe cases, and sodium nitroprusside is usually reserved for hypertensive emergencies.

Examples of vasodilators include:

> hydralazine (Apresoline)
> minoxidil (Loniten, Minodyl)
> nitroprusside sodium (Nipride, Nitropress)

Anti-adrenergic agents

Centrally acting drugs

Drugs in this group act on the sympathetic nervous system which controls involuntary responses to stressful situations. They can cause dry mouth, drowsiness, depression, excessive dreaming, diarrhea and nausea.

Examples of centrally acting anti-adrenergic drugs:

> clonidine (Catapres)
> guanabenz (Wytensin)
> guanfacine (Tenex)
> methyldopa (Aldomet)

These medications are all generally inexpensive and may cause small, beneficial changes in blood cholesterol levels. And, an added benefit: Clonidine is available in a band-aid-type patch that you apply just once a week.

The medication is absorbed through the skin throughout the week. Using the patch is helpful for people who have trouble remembering to take their medicine every day, and it is helpful for elderly people who have difficulty swallowing pills.

However, according to a recent report, clonidine can slow down a person's recovery after a stroke.

Dr. Larry B. Goldstein and his colleagues at Duke University Medical Center studied the records of 58 people who had a stroke to determine the effects of different drugs on recovery.

Of the 58 patients, 24 took clonidine at the time of their stroke or during their treatment.

Patients who did not take clonidine improved more quickly than those who did.

Peripherally acting drugs
These drugs act in various ways on the sympathetic nerve endings to dilate blood vessels and are used to treat severe hypertension.

Guanethidine-type drugs can cause low blood pressure and a loss of balance when you stand quickly. Drinking alcohol, exercising or hot weather can aggravate this side effect.

Diarrhea, fluid retention, stuffy nose, dry mouth and sexual problems in men also are common. People with a history of depression should not take reserpine, since it can cause severe depression even in someone without a history of depression.

Drugs in this group include:

doxazosin (Cardura)
guanadrel (Hylorel)
guanethidine (Ismelin)
prazosin (Minipress)
rescinnamine (Moderil)
reserpine (Serpalan, Serpasil)
terazosin (Hytrin)

Calcium channel blockers

These medicines interfere with the movement of calcium into the heart, artery and vein muscle cells. Calcium inside a cell causes it to contract.

Therefore, the medicine causes the veins and arteries to enlarge (vasodilate) and reduces the heart rate and blood pressure. Calcium channel blockers are used mostly to treat chest pain. However, some calcium channel blockers also are used in the management of high blood pressure.

Dizziness, light-headedness, flushing and fluid retention are just some of the side effects of this class of drugs.

Calcium channel blockers lower the risk of coronary artery disease in people with high blood pressure, suggests Dr. James Sowers. Dr. Sowers is a professor of medicine and physiology and the director of the endocrinology and hypertension division at Wayne State University School of Medicine.

Most high blood pressure drugs do not sufficiently lower the risk of coronary artery disease because of their effect on cholesterol and other blood fats.

In human and animal studies, some calcium channel blockers have been found to inhibit the development of atherosclerosis.

Doctors are decreasing their use of calcium channel

blockers after a heart attack. Results of a study of diltiazem showed the drug can help lower the rates of second heart attack and death in some people. However, for many people, particularly those with pulmonary (lung) congestion, diltiazem can increase the risks.

But calcium channel blockers can help protect your kidneys, say researchers. These drugs can open up constricted veins, cause the kidneys to flush out sodium faster and protect against kidney failure.

They are even thought to protect transplanted kidneys against damage. People with high blood pressure seem to be more sensitive to the beneficial effects of calcium channel blockers on the kidneys than people with normal blood pressure levels. This is all good news for people with high blood pressure caused by kidney problems.

Taking beta blockers at the same time as calcium channel blockers is usually well-tolerated, but calcium channel blockers may cause heart failure in people with aorta problems who also are taking beta blockers.

Don't withdraw suddenly from beta blockers before or during calcium channel blocker therapy. Some calcium channel blockers should be used with caution in people with congestive heart failure.

Prescriptions for calcium channel blockers include:

diltiazem (Cardizem, Cardizem SR, Cardizem CD)
felodipine (Plendil)
isradipine (DynaCirc)
nicardipine (Cardene, Cardene SR)
nifedipine (Procardia XL)
verapamil (Calan, Calan SR, Isoptin, Isoptin SR,
    Verelan)

Calcium channel blockers have no effect on insulin or sugar levels in the blood, so they are good medications for people with diabetes and high blood pressure.

Also, they work equally well in black and white, young and old people.

Diuretics

Diuretics are probably the most commonly recommended high blood pressure drugs, with thiazides comprising the largest group in this class.

Often called water pills, diuretics are chemicals which act on the kidneys, causing them to flush salt and water from the body. To understand how these drugs lower blood pressure, you must remember how important our kidneys are to our health.

One of the main jobs of the kidneys is to flush out excess salt and minerals from our bodies each day.

However, if over the years we've eaten too much salt or are salt-retentive, the kidneys can't take salt out fast enough, and it builds up in our bodies. We then retain extra fluid to dilute the salt

Our bodies begin to sense a problem — there's too much salt and fluid building up in the system. To solve the problem our blood pressure rises, forcing the kidneys to flush out the extra salt and fluids.

The function of the diuretics is to help the kidneys take out the excess salt and fluid so that our blood pressure doesn't have to rise to do the job. As fluid volume in the blood vessels drops, the blood pressure goes down.

Diuretics also are prescribed to add to the effectiveness of other blood-pressure-reducing drugs.

One problem with this type of drug is that it's hard to find the right one. Either they simply aren't effective or they are too potent and make you run to the bathroom continually. To find the right drug at the right dose for you can be very difficult.

Also, if you continue to eat a lot of salt and you are taking a diuretic, the drug will be flushing out too many other minerals from your body, like potassium.

It has been estimated that the majority of people taking diuretics exhibit one or more of the signs and symptoms of low potassium.

Therefore, potassium supplements are usually prescribed as well, unless the patient is receiving potassium-sparing diuretics.

Thiazide diuretics should be used with caution by people with poor kidney function or progressive liver disease. Sensitivity reactions are most likely to occur in people with allergies or bronchial asthma.

Thiazide diuretics can result in severe sunburn with modest exposure to the sun. Insulin requirements may have to be adjusted.

Pain relievers and barbiturates may cause increased effects of the diuretics and should be avoided if possible. Thiazide diuretics also interact with digitalis and related drugs, adrenocorticoids and tricyclic antidepressant drugs.

Loop diuretics are so called because they work in the loop of Henle, a part of the kidney, which helps make them much more effective.

Dosages should be individualized and carefully monitored.

Although diuretics are often prescribed, they are not without serious drawbacks.

One recent study showed that people with unstable angina who received thiazide diuretics had higher death rates than those who didn't take thiazide diuretics.

Commonly prescribed diuretic drugs include:

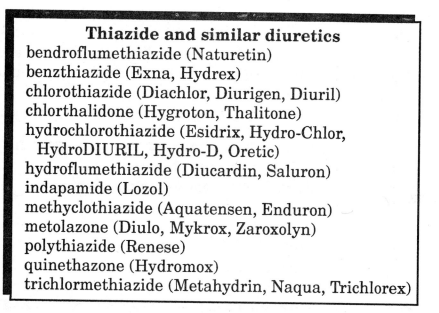

Thiazide and similar diuretics
bendroflumethiazide (Naturetin)
benzthiazide (Exna, Hydrex)
chlorothiazide (Diachlor, Diurigen, Diuril)
chlorthalidone (Hygroton, Thalitone)
hydrochlorothiazide (Esidrix, Hydro-Chlor,
  HydroDIURIL, Hydro-D, Oretic)
hydroflumethiazide (Diucardin, Saluron)
indapamide (Lozol)
methyclothiazide (Aquatensen, Enduron)
metolazone (Diulo, Mykrox, Zaroxolyn)
polythiazide (Renese)
quinethazone (Hydromox)
trichlormethiazide (Metahydrin, Naqua, Trichlorex)

Loop diuretics
bumetanide (Bumex)
ethacrynic acid
  (Edecrin)
furosemide (Lasix)

**Potassium-sparing
diuretics**
amiloride (Midamor)
spironolactone (Aldactone)
triamterene (Dyrenium)

These medications are generally the first medication tried
when a person is newly diagnosed with high blood pressure

Combination drugs

Combinations of different types of drugs are sometimes
used to make it easier for people to remember to take their

medication and to have the most efficient use of the drugs in the body.

They are not usually given as the initial treatment for high blood pressure because the individual doses of each drug need to be adjusted separately before the right combination for each person can be determined.

Here are some combinations that are often prescribed:

Diuretic combinations

amiloride and hydrochlorothiazide (Moduretic)
spironolactone and hydrochlorothiazide
(Aldactazide, Spirozide)
triamterene and hydrochlorothiazide
(Dyazide, Maxzide)

Antihypertensive combinations

bendroflumethiazide and nadolol (Corzide)
chlorothiazide and methyldopa (Aldoclor)
chlorothiazide and reserpine (Diupres)
chlorthalidone and atenolol (Tenoretic)
chlorthalidone and clonidine (Combipres)
chlorthalidone and reserpine (Demi-Regroton, Regroton)
hydrochlorothiazide and deserpidine (Oreticyl)
hydrochlorothiazide and hydralazine (Apresazide,
Apresoline-Esidrix, Hydra-Zide)
hydrochlorothiazide, hydralazine and reserpine (Cam-ap-
es, H-H-R, Ser-A-Gen, Seralazide, Ser-Ap-Es, Serpazide,
Tri-Hydroserpine, Unipres)
hydrochlorothiazide and reserpine (Hydropres, Hydro-
Serp, Hydroserpine, Serpasil-Esidrix)
hydrochlorothiazide and captopril (Capozide)

Antihypertensive combinations
hydrochlorothiazide and enalapril (Vaseretic)
hydrochlorothiazide and guanethidine monosulfate (Esimil)
hydrochlorothiazide and labetalol (Normozide, Trandate)
hydrochlorothiazide and methyldopa (Aldoril)
hydrochlorothiazide and metoprolol (Lopressor HCT)
hydrochlorothiazide and propranolol HCl (Inderide,
  Inderide LA)
hydrochlorothiazide and timolol maleate (Timolide)
hydroflumethiazide and reserpine (Hydropine, Salutensin,
  Salutensin-Demi)
methychlothiazide and deserpidine (Enduronyl)
methychlothiazide and reserpine (Diutensen-R)
polythiazide and prazosin (Minizide)
polythiazide and reserpine (Renese-R)
quinethazone and reserpine (Hydromox R)
trichlormethiazide and reserpine (Diurese-R, Metatensin,
  Naquival)

MAO inhibitors
Another group of drugs that works by inhibiting a normal body action is the monoamine oxidase (MAO) inhibitors. They stop the body from producing certain chemicals in the brain and nerves. MAO inhibitors are antidepressant drugs and have many side effects like dizziness and weakness. Lowering blood pressure is really just one more side effect. For that reason, some MAO inhibitors have been used in the past to treat high blood pressure.

MAO inhibiting drugs can have more serious side effects. We have not listed these drugs because they are not normally used in the treatment of high blood pressure. However, people using these drugs should exercise caution because of the effects they can have on blood pressure.

Potassium supplements

Extra potassium is needed to offset the side effects of certain blood-pressure-reducing drugs that lower the body's potassium to below-normal levels.

And a low potassium level is itself a risk factor for high blood pressure.

Potassium supplements are often needed because it would be difficult to eat enough potassium-rich foods to compensate for the loss. Tablet forms of potassium salts can cause stomach irritation or even ulcers in some people. Liquid forms are usually safest.

Forms of potassium available include:

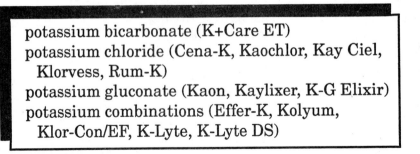

> potassium bicarbonate (K+Care ET)
> potassium chloride (Cena-K, Kaochlor, Kay Ciel, Klorvess, Rum-K)
> potassium gluconate (Kaon, Kaylixer, K-G Elixir)
> potassium combinations (Effer-K, Kolyum, Klor-Con/EF, K-Lyte, K-Lyte DS)

What drugs work best?

In general, African-Americans who suffer from high blood pressure are more responsive to diuretics and calcium channel blockers than to beta blockers or ACE inhibitors.

Elderly people with high blood pressure are generally responsive to all classes of high blood pressure medications. These drugs are equally effective for both men and women.

In order to maximize the effects of your medications, be sure you know and monitor the drug or drugs you are taking so that you can advise your doctor of any side effects. Also, you can help him determine if the drug is doing what it's supposed to do.

Average costs of high blood pressure medication

Medication	Usual maintenance range	Average wholesale price*
ACE inhibitors		
benazepril (Lotensin)	10 mg every day	$19.09
captopril (Capoten)	25 mg twice daily or 50 mg 3 times daily	$40.82 to $141.52
enalapril (Vasotec)	5 mg daily or 20 mg twice daily	$26.46 to $79.03
fosinopril (Monopril)	10 mg to 20 mg daily	$21.26 to $22.75
lisinopril (Pinivl, Zestril)	5 to 20 mg daily	$23.62 to $25.09
quinapril (Accupril)	10 to 20 mg daily	$23.49
Anti-adrenergic agents		
prazosin (Minipress)	1 to 2 mg twice daily	$11.71 to $32.60
terazosin (Hytrin)	1 to 2 mg daily	$35.30
doxazosin (Cardura)	1 to 4 mg daily	$25.58 to $26.83
Beta blockers		
atenolol (Tenormin)	25 to 50 mg daily	$24.52 to $25.02
betaxolol (Kerlone)	10 to 20 mg daily	$20.81 to $31.21
metoprolol (Lopressor)	50 mg daily or 100 mg twice daily	$14.87 to $44.69
nadolol (Corgard)	40 mg twice daily or 40 mg 3 times daily	$60.87 to $120.13
propranolol (Inderal LA)	80 to 120 mg daily	$25.29 to $31.36
timolol (Blocadren)	10 to 20 mg twice daily	$30.01 to $55.35

Medication	Usual maintenance range	Average wholesale price*
Calcium channel blockers		
diltiazem (Cardizem CD)	240 mg daily	$50.40
verapamil (Calan SR, Verelan)	240 mg daily	$37.30
felodipine (Plendil)	5 to 10 mg daily	$26.06 to $46.24
nicardipine (Cardene SR)	30 to 45 mg twice daily	$36.72 to $58.32
nifedipine (Procardia XL)	30 to 90 mg daily	$29.92 to $77.66
Thiazide diuretics		
chlorothiazide (Diuril)	250 to 500 mg daily	$3.83 to $6.07
hydrochlorothiazide (Esidrix)	25 to 50 mg daily	$3.47 to $5.50
chlorthalidone (Hygroton)	25 to 50 mg daily	$18.95 to $23.36
indapamide (Lozol)	2.5 mg daily	$23.98
Loop diuretics		
bumetanide (Bumex)	0.5 to 2 mg daily	$8.11 to $19.28
furosemide (Lasix)	20 to 40 mg daily	$4.04 to $5.69

*Estimated cost of one month's medication. These prices are wholesale. The consumer can expect to pay slightly higher prices.

Some drugs affect sex drive

One of the questions doctors get asked most by men with high blood pressure is, "Can I still have a regular sex life?" In most cases, patients with high blood pressure can continue their sexual relations with their spouse without any problems.

If you do experience unusual symptoms like shortness of breath or chest pain following sex, see your doctor as soon as possible to discuss these problems.

Some drugs prescribed for high blood pressure can cause a reduced sex drive and make it difficult to maintain an erection. However, in a recent study by the University of Connecticut Health Center, Boston University and several other centers, three drugs were compared for their sex-related side effects.

Propranolol and methyldopa were found to cause a decrease in sex drive and made it difficult to maintain an erection. Sexual problems were the worst in men over 51 who were taking methyldopa or propranolol and a diuretic. Captopril, the third drug in the study, did not seem to have any effect on either problem, making it the best choice to avoid sexual problems.

Since doctors believe that some men avoid treatment for high blood pressure because they worry about losing their sex drive, this study is very reassuring.

If you are taking prescription drugs for blood pressure and you think the drugs might be affecting your sex drive, be sure to discuss this with your doctor to see if an alternative drug might work better for you.

25 || Low-Fat Substitutions

D on't want to give up your favorite family recipes? You may not have to, if you're willing to do a little substituting. Use our low-fat food substitution chart to make your snacks and dinners healthier.

The chart makes it easy to count the fat and calories you'll save. You may not even miss the extra fat.

Food	Portion	Calories	Fat (g)	Substitute Food	Portion	Calories	Fat (g)	Calorie Savings	Fat (g) Savings
baking chocolate	1 sq.	185	16	cocoa	3 Tbsp.	122	12	63	4
buttered bread crumbs	1 cup	392	5	crushed corn flakes	1 cup	110	0	282	5
cabbage, boiled with 2 Tbsp. melted butter	1/2 cup	232	12	cabbage, boiled with 2 Tbsp. melted nonfat margarine or 2 tsp. butter-flavored seasoning	1/2 cup	26	0	206	12
cheddar cheese	1 oz.	114	9	reduced fat cheddar cheese	1 oz.	80	5	34	4

Food	Portion	Calories	Fat (g)	Substitute Food	Portion	Calories	Fat (g)	Calorie Savings	Fat (g) Savings
cheddar cheese, cubed for sauces	1 cup	457	38	reduced fat cheddar sauce (1/2 cup low-fat cottage cheese, pureed, + 1/2 cup cheddar, cubed)	1 cup	311	20	146	18
chicken breast, with skin	3 oz.	165	7	chicken breast, skinless	3 oz.	140	3	25	4
chocolate sandwich cookies	2 items	98	4	graham crackers	2 items	60	1	38	3

Food	Portion	Calories	Fat (g)	Substitute Food	Portion	Calories	Fat (g)	Calorie Savings	Fat (g) Savings
cinnamon roll	1 item	154	7	whole wheat toast	1 item	72	1	82	6
cola, with sugar	12 oz.	160	0	cola, sugar-free	12 oz.	0	0	160	0
cream cheese	2 Tbsp.	99	10	cream cheese, light	2 Tbsp.	62	5	37	5
creamed cottage cheese	1 cup	217	10	cottage cheese, low-fat (1% fat)	1 cup	164	2	53	8
croissant	1 item	235	12	dinner roll	1 item	85	2	150	10
dessert topping, non-dairy whipped	1 cup	224	4	evaporated skim milk, partially frozen whipped	1 cup	215	1	9	3
doughnut	1 item	105	6	bagel	1 item	163	1	0	5

Food	Portion	Calories	Fat (g)	Substitute Food	Portion	Calories	Fat (g)	Calorie Savings	Fat (g) Savings
egg	1 whole	79	6	egg	2 whites only	32	0	47	6
ham, cubed (used in baked beans)	1 cup	255	15	dried tomatoes	1 cup	139	2	116	13
hamburger, regular ground beef baked	3.5 oz. patty	289	21	ground turkey, baked	3.5 oz. patty	225	12	64	9
hot dog, regular	1 item	214	14	hot dog, low-fat	1 item	50	2	164	12
ice cream, premium	1 cup	350	24	sorbet	1 cup	190	0	160	24
Italian salad dressing	1 Tbsp.	70	8	no-oil Italian salad dressing	1 Tbsp.	6	0	64	8

Food	Portion	Calories	Fat (g)	Substitute Food	Portion	Calories	Fat (g)	Calorie Savings	Fat (g) Savings
mayonnaise, regular	1 Tbsp.	102	11	mayonnaise, nonfat	1 Tbsp.	12	0	90	11
milk, evaporated whole	4 oz.	169	10	milk, evaporated skim	4 oz.	99	0	70	10
milk, whole	8 oz.	150	8	milk, skim	8 oz.	86	0	64	8
nachos, with cheese **12 tortilla chips &1/4 cup cheese	**	285	19	raw vegetables (celery, zucchini sticks and cherry tomatoes)	1 platter	30	0	255	19
New England clam chowder	1 cup	165	7	Manhattan clam chowder	1 cup	80	2	85	5

Food	Portion	Calories	Fat (g)	Substitute Food	Portion	Calories	Fat (g)	Calorie Savings	Fat (g) Savings
orange juice	6 oz.	80	0	tomato juice (high in sodium)	6 oz.	30	0	50	0
pizza, cheese with everything *1/8 of medium thin crust	1 slice *	240	12	pizza, cheese with vegetable toppings	1 slice*	165	5	75	7
popcorn, popped in oil	3 cups	100	6	popcorn, air popped	3 cups	75	2	25	4
potato chips	10 chips	105	7	pretzel sticks	2/3 cup	100	0	5	7
pound cake	1 slice	146	7	angel food cake	1 slice	192	0	0	7
prime rib	3 oz.	360	31	round roast of beef	3 oz.	155	6	205	25

Food	Portion	Calories	Fat (g)	Substitute Food	Portion	Calories	Fat (g)	Calorie Savings	Fat (g) Savings
Ricotta whole milk cheese	1/2 cup	216	16	Ricotta part skim cheese	1/2 cup	171	10	45	6
sausage	1 3-in. patty	200	17	Canadian bacon	2 slices	85	4	115	13
shortening, for baked goods	1/2 cup	848	96	applesauce or fruit puree (substitute for half of shortening)	1/2 cup	97	0	751	96
sirloin steak	3.5 oz. piece	280	18	flank steak	3.5 oz. piece	243	15	37	3
solid shortening, for greasing pans	1 Tbsp.	100	11	nonstick cooking spray, for pans	3 sec. spray	6	1	94	10

Food	Portion	Calories	Fat (g)	Substitute Food	Portion	Calories	Fat (g)	Calorie Savings	Fat (g) Savings
sour cream, for baked goods	1 cup	493	48	yogurt, low-fat	1 cup	144	0	349	48
sour cream, regular	2 Tbsp.	60	6	sour cream, nonfat	2 Tbsp.	35	0	25	6
sour cream, regular	1 Tbsp.	30	3	sour cream, light	1 Tbsp.	18	1	12	2
Swiss cheese	1 oz.	107	8	mozzarella, part-skim	1 oz.	79	5	28	3
Thousand Island salad dressing	1 Tbsp.	59	6	reduced calorie Thousand Island salad dressing	1 Tbsp.	24	2	35	4
vanilla butter cream icing	for 1/12 cake	158	7	vanilla egg white icing	for 1/12 cake	60	0	98	7

Food	Portion	Calories	Fat (g)	Substitute Food	Portion	Calories	Fat (g)	Calorie Savings	Fat (g) Savings
vegetables, sauteed	1 cup	292	14	vegetables, steamed	1 cup	54	0	238	14
vinaigrette dressing	1 Tbsp.	70	8	vinaigrette dressing with fruit juice (1/4 cup of juice replaces 1/4 cup oil per 1 cup of dressing)	1 Tbsp.	54	6	16	2

26 | High-Fiber Foods

A high-fiber diet of beans, grains, vegetables and fruits can help you maintain a healthy weight, avoid high blood pressure and high cholesterol, and keep you regular. The typical American eats too many highly processed foods that have lost most of their natural fiber.

Use the following chart to find high-fiber breads, grains and pasta, cereals, desserts, fruits, nuts and seeds, sauces and dips, and vegetables.

We've included the fat content of the foods as well as the fiber content to help you keep your fat intake low. Granola, for instance, has lots of fiber, but is also high in fat. You'll probably want to choose the low-fat version.

Food	Portion	Dietary Fiber (g)	Fat (g)
Breads, Grains & Pasta			
bread			
bagel (plain)	1 bagel	1.5	1.1
biscuit	1 biscuit	0.9	4.0
biscuit (low-fat)	1 biscuit	0.9	1.1
black	1 slice	3.0	3.1
breadstick	1 stick	0.3	1.1
cheese	1 slice	0.5	1.4
cornbread	1 serving	1.1	2.0
croissant	1 serving	0.3	6.1
French	1 slice	0.7	0.8
honey wheat	1 slice	0.7	0.9
Italian	1 ounce	2.7	0.2
mixed grain	1 slice	0.2	1.0
oatmeal	1 slice	0.3	2.0
pita	1 ounce	1.6	0.4
pumpernickle	1 ounce	2.8	0.3
raisin	1 ounce	2.9	0.8
rye	1 ounce	1.7	0.3
white	1 slice	0.6	0.9

Food	Portion	Dietary Fiber (g)	Fat (g)
whole wheat	1 slice	2.9	1.8
breakfast items			
buckwheat pancake	1 item	0.7	2.3
buttermilk pancake	1 item	0.1	2.0
doughnut	1 whole	1.3	13.7
French toast	1 slice	1.6	3.6
waffle	1 item	0.3	4.0
wheat pancake	1 item	0.8	4.0
crackers			
bran	1 serving	0.8	3.0
brown rice cakes	1 cake	0.4	0.2
butter	1 serving	0.7	4.0
cheese	1 piece	0.1	0.3
club	1 serving	0.8	3.0
graham	1 piece	0.1	0.7
herb	1 serving	0.7	4.0
Holland Rusk	1 ounce	5.1	2.5
melba toast	1 slice	0.3	0.0
oyster	1 piece	0.2	0.1
popcorn cakes	1 cake	0.3	0.3

Food	Portion	Dietary Fiber (g)	Fat (g)
pretzel chips	1 serving	0.8	3.0
Ritz	1 piece	0.3	1.0
rye	1 piece	0.1	0.0
rye wafers	1 cup	5.1	0.6
saltine	1 piece	0.1	0.4
sesame	1 piece	0.2	0.4
Triscuit	1 piece	0.2	0.8
Wasa chips	1 slice	0.3	1.5
wheat	1 piece	0.1	0.4
zwieback toast	1 toast	0.4	1.4
grains (cooked)			
barley	1 cup	6.0	0.7
brown and wild rice	1 cup	2.1	2.8
bulgar	1 cup	8.2	0.4
millet	1 cup	3.1	2.4
white rice	1 cup	0.7	0.5
miscellaneous			
chicken stuffing	1 serving	0.3	1.0
chow mein noodles	1 cup	1.8	13.8
corn tortilla	1 item	1.1	2.5

Food	Portion	Dietary Fiber (g)	Fat (g)
cornbread stuffing	1 serving	0.3	1.0
couscous	1 cup	2.5	0.3
croutons	1 cup	2.0	1.8
dumplings	1 ounce	2.0	3.2
pizza crust	1 serving	0.8	1.0
pretzels	10 pieces	1.9	2.1
rice stuffing	1 serving	0.4	1.0
muffins			
blueberry	1 item	2.0	3.7
bran	1 item	4 0	6.0
corn	1 item	0 1	4.0
English	1 item	2 0	0.7
whole wheat English	1 item	4.2	1.4

Food	Portion	Dietary Fiber (g)	Fat (g)
pasta			
angel hair	1 cup	1.3	0.9
egg noodles	1 cup	1.0	1.6
macaroni	1 cup	1.8	0.9
rotini	1 cup	2.0	1.3
spaghetti	1 cup	2.0	1.3
spinach spaghetti	1 cup	9.0	1.3
ziti	1 cup	2.5	1.7
rolls			
cinnamon	1 item	0.3	4.2
dinner	1 item	0.1	2.0
dinner wheat	1 item	1.4	1.5
hard	1 ounce	3.5	0.9
hoagie (submarine)	1 item	0.1	4.0

Food	Portion	Dietary Fiber (g)	Fat (g)
Cereals			
100% Bran	1/2 cup	9.8	1.7
40% Bran Flakes	1 cup	6.9	0.7
All Bran	1/3 cup	10.1	0.5
Alpha Bits	1 cup	1.0	1.1
Apple Jacks	1 cup	0.5	0.1
Basic Four	1 serving	2.0	2.0
Booberry Cereal	1 ounce	0.5	1.0
Bran Buds	1 cup	31.4	2.0
Bran Chex	1 cup	7.9	1.4
Bran Flakes & Fruit	1 cup	4.7	0.7
C.W. Post	1 cup	2.2	15.2
Cap'N Crunch	1 cup	0.4	3.4
Cheerios	1 cup	1.4	1.6
Cinnamon Mini Buns	1 ounce	1.0	1.0
Cinnamon Toast Crunch	1 cup	0.7	3.9
Clusters	1 ounce	2.0	2.0
Coco Crunchies	1 cup	0.6	0.7
Cocoa Krispies	1 cup	0.2	0.5
Cocoa Pebbles	1 cup	0.7	1.9

Food	Portion	Dietary Fiber (g)	Fat (g)
Cocoa Puffs	1 cup	0.2	0.6
Common Sense Oat Bran	1 cup	5.4	1.2
Complete Bran Flakes	1 cup	7.5	0.0
Cookie Crisp	1 cup	0.4	1.1
Corn Chex	1 cup	0.5	0.1
Corn Flakes	1 cup	0.7	0.1
Corn Pops	1 cup	0.1	0.1
Count Chocula	1 cup	0.6	0.4
Cracklin Bran	1 cup	10.8	8.6
Cracklin Oat Bran	1 cup	8.2	7.7
Cream Of Rice	1 cup	0.4	0.2
Cream Of Wheat	1 cup	5.7	2.5
Crispix	1 cup	0.6	0.1
Crispy Rice	1 cup	0.3	0.1
Crispy Wheats 'N' Raisins	1 cup	2.9	0.7
Farina	1 cup	3.3	0.9
Fiber 7 Flakes	1 ounce	5.0	1.0
Fiber One Plus	1 ounce	13.0	1.0
Frankenberry	1 ounce	0.5	1.0
Froot Loops	1 cup	1.0	1.0

Food	Portion	Dietary Fiber (g)	Fat (g)
Frosted Bran	1 cup	4.5	0.0
Frosted Flakes	1 cup	0.6	0.1
Frosted Mini Wheats	1 cup	6.0	0.0
Frosted Rice Krispies	1 cup	0.1	0.1
Fruit & Fiber	1 serving	4.6	2.5
Fruit & Nut	1 ounce	1.0	5.0
Fruitful Bran	1 cup	7.5	0.0
Fruity Marshmallow Krispies	1 cup	0.2	0.1
Fruity Pebbles	1 cup	0.7	1.8
Golden Grahams	1 cup	1.4	1.5
granola	1 cup	4.2	19.6
granola, fat free	1 ounce	3.0	0.0
granola, homemade	1 cup	12.8	33.2
granola, low fat	1 ounce	2.0	2.0
granola, low fat with raisins	1 cup	6.0	6.0
Grape Nuts	1/4 cup	2.8	0.1
Grape Nuts Flakes	1 cup	2.4	0.7
grits	1 cup	0.5	0.5
Harvest Crunch	1 cup	5.7	22.2
Heartland Natural	1 cup	5.4	17.7

Food	Portion	Dietary Fiber (g)	Fat (g)
Shredded Wheat	2 biscuits	6.1	0.0
Wheat Chex	1 cup	4.1	1.2
whole wheat-natural	1 cup	8.9	1.9

Food	Portion	Dietary Fiber (g)	Fat (g)
Desserts			
bread pudding	1/2 cup	0.0	7.4
butter cookies	1 item	0.1	0.9
caramel-flavored popcorn	1 cup	1.8	4.5
chocolate chip cookies	1 item	0.2	2.3
chocolate pudding	1 cup	0.3	8.4
chocolate-coated peanuts	1 cup	6.3	49.9
chocolate-coated raisins	1 cup	8.0	28.1
fig cookie	1 item	0.7	1.2
fruit streusel	1 slice	0.8	12.3
fudge brownie	1 item	1.4	15.4
gingerbread	1 square	1.1	5.0
gingersnap cookies	1 item	0.2	0.7
oatmeal cookies	1 item	0.6	3.3
peanut butter cookies	1 item	0.5	7.6
pecan pie	1 slice	1.4	22.8
pumpkin pie	1 slice	1.9	8.5

Food	Portion	Dietary Fiber (g)	Fat (g)
Fruit			
apple ring, dried	1 ring	0.6	0.0
apple slices	1 cup	3.0	0.4
applesauce	1 cup	3.1	0.5
apricot, in juice	1 cup	3.2	0.1
apricot, sliced	1 cup	0.8	0.1
avocado	1 item	6.8	30.0
banana, sliced	1/2 cup	2.7	0.6
blackberries	1 cup	7.2	0.6
blueberries	1 cup	3.9	0.6
boysenberries	1 cup	5.2	0.3
cantaloupe, cubed	1 cup	1.1	0.4
cherries, in juice	1 cup	1.8	0.0
coconut, toasted	1/2 cup	3.5	24.4
cranberries	1 cup	4.6	0.2
cranberry sauce	1 cup	2.8	0.4
currants	1 cup	4.8	0.2
date	1 item	0.7	0.0
elderberries	1 cup	10.2	0.7
fig	1/4 cup	1.6	0.2

Food	Portion	Dietary Fiber (g)	Fat (g)
fruit bar, fat free	1 bar	3.4	0.0
fruit cocktail	1 cup	2.7	0.0
fruit salad	1 cup	2.8	0.2
grapefruit, in juice	1 cup	1.0	0.2
guava	1/2 cup	4.9	0.5
honeydew, cubed	1 cup	1.5	0.2
jam, most flavors	1 Tbsp.	0.2	0.0
juice, apple	1 cup	0.2	0.2
juice, cranberry cocktail	1 cup	0.2	0.0
juice, grapefruit	1 cup	0.4	0.2
juice, orange	1 cup	2.0	0.5
juice, pineapple	1 cup	0.3	0.1
juice, prune	1 cup	2.6	0.1
kiwifruit	1 item	3.0	0.4
kumquat	1 item	1.2	0.0
lemonade	1 cup	0.6	0.0
mango	1 item	4.8	0.6
mixed fruit	1 cup	2.9	0.3
nectarine	1 item	1.6	0.6
orange	1 item	3.5	0.4

Food	Portion	Dietary Fiber (g)	Fat (g)
orange, mandarin	1/2 cup	1.9	0.2
papaya	1 item	8.3	0.6
peach, slices	1 cup	3.4	0.2
pears	1 cup	4.0	0.7
pears, canned in syrup	1 cup	5.2	0.3
persimmon	1 item	7.2	0.1
pineapple, bits	1 cup	2.0	0.2
plantain	1 item	4.1	0.7
plums	1 cup	3.5	1.8
pomegranate	1 item	1.1	0.5
pricklypear	1 item	4.9	0.7
prunes	1 ounce	0.6	0.0
raisins, seedless	1 cup	5.8	0.7
raspberries	1 ounce	2.1	0.0
rhubarb	1 cup	6.5	0.7
strawberries	1 cup	2.7	0.6
tangerine	1 item	1.9	0.2
watermelon	1 cup	0.6	0.7

Food	Portion	Dietary Fiber (g)	Fat (g)
Nuts & Seeds			
nuts			
almonds	1 ounce	2.5	13.8
beechnuts	1 ounce	2.6	14.2
Brazil	1 cup	10.8	92.7
cashews	1 cup	4.9	62.7
coconut, flaked	1 cup	4.4	24.4
ginkgonuts	1 cup	14.4	2.5
hazel	1 cup	12.2	95.5
hickory	1 cup	8.0	80.5
macadamia	1 cup	12.5	98.8
mixed nuts	1 cup	11.6	70.5
peanut butter	1 Tbsp	1.0	8.0
peanuts	1 cup	10.7	71.0
pecans	1 cup	8.2	73.0
pignolia (pine nuts)	1 Tbsp	0.4	5.1
pistachio	1 cup	13.8	67.6
trail mix	1 cup	10.8	44.1
walnuts	1 cup	3.0	45.3

Food	Portion	Dietary Fiber (g)	Fat (g)
seeds			
caraway	1 Tbsp	2.6	1.0
celery	1 Tbsp	0.8	1.6
pumpkin	1 ounce	0.5	15.6
sesame	1 ounce	5.3	13.6
soybean kernels	1 cup	9.2	25.9
sunflower	1 cup	9.2	77.6

Food	Portion	Dietary Fiber (g)	Fat (g)
Sauces & Dips			
barbecue sauce	1 cup	3.0	4.5
black bean sauce	1/2 cup	2.2	6.9
chutney	1 Tbsp	0.5	0.1
guacamole dip	1 cup	5.6	33.9
hollandaise sauce	1/4 cup	0.3	5.1
pesto sauce	1/2 cup	1.8	56.4
picante sauce	1 cup	3.4	27.3
salsa	1/4 cup	0.9	0.2
spaghetti sauce	1 cup	8.5	11.9

Food	Portion	Dietary Fiber (g)	Fat (g)
Vegetables and Vegetable Dishes			
alfalfa sprouts	1 cup	0.8	0.2
artichoke hearts	1/2 cup	4.5	0.1
asparagus spears	4 spears	1.2	0.1
bamboo shoots	1 cup	2.0	0.5
bean sprouts	1 cup	1.3	0.2
beans, baby lima	1 cup	12.7	0.7
beans, baked	1 cup	19.6	1.1
beans, black	1 cup	15.0	0.9
beans, Great Northern	1 cup	9.7	0.8
beans, green	1 cup	2.6	0.1
beans, Italian green	1 cup	3.4	0.2
beans, kidney	1 cup	13.3	0.8
beans, mung	1 cup	15.4	0.8
beans, navy	1 cup	10.1	1.0
beans, pinto	1 cup	12.7	0.9
beans, refried	1 cup	11.6	2.7
beans, shellie	1 cup	12.0	0.5
beans, snap	1 cup	2.3	0.4
beans, vegetarian (canned)	1 ounce	1.6	0.1

Food	Portion	Dietary Fiber (g)	Fat (g)
beans, white	1 cup	11.3	0.6
beets	1 cup	4.2	0.2
bok choy	1 cup	0.7	0.1
broccoli	1 cup	5.4	0.5
brussels sprouts	1 cup	6.4	0.6
cabbage, fresh	1 cup	3.4	0.4
carrot	1 item	1.8	0.1
carrot juice	1 cup	5.9	0.4
carrots	1 cup	5.1	0.4
cauliflower	1 cup	3.2	0.4
celery	1 stalk	0.6	0.1
chard	1 cup	3.7	0.1
chickpea	1 cup	10.6	2.7
chicory greens, chopped	1 cup	4.3	0.5
chives	1 Tbsp	0.1	0.0
chop suey vegetables	1 cup	0.0	0.1
clamato juice	1 cup	1.5	0.2
collards, chopped	1 cup	6.9	0.4
corn on the cob	1 ear	2.7	0.9
corn, sweet	1 cup	3.1	1.7

Food	Portion	Dietary Fiber (g)	Fat (g)
cowpeas	1 cup	15.0	0.9
cucumber	1 cup	2.0	0.3
dandelion greens	1 cup	4.1	0.6
eggplant	1 ounce	0.3	0.0
endive, chopped	1/2 cup	0.8	0.0
garlic, clove	1 item	0.1	0.0
ginger root, sliced	1 cup	0.7	0.7
hominy, canned	1 cup	1.0	1.4
kale	1 cup	4.3	0.5
kohlrabi	1 cup	3.3	0.2
leeks	1 item	4.0	0.2
lentils	1 cup	9.8	0.7
lettuce, iceberg	1 cup	0.6	0.1
lettuce, romaine	1 cup	1.0	0.1
mixed chinese vegetables	1 cup	0.3	0.1
mixed vegetables	1 cup	6.9	0.3
mushrooms, fresh chopped	1 cup	0.9	0.3
mustard greens	1 cup	2.7	0.3
okra	1 cup	2.6	0.3
olives, green	1 cup	6.5	18.7

Food	Portion	Dietary Fiber (g)	Fat (g)
olives, ripe	1 item	0.1	0.7
onion, young green	1 item	0.1	0.0
onions, chopped	1 cup	2.7	0.3
onions, dried flakes	1 Tbsp	0.5	0.0
parsnips, sliced	1 cup	7.6	0.5
peas & carrots, canned	1 cup	8.6	0.7
peas, blackeye	1 cup	7.9	1.3
peas, green	1 cup	7.7	0.6
peas, split	1 cup	10.5	1.0
peas, sugar snap	1 cup	4.0	0.0
pepper, black	1 Tbsp	1.7	0.2
pepper, cayenne	1 Tbsp	1.3	0.9
peppers, hot red	1 tsp	0.7	0.0
peppers, sweet	1 cup	3.8	0.4
pickle, sweet gherkin	1 item	0.2	0.0
pickle, whole cucumber dill	1 item	0.7	0.1
potato chips	1 cup	0.7	6.4
potato puff	1 item	0.2	0.8
potato, baked	1 item	5.1	0.2
potato, sweet, baked	1 item	3.4	0.1

Food	Portion	Dietary Fiber (g)	Fat (g)
potatoes au gratin	1 ounce	0.5	1.2
potatoes, French fried	1 cup	2.4	6.0
potatoes, hash brown	1 cup	3.1	21.7
potatoes, scalloped	1 cup	4.4	9.0
pumpkin, canned	1 cup	7.1	0.7
purslane	1 ounce	0.6	0.1
radishes	1 item	0.1	0.0
rutabagas	1 cup	5.1	0.5
sauerkraut	1 cup	6.1	0.3
soup, bean and bacon	1 cup	6.0	0.7
soup, black bean	1 cup	4.4	1.5
soup, green pea	1 cup	2.8	2.9
soybeans, boiled	1 cup	7.5	15.4
spinach	1 ounce	2.5	0.1
squash, acorn	1 cup	4.3	0.3
squash, butternut	1 cup	3.5	0.2
squash, summer	1 cup	2.5	0.6
squash, winter	1 cup	5.7	1.3
squash, zucchini	1 cup	1.2	0.2
tofu, soybean curd	1 piece	1.4	5.6

Food	Portion	Dietary Fiber (g)	Fat (g)
tomato juice	1 cup	2.9	0.1
tomato paste	1 Tbsp	0.5	0.5
tomato puree	1 cup	5.8	0.3
tomato, green	1 item	0.6	0.2
tomatoes, whole, canned	1 cup	1.7	0.6
turnip greens	1 cup	4.5	0.3
turnips	1 cup	3.1	0.1
vegetable juice	1 cup	2.7	0.2
water chestnuts	1 cup	3.3	0.2
watercress	1 cup	0.4	0.0
yams	1 cup	3.3	0.2

27 ‖ Calorie Counter

How many calories do you take in every day? You may have no idea, especially if most of the food you eat isn't prepackaged and stamped with a handy label. Our calorie counter is certainly not all-inclusive, but it can help you estimate how much "energy" you consume in a day. You'll be surprised at how all the little extras, such as a pat of butter or a handful of peanuts, add up.

Food	Portion	Approx. Equivalent	Calories	Fat Calories (%)	Cholesterol (mg)
Alcohol					
100 proof whisky	1 1/2 oz.	jigger	94	0	0
beer	12 oz.	can	146	0	0
Bloody Mary	8 oz.		177	0	0
gin and tonic	7 1/2 oz.		161	0	0
wine, dessert	6 oz.		233	0	0
wine, red	6 oz.		122	0	0
wine, white	6 oz.		116	0	0
Beverages					
coffee (black)	6 oz.		2	0	0
coffee (cream and sugar)	6 oz.		68	40	11
coffee (cream)	6 oz.		36	75	11

Food	Portion	Approx. Equivalent	Calories	Fat Calories (%)	Choles- terol (mg)
fruit punch drink	8 oz.		106	0	0
grapefruit drink	6 oz.		92	0	0
grapefruit juice	6 oz.		66	0	0
hot cocoa	8 oz.		197	37	30
juice, apple	6 oz.		71	0	0
juice, carrot	6 oz.		68	0	0
juice, cranberry	8 oz.		131	0	0
juice, cranberry-apple	8 oz.		152	0	0
juice, grape	8 oz.		138	0	0
juice, orange, fresh	6 oz.		77	0	0
juice, pineapple	6 oz.		95	0	0
juice, prune	6 oz.		121	0	0

Food	Portion	Approx. Equivalent	Calories	Fat Calories (%)	Cholesterol (mg)
juice, vegetable	6 oz.		32	0	0
lemonade	8 oz.		100	0	0
soda, club	8 oz.		0	0	0
soda, cola, etc.	12 oz.		133	0	0
soda, cream	12 oz.		146	0	0
tea, brewed	8 oz.		2	0	0
water	8 oz.		0	0	0
water, tonic	4 oz.		39	0	0
Breads					
bagel	2 oz.	1 small	152	6	0
biscuits	1 oz.	1 biscuit	104	43	5
bread, corn	2 1/2 oz.	2 in. square	148	31	58

Food	Portion	Approx. Equivalent	Calories	Fat Calories (%)	Choles- terol (mg)
bread, French	1 oz.	1 slice	82	11	1
bread, Italian	1 oz.	1 slice	78	0	0
bread, pita	2 oz.	1 small loaf	134	0	0
bread, pumpernickel	1 oz.	1 slice	70	0	0
bread, raisin	1 oz.	1 slice	74	12	1
bread, rye	1 oz.	1 slice	70	0	0
bread, Vienna	1 oz.	1 slice	82	11	1
bread, white	1 oz.	1 slice	76	12	1
bread, whole wheat	1 oz.	1 slice	69	13	1
croissant	2 oz.	1 pastry	233	46	13
danish pastry	2 oz.	1 pastry	239	49	36
dinner roll	1 oz.	1 roll	84	21	2

Food	Portion	Approx. Equivalent	Calories	Fat Calories (%)	Choles- terol (mg)
doughnut, cake	2 oz.	1 serving	221	45	34
doughnut, glazed	2 oz.	1 serving	229	51	14
French toast	3 1/2 oz.	2 slices	177	27	165
muffin, blueberry	2 1/2 oz.	1 muffin	149	30	44
muffin, bran	2 1/2 oz.	1 muffin	139	32	55
muffin, corn	2 oz.	1 muffin	133	27	25
muffin, English	2 1/2 oz.	1 muffin	151	7	0
roll, sweet	2 oz.	1 roll	178	30	6
waffle	2 items		180	30	6
Candy					
butterscotch	1 oz.		112	8	3
caramel	1 oz.		113	24	1

Food	Portion	Approx. Equivalent	Calories	Fat Calories (%)	Choles- terol (mg)
chocolate coated peanuts	1 oz.		159	68	0
chocolate coated raisins	1 oz.		120	38	3
fudge	1 oz.		113	24	0
hard candy	1 oz.		109	0	0
jelly beans	1 oz.		104	0	0
marshmallows	1 oz.		90	0	0
Condiments					
apple butter	1 Tbsp.		26	0	0
apple jelly	2 Tbsp.		78	0	0
barbeque sauce	2 Tbsp.		22	0	0
cherry jelly	1 Tbsp.		39	0	0
chili sauce	2 oz.		59	4	0

Food	Portion	Approx. Equivalent	Calories	Fat Calories (%)	Choles-terol (mg)
cocktail sauce	2 Tbsp.		28	0	0
grape jam	1 Tbsp.		39	0	0
guacamole dip	1 oz.		47	96	0
horseradish	1 Tbsp.		5	0	0
ketchup	1 Tbsp.		15	0	0
maple syrup	2 Tbsp.		72	0	0
Mexican salsa	4 Tbsp.		12	0	0
mint flavored apple jelly	1 Tbsp.		39	0	0
mustard	1 Tbsp.		11	82	0
orange marmalade	1 Tbsp.		36	0	0
peach preserves	1 Tbsp.		39	0	0
pickle relish, sweet	1 Tbsp.		20	0	0

Food	Portion	Approx. Equivalent	Calories	Fat Calories (%)	Choles- terol (mg)
salad dressing, French	1 Tbsp.		61	89	8
salad dressing, Italian	1 Tbsp.		66	95	0
salad dressing, Thousand Island	1 Tbsp.		53	85	4
salad dressing, vinegar and oil	1 Tbsp.		64	98	0
sorghum syrup	2 Tbsp.		72	0	0
soy sauce	2 Tbsp.		18	0	0
tartar sauce	1 Tbsp.		75	96	7
teriyaki sauce	2 Tbsp.		24	0	0
Cooking Ingredients					
egg noodles (cooked)	2 oz.		71	13	18
flour, all purpose wheat	1 oz.	1/4 cup	103	0	0
honey	1 Tbsp.		43	0	0

Food	Portion	Approx. Equivalent	Calories	Fat Calories (%)	Choles- terol (mg)
icing, chocolate	1 oz.		106	34	5
icing, white	1 oz.		106	17	6
lemon juice	1 Tbsp.		4	0	0
marshmallow creme	1 oz.		90	0	0
molasses	2 Tbsp.		66	0	0
pasta, spaghetti	2 oz.		84	5	0
peanut butter	1 Tbsp.		84	75	0
sugar, granulated	2 oz.	1/4 cup	190	0	0
syrup, corn	2 Tbsp.		82	0	0
vinegar	1 Tbsp.		2	0	0

Food	Portion	Approx. Equivalent	Calories	Fat Calories (%)	Choles- terol (mg)
Dairy					
butter	1 Tbsp.	1/2 oz.	100	103	31
buttermilk, cultured	8 oz.	1 cup	99	20	9
cheese, American processed	1 oz.	1 slice	106	76	27
cheese, Brie	1 oz.	1 slice	95	76	28
cheese, cheddar	1 oz.	1 slice	114	71	30
cheese, colby	1 oz.	1 slice	112	72	27
cheese, cream	1 oz.	2 Tbsp.	99	91	31
cheese, edam	1 oz.		101	71	25
cheese, feta	1 oz.		75	72	25
cheese, gouda	1 oz.		101	71	32
cheese, Monterey Jack	1 oz.	1 slice	105	73	25

Food	Portion	Approx. Equivalent	Calories	Fat Calories (%)	Cholesterol (mg)
cheese, mozzarella	1 oz.		80	68	22
cheese, mozzarella, part skim	1 oz.		79	57	16
cheese, mozzarella, skim	1 oz.		72	63	15
cheese, Neufchatel	1 oz.		74	85	22
cheese, Parmesan grated	1 Tbsp.		26	69	4
cheese, pimento	1 oz.		106	76	27
cheese, provolone	1 oz.		99	73	20
cheese, ricotta	4 oz.	1/4 lb.	196	73	252
cheese, ricotta (part skim)	4 oz.	1/4 lb.	156	46	152
cheese, Swiss	1 oz.	1 slice	106	68	26
cottage cheese, 1% low-fat	4 oz.	1/2 cup	82	11	5
cottage cheese, 2% low-fat	4 oz.	1/2 cup	102	18	10

Food	Portion	Approx. Equivalent	Calories	Fat Calories (%)	Choles- terol (mg)
cottage cheese, creamed	4 oz.	1/2 cup	117	38	16
cream, 25% fat	1 Tbsp.		35	103	13
cream, half and half	1 Tbsp.		18	100	6
cream, light	1 Tbsp.		28	96	10
cream, whipping, heavy	1 Tbsp.		49	92	21
cream, whipping, light	1 Tbsp.		41	88	17
egg whites	1 med.		14	0	0
egg yolk	1 med.		52	87	272
eggnog	6 oz.		230	50	112
eggs, fried	2 oz.	1 egg	90	70	246
eggs, poached	2 oz.	1 egg	89	61	273
eggs, scrambled	2 oz.	1 egg	108	67	248

Food	Portion	Approx. Equivalent	Calories	Fat Calories (%)	Cholesterol (mg)
hot cocoa	6 oz.		148	37	25
ice cream, vanilla, 10% fat	5 oz.	1 cup	269	47	59
ice milk, hard vanilla	5 oz.	1 cup	182	30	18
margarine, hard	1/2 oz.	1 Tbsp.	100	102	0
milk shake, chocolate (whole milk)	8 oz.	1 cup	230	35	35
milk shake, vanilla (whole milk)	8 oz.	1 cup	230	35	35
milk, chocolate, whole	8 oz.	1 cup	208	37	30
milk, evaporated skim	6 oz.	2/3 cup	150	4	6
milk, evaporated whole	6 oz.	2/3 cup	252	51	54
milk, low-fat (1%)	8 oz.	1 cup	102	23	10
milk, skim	8 oz.	1 cup	86	4	4
milk, sweetened condensed	4 oz.	1/2 cup	492	24	52

Food	Portion	Approx. Equivalent	Calories	Fat Calories (%)	Choles- terol (mg)
sherbert, orange	5 oz.	1 cup	193	13	10
sour cream	8 oz.	1 cup	485	89	80
sour cream, imitation	8 oz.	1 cup	471	84	0
yogurt, frozen	7 oz.	regular size	175	9	12
yogurt, frozen, nonfat	7 oz.	regular size	158	0	0
yogurt, low-fat fruit	8 oz.	small carton	236	14	9
yogurt, plain	8 oz.	small carton	140	26	15
Desserts					
brownies with nuts	1 oz.	1 serving	96	56	16
cake, angel food	2 oz.	1 serving	152	0	0
cake, carrot	4 oz.	1 serving	455	47	87
cake, cheese	4 oz.	1 serving	342	58	210

Food	Portion	Approx. Equivalent	Calories	Fat Calories (%)	Choles-terol (mg)
cake, chocolate	3 oz.	1 serving	311	43	49
cake, chocolate with chocolate icing	4 oz.	1 serving	407	40	75
cake, coffee	3 oz.	1 serving	273	26	53
cake, fruit	3 oz.	1 serving	320	37	22
cake, pound	3 oz.	1 serving	349	36	161
cake, yellow with chocolate icing	4 oz.	1 serving	413	33	50
chocolate syrup, fudge type	1 Tbsp.		47	38	0
cookie, butter	1 item		23	333	0
cookie, chocolate chip	1 item		50	40	0
cookie, gingersnap	1 item		36	25	3
cookie, oatmeal raisin	1 item		59	31	0
cookie, peanut butter	1 item		50	47	0

Food	Portion	Approx. Equivalent	Calories	Fat Calories (%)	Choles- terol (mg)
cookie, sandwich type	1 item		70	39	6
cookie, shortbread	1 item		42	43	3
cookie, sugar wafer	1 item		41	44	3
cookie, vanilla wafer	1 item		13	0	1
cookies, fig bar	1 item		51	18	6
eclair	4 oz.	1 pastry	237	49	135
gelatin dessert	4 oz.	1 serving	67	0	0
graham crackers, chocolate coated	2 sq.		67	40	0
lime ice	8 oz.		247	0	0
pie, apple	4 oz.	1 serving	290	40	0
pie, chocolate meringue	4 oz.	1 serving	285	44	70
pie, coconut custard	4 oz.	1 serving	266	47	116

Food	Portion	Approx. Equivalent	Calories	Fat Calories (%)	Choles-terol (mg)
pie, custard	4 oz.	1 serving	247	47	122
pie, lemon meringue	4 oz.	1 serving	289	37	113
pie, pecan	4 oz.	1 serving	473	49	71
pie, pumpkin	4 oz.	1 serving	239	49	69
pie, sweet potato	4 oz.	1 serving	241	49	61
pudding, bread with raisins	1 oz.	1 serving	53	34	19
pudding, chocolate	4 oz.	1 serving	168	27	12
pudding, rice	4 oz.	1 serving	175	21	17
pudding, tapioca	1 oz.	1 serving	28	34	4
Fish					
anchovy	4 oz.		199	54	62
bass, fried	3 1/2 oz.		194	39	63

Food	Portion	Approx. Equivalent	Calories	Fat Calories (%)	Choles- terol (mg)
bluefish	3 1/2 oz.		123	31	58
bluefish, baked or broiled	3 1/2 oz.		158	30	0
cod, broiled	3 1/2 oz.		104	8	55
crab, steamed	8 oz		211	17	227
fish cakes, fried	8 oz.		390	42	95
flounder, baked	8 oz.		458	37	204
haddock, fried	8 oz.		374	34	145
herring, smoked	4 oz.		239	56	123
mackerel, broiled	8 oz.		593	61	170
ocean perch, fried	8 oz.		514	53	131
oysters, fried	8 oz.		541	52	102
oysters, raw	2 oz.		40	45	32

Food	Portion	Approx. Equivalent	Calories	Fat Calories (%)	Choles- terol (mg)
salmon, broiled or baked	8 oz.		412	37	106
sardines, canned in oil	4 oz.		236	50	161
scallops, steamed	8 oz.		254	11	120
shrimp cocktail	4 oz.		108	8	59
shrimp, fried	8 oz.		510	42	340
sturgeon, steamed	8 oz.		306	35	174
swordfish, broiled	8 oz.		351	31	113
trout	8 oz.		267	27	129
Fruits					
applesauce, sweetened	4 oz.		86	0	0
apricots	1 oz.		18	0	0
avocado	10 oz.		456	85	0

Food	Portion	Approx. Equivalent	Calories	Fat Calories (%)	Cholesterol (mg)
banana	4 oz.	1 medium	104	6	0
blackberries	5 oz.		74	12	0
blueberries	5 oz.		79	11	0
cantaloupe	1/4 melon		92	7	0
cherries	1 cup	4 ounces	57	0	0
coconut	1 oz.		100	81	0
cranberries	1 cup	3 ounces	42	0	0
dates	1 date		23	0	0
dried fruit	1 oz.		69	0	0
fig	1 item	2 ounces	42	0	0
grapes	5 oz.		89	0	0
honeydew melon	1/4 melon		208	2	0

Food	Portion	Approx. Equivalent	Calories	Calories from Fat (%)	Cholesterol (mg)
kiwifruit	1 item	3 ounces	52	0	0
kumquat	1 oz.		12	0	0
mango	7 1/2 oz.	1 1/4 cup	138	5	0
maraschino cherries	1 oz.		33	0	0
nectarine	5 oz.		69	13	0
orange	7 oz.		93	0	0
papayas	16 oz.		177	0	0
peaches	5 oz.		61	0	0
persimmon	1 oz.		36	0	0
pineapple	4 oz.	1 cup	55	0	0
plums	3 oz.		47	19	0
raisins	5 oz.	1 cup	425	2	0

Food	Portion	Approx. Equivalent	Calories	Fat Calories (%)	Choles- terol (mg)
raspberries	5 oz.		69	13	0
strawberries	8 oz.	1 cup	64	0	0
watermelon	8 oz.		72	0	0
Main Dishes and Side Dishes					
bean burrito	4 oz.	1 serving	213	25	8
beef and bean burrito	4 oz.	1 serving	238	38	35
beef enchiladas	8 oz.		713	38	82
beef potpie	8 oz.		435	46	41
beef ravioli	8 oz.		233	35	20
beef stroganoff	8 oz.		408	51	80
beef teriyaki	8 oz.		598	62	142
cannelloni (tomato sauce/cheese)	8 oz.	1 serving	236	31	7

Food	Portion	Approx. Equivalent	Calories	Fat Calories (%)	Choles-terol (mg)
cheese omelet	8 oz.		446	71	744
cheese ravioli	8 oz.		236	31	7
cheese souffle	1 oz.		62	73	52
chicken a la king	8 oz.	1 serving	433	67	172
chicken and rice casserole	8 oz.	1 serving	258	17	47
chicken chow mein	8 oz.		231	35	70
chicken dijon	8 oz.	1 serving	437	41	161
chicken enchiladas	8 oz.		677	32	82
chicken kiev	8 oz.	1 serving	775	60	385
chicken parmesan	8 oz.		464	50	131
chili con carne with beans	8 oz.	1 serving	301	42	39
chili con queso	8 oz.	1 serving	553	72	139

Food	Portion	Approx. Equivalent	Calories	Fat Calories (%)	Choles- terol (mg)
chop suey with meat	8 oz.	1 serving	272	50	91
corned beef hash	4 oz.	1 serving	205	57	37
crab imperial	1 oz.	1 serving	42	43	40
egg rolls	4 oz.	1 serving	220	53	4
fettucini alfredo	8 oz.	1 serving	557	68	137
green bean casserole	4 oz.	1 serving	83	43	0
lasagne	8 oz.	1 serving	408	33	57
linguini with white clam sauce	8 oz.	1 serving	347	29	38
macaroni & cheese	4 oz.	1 serving	243	48	39
manicotti	8 oz.	1 serving	304	36	46
mushroom pizza (19 in.)	5 oz.	1/4 pie	298	30	23
nachos	1 oz.	1 serving	110	57	13

Food	Portion	Approx. Equivalent	Calories	Fat Calories (%)	Choles- terol (mg)
nachos grande	6 oz.	1 serving	401	61	56
pasta salad	4 oz.	1 serving	331	73	20
pasta with carbonara sauce	4 oz.	1 serving	442	49	171
pepperoni pizza (19 in.)	5 oz.	1/4 pie	373	42	35
quesadillas	2 oz.	1 serving	222	41	28
quiche lorraine	4 oz.	1 serving	377	76	187
shrimp creole	8 oz.	1 serving	159	6	187
spaghetti with meat sauce	8 oz.	1 cup	304	33	68
spaghetti with tomato sauce	8 oz.	1 cup	213	18	0
spinach souffle	4 oz.	1 serving	182	74	153
tacos	4 oz.	1 serving	281	58	32
tuna noodle casserole	8 oz.	1 serving	396	41	76

Food	Portion	Approx. Equivalent	Calories	Fat Calories (%)	Cholesterol (mg)
turkey potpie	8 oz.	1 serving	550	51	70
veal parmesan	8 oz.	1 serving	691	66	89
veal scaloppine	8 oz.	1 serving	591	55	207
veal scaloppine (with cheese)	8 oz.	1 serving	632	57	207
western omelet	8 oz.	1 serving	365	67	611
Meat					
bacon	4 oz.		652	77	0
bacon, Canadian	4 oz.		210	43	0
beef, flanksteak	6 oz.		384	49	116
beef, hamburger	4 oz.		328	65	102
beef, lean chuck	6 oz.		364	41	155
beef, lean flanksteak	6 oz.		352	44	114

Food	Portion	Approx. Equivalent	Calories	Fat Calories (%)	Cholesterol (mg)
beef, sirloin steak	6 oz.		457	56	153
beef, T-bone steak	6 oz.		506	64	141
corned beef	3 1/2 oz.		249	70	97
ham, lean	4 oz.		137	35	43
hot dog	2 oz.		145	81	23
lamb, leg (lean)	8 oz.		421	34	0
meatloaf (beef)	4 oz.		303	58	129
meatloaf (pork sausage)	4 oz.		227	59	0
pork centerloin, lean	8 oz.		528	41	224
pork tenderloin, lean	8 oz.		379	26	213
pork, spareribs	8 oz.		907	69	277
salami	4 oz.		283	73	74

Food	Portion	Approx. Equivalent	Calories	Fat Calories (%)	Cholesterol (mg)
sausage, bratwurst	4 oz.		341	77	68
sausage, Italian (pork)	4 oz.		366	71	88
sausage, pepperoni	4 oz.		563	80	89
sausage, Polish (pork)	4 oz.		369	80	79
sausage, pork (brown and serve)	4 oz.		445	83	70
veal, flank	3 1/2 oz.		386	74	100
veal, foreshank	3 1/2 oz.		214	44	100
Nuts and Seeds					
almonds, dry roasted	1 oz.	1/4 cup	166	79	0
black walnuts	2 oz.		344	84	0
brazil nuts	1 oz.		186	91	0
cashews, dry roasted	1 oz.		163	73	0

Food	Portion	Approx. Equivalent	Calories	Fat Calories (%)	Cholesterol (mg)
chestnuts, roasted	1 oz.		69	8	0
English walnuts	1 oz.		182	87	0
macadamia nuts	1 oz.		199	94	0
mixed nuts, dry roasted	1 oz.		168	78	0
peanuts	1 oz.		161	78	0
pecans, dry roasted	1 oz.		187	88	0
pistachio nuts, dry roasted	1 oz.		172	79	0
pumpkin seeds, roasted	2 oz.		296	73	0
sunflower seeds, dry roasted	1 oz.		165	76	0
Oils and Shortenings					
lard	1 Tbsp.		128	98	13
margarine, corn oil	4 oz.		814	101	0

Food	Portion	Approx. Equivalent	Calories	Fat Calories	Calories (%)	Choles- terol (mg)
margarine, corn oil (soft)	1 Tbsp.		101	98		0
margarine, imitation	1 Tbsp.		49	92		0
mayonnaise	1 Tbsp.		102	97		8
mayonnaise, imitation	1 Tbsp.		68	93		0
shortening	2 oz.	1/4 cup	501	102		0
vegetable oil	2 oz.		501	102		0
Poultry						
chicken breast, skinless, roasted	3.5 oz.	1 serving	163	19		84
chicken breast, with skin, fried	3.5 oz.	1 serving	258	45		84
chicken breast, with skin, roasted	3.5 oz.	1 serving	195	38		83
chicken leg, skinless, roasted	3.5 oz.	1 serving	189	42		93
chicken leg, with skin, fried	3.5 oz.	1 serving	270	52		89

Food	Portion	Approx. Equivalent	Calories	Fat Calories (%)	Cholesterol (mg)
chicken leg, with skin, roasted	3.5 oz.	1 serving	230	51	91
duck meat, with skin, roasted	3.5 oz.	1 serving	334	75	83
duck, skinless, roasted	3.5 oz.	1 serving	199	49	88
frankfurter, turkey	2 oz.	1 serving	102	71	48
turkey breast, with skin, roasted	8 oz.		428	36	168
turkey leg, with skin, roasted	8 oz.		471	42	193
turkey, fresh ground	4 oz.		159	45	68
Sauces and Dips					
chip dip, sour cream & onion	2 oz.		120	75	20
clam sauce, red	8 oz.		79	11	16
clam sauce, white	8 oz.		369	66	103
gravy, au jus	2 oz.		10	0	0

Food	Portion	Approx. Equivalent	Calories	Fat Calories (%)	Choles-terol (mg)
gravy, beef	2 oz.		25	36	2
gravy, mushroom	2 oz.		21	39	0
gravy, turkey	2 oz.		26	42	2
tomato sauce	8 oz.		68	0	0
white sauce	8 oz.		367	69	93
Snacks					
cheese puffs	1 oz.		160	62	1
chips, corn	1 oz.		153	52	0
chips, potato	1 oz.		148	61	0
chips, tortilla	1 oz.		150	48	0
corn chips	1 oz.		153	52	0
cracker, butter	1 item		18	51	0

Food	Portion	Approx. Equivalent	Calories	Fat Calories (%)	Choles- terol (mg)
crackers, saltines	2 items		26	21	0
crackers, wheat thin	8 items		70	39	0
crackers, whole wheat	5 items		70	39	0
graham crackers, plain	2 sq.		60	23	0
popcorn with vegetable oil & salt	3 cups		123	44	0
popcorn, popped, plain	3 cups		69	12	0
popcorn, sugar coated	1 cup		134	8	0
potato skins w/cheese & bacon	4 oz.		335	43	41
potato sticks	1 oz.		148	61	0
pretzels	1 oz.		110	8	0
Vegetables					
alfalfa	1 oz.		8	0	0

Food	Portion	Approx. Equivalent	Calories	Fat Calories (%)	Cholesterol (mg)
artichokes	4 oz.		58	0	0
asparagus	4 oz.		25	0	0
bamboo shoots	1 oz.		8	0	0
beans, baked	4 oz.		138	20	5
beans, green	4 oz.		35	0	0
beans, lima	4 oz.		128	7	0
beans, pinto	1 oz.		99	0	0
beets	1 oz.		12	0	0
broccoli	4 oz.		32	0	0
brussels sprouts	4 oz.		49	0	0
cabbage	1 oz.		7	0	0
carrots	1 oz.	1/4 cup	12	0	0

Food	Portion	Approx. Equivalent	Calories	Fat Calories (%)	Choles- terol (mg)
cauliflower	4 oz.		27	0	0
celery	1 oz.		5	0	0
chives	1 oz.		7	0	0
coleslaw	4 oz.		78	35	9
collards	1 oz.		5	0	0
corn on the cob	5 oz.	1 ear	122	15	0
cucumber	1 oz.		4	0	0
eggplant	1 oz.		7	0	0
garden salad (no dressing)	6 oz.		26	0	0
greens, turnip	1 oz.		8	0	0
kale	1 oz.		14	0	0
lentils	1 oz.		30	0	0

Food	Portion	Approx. Equivalent	Calories	Fat Calories (%)	Choles- terol (mg)
lettuce, iceberg	1 oz.	1/4 cup	4	0	0
lettuce, romain	1 oz.	1/4 cup	5	0	0
mushrooms	1 oz.		7	0	0
okra	1 oz.		11	0	0
olives, green	1 cup	5 oz.	164	99	0
olives, ripe	1 cup	5 oz	260	97	0
onion rings	4 oz.		292	49	0
onions	1 oz.	3 Tbsp.	10	0	0
parsnips	1 oz.		21	0	0
pea pods	1 oz.		12	0	0
peas, chick	1 oz.		102	9	0
peas, green	4 oz.		92	0	0

Food	Portion	Approx. Equivalent	Calories	Fat Calories (%)	Choles- terol (mg)
peppers, chili, hot	1 oz.		11	0	0
peppers, green (bell peppers)	2 Tbsp.		3	0	0
peppers, jalapeno	0.5 cup		17	21	0
potato puffs	4 oz.		251	43	0
potatoes, au gratin	4 oz.		149	54	26
potatoes, boiled	4 oz.		99	0	0
potatoes, French fried	4 oz.		357	48	0
potatoes, mashed	4 oz.		120	38	2
potatoes, sweet	1 oz.		30	0	0
radishes	1 oz.		5	0	0
rice, brown	4 oz.		135	7	0
rice, Chinese fried	8 oz.		299	33	114

Food	Portion	Approx. Equivalent	Calories	Fat Calories (%)	Choles- terol (mg)
rice, Spanish	4 oz.		99	18	0
rice, white	4 oz		123	0	0
rutabagas	1 oz.		10	0	0
soybeans	1 oz.		42	43	0
spinach	4 oz.		25	0	0
squash, butternut	4 oz.		51	0	0
squash, summer	4 oz.		23	0	0
squash, zucchini	4 oz.		16	0	0
succotash	4 oz.		112	8	0
tomato	1 med.	5 oz.	27	0	0
turnips	1 oz.		8	0	0
yams	1 oz.		33	0	0

28 ‖ Fat Calculator

The new food labels are perfect for men and active women on a 2,000-calorie-a-day diet. The Percent Daily Value for Total Fat tells you what percentage of fat one serving of the food contributes to your daily allowance, *if* you can eat 2,000 calories a day and *if* you are trying to get only 30 percent of your calories from fat.

What if you are only allowed 1,500 calories a day? And what if you want to get less than 20 percent of your calories from fat? You now need a math formula and a calculator.

The following chart does the figuring for you. If you are trying to eat only foods with less than 20 percent calories from fat, go to that column. Suppose one serving of your food has 100 calories. According to the chart, it must have 2.2 grams of fat per serving or less to qualify as an "under-20-percent-fat" food.

How to Select Foods with 10% Fat

Calories	Fat Grams	Calories	Fat Grams	Calories	Fat Grams	Calories	Fat Grams
5	0.1	150	1.7	295	3.3	440	4.9
10	0.1	155	1.7	300	3.3	445	4.9
15	0.2	160	1.8	305	3.4	450	5.0
20	0.2	165	1.8	310	3.4	455	5.1
25	0.3	170	1.9	315	3.5	460	5.1
30	0.3	175	1.9	320	3.6	465	5.2
35	0.4	180	2.0	325	3.6	470	5.2
40	0.4	185	2.1	330	3.7	475	5.3
45	0.5	190	2.1	335	3.7	480	5.3
50	0.6	195	2.2	340	3.8	485	5.4
55	0.6	200	2.2	345	3.8	490	5.4
60	0.7	205	2.3	350	3.9	495	5.5
65	0.7	210	2.3	355	3.9	500	5.6
70	0.8	215	2.4	360	4.0	505	5.6
75	0.8	220	2.4	365	4.1	510	5.7
80	0.9	225	2.5	370	4.1	515	5.7
85	0.9	230	2.6	375	4.2	520	5.8
90	1.0	235	2.6	380	4.2	525	5.8
95	1.1	240	2.7	385	4.3	530	5.9
100	1.1	245	2.7	390	4.3	535	5.9
105	1.2	250	2.8	395	4.4	540	6.0
110	1.2	255	2.8	400	4.4	545	6.1
115	1.3	260	2.9	405	4.5	550	6.1
120	1.3	265	2.9	410	4.6	555	6.2
125	1.4	270	3.0	415	4.6	560	6.2
130	1.4	275	3.1	420	4.7	565	6.3
135	1.5	280	3.1	425	4.7	570	6.3
140	1.6	285	3.2	430	4.8	575	6.4
145	1.6	290	3.2	435	4.8	580	6.4

How to Select Foods with 20% Fat

Calories	Fat Grams	Calories	Fat Grams	Calories	Fat Grams	Calories	Fat Grams
5	0.1	150	3.3	295	6.6	440	9.8
10	0.2	155	3.4	300	6.7	445	9.9
15	0.3	160	3.6	305	6.8	450	10.0
20	0.4	165	3.7	310	6.9	455	10.1
25	0.6	170	3.8	315	7.0	460	10.2
30	0.7	175	3.9	320	7.1	465	10.3
35	0.8	180	4.0	325	7.2	470	10.4
40	0.9	185	4.1	330	7.3	475	10.6
45	1.0	190	4.2	335	7.4	480	10.7
50	1.1	195	4.3	340	7.6	485	10.8
55	1.2	200	4.4	345	7.7	490	10.9
60	1.3	205	4.6	350	7.8	495	11.0
65	1.4	210	4.7	355	7.9	500	11.1
70	1.6	215	4.8	360	8.0	505	11.2
75	1.7	220	4.9	365	8.1	510	11.3
80	1.8	225	5.0	370	8.2	515	11.4
85	1.9	230	5.1	375	8.3	520	11.6
90	2.0	235	5.2	380	8.4	525	11.7
95	2.1	240	5.3	385	8.6	530	11.8
100	2.2	245	5.4	390	8.7	535	11.9
105	2.3	250	5.6	395	8.8	540	12.0
110	2.4	255	5.7	400	8.9	545	12.1
115	2.6	260	5.8	405	9.0	550	12.2
120	2.7	265	5.9	410	9.1	555	12.3
125	2.8	270	6.0	415	9.2	560	12.4
130	2.9	275	6.1	420	9.3	565	12.6
135	3.0	280	6.2	425	9.4	570	12.7
140	3.1	285	6.3	430	9.6	575	12.8
145	3.2	290	6.4	435	9.7	580	12.9

How to Select Foods with 30% Fat

Calories	Fat Grams	Calories	Fat Grams	Calories	Fat Grams	Calories	Fat Grams
5	0.2	150	5.0	295	9.8	440	14.7
10	0.3	155	5.2	300	10.0	445	14.8
15	0.5	160	5.3	305	10.2	450	15.0
20	0.7	165	5.5	310	10.3	455	15.2
25	0.8	170	5.7	315	10.5	460	15.3
30	1.0	175	5.8	320	10.7	465	15.5
35	1.2	180	6.0	325	10.8	470	15.7
40	1.3	185	6.2	330	11.0	475	15.8
45	1.5	190	6.3	335	11.2	480	16.0
50	1.7	195	6.5	340	11.3	485	16.2
55	1.8	200	6.7	345	11.5	490	16.3
60	2.0	205	6.8	350	11.7	495	16.5
65	2.2	210	7.0	355	11.8	500	16.7
70	2.3	215	7.2	360	12.0	505	16.8
75	2.5	220	7.3	365	12.2	510	17.0
80	2.7	225	7.5	370	12.3	515	17.2
85	2.8	230	7.7	375	12.5	520	17.3
90	3.0	235	7.8	380	12.7	525	17.5
95	3.2	240	8.0	385	12.8	530	17.7
100	3.3	245	8.2	390	13.0	535	17.8
105	3.5	250	8.3	395	13.2	540	18.0
110	3.7	255	8.5	400	13.3	545	18.2
115	3.8	260	8.7	405	13.5	550	18.3
120	4.0	265	8.8	410	13.7	555	18.5
125	4.2	270	9.0	415	13.8	560	18.7
130	4.3	275	9.2	420	14.0	565	18.8
135	4.5	280	9.3	425	14.2	570	19.0
140	4.7	285	9.5	430	14.3	575	19.2
145	4.8	290	9.7	435	14.5	580	19.3

29 || Herbs

More and more people are using herbs and herbal remedies these days. Using herbs can make you feel stronger, more energetic and more in control of your own health. And they can be an inexpensive addition to your normal medical treatment.

Of course, herbs can be powerful medicine, too. Some are safe and effective. Some are neither. And some can have serious side effects.

Use the following charts to find some safe, helpful herbs that seem to work to lower blood pressure and cholesterol and relieve stress. If you use caution and stay on the lookout for side effects or allergic reactions, you'll be glad you tapped into some of nature's best healing secrets.

Helpful Herbs

Herb	Source	Part Used
Alfalfa	*Medicago sativa*	leaves and tops
Bran	*Triticum aestivum*	outer seed coat
Chamomiles and Yarrow	*Matricaria recutita* *Chamaemelum nobile* *Achillea millefolium*	flower heads flower heads flowering herb
Evening Primrose	*Oenothera biennis*	seed oil
Garlic and other alliums	*Allium sativum* (garlic) *Allium cepa* (onion) *Allium ampeloprasum* (leek) *Allium ascalonicum* (scallion)	bulbs and occasionally leaves
Ginkgo	*Ginkgo biloba*	leaf extract
Hawthorn	*Crateagus laevigata*	fruits (haws), leaves, flowers
Kelp	*Laminaria, Macrocystis, Nereocystis* and *Fucus*	entire plant
Suma	*Hebanthe paniculata*	root

Remember, high blood pressure is a serious condition. Do not self-medicate with herbs without consulting your doctor.

Use	Considered Effective*	Considered Safe*
Lowers cholesterol	No	Yes
Increases dietary fiber	Yes	Yes
Cure-all, aids digestion, inflammation, infections, minor illnesses	Yes	Yes
Lowers blood pressure	Maybe (unproven)	Maybe (not tested for long-term use)
Improves atherosclerosis, lowers high blood pressure, lowers cholesterol	Yes	Yes
Dilates blood vessels, improves blood flow	Yes	Yes
Dilates blood vessels, strengthens heart, improves high blood pressure	Yes	Yes
Controls obesity, atherosclerosis	No (Does work well as a laxative, however)	Maybe
Cure-all	No	Maybe

*by herbal expert Varro E. Tyler, PhD

Safe Stress Relievers

Herb	Source	Part Used
Catnip	*Nepeta cataria*	leaves and tops
Chicory	*Cichorium intybus*	root
Ginseng and related herbs	*Panax ginseng* (Oriental ginseng) *Panax quinquefolius* (American ginseng) *Panax pseudo-ginseng* (San qui ginseng) *Eleutherococcus senticosus* (Eleuthero)	roots
Honey	*Apis mellifera*	saccharine secretion
Passion Flower	*Passiflora incarnata*	flowering and fruiting top
Valerian	*Valeriana officinalis*	rhizome and roots

Unsafe Herbs That Reduce Blood Pressure

Herb	Source	Part Used
Mistletoe, European	*Viscum album*	leaves

Remember, high blood pressure is a serious condition.
Do not self-medicate with herbs without consulting your doctor.

Use	Considered Effective*	Considered Safe*
Sleep-aid, aids digestion	Maybe	Yes
Calming, caffeine-free beverage	Yes	Yes
Relieves stress	Maybe	Yes
Sedative, relieves stress	Maybe	Yes
Relieves stress, calming	Yes	Yes
Calms nerves	Yes	Yes

Use	Considered Effective*	Considered Safe*
Reduces blood pressure	Maybe	No (may be slightly poisonous)

*by herbal expert Varro E. Tyler, PhD

Herbs That May Raise Blood Pressure

Herb	Source	Part Used
Caffeine-Containing Plants:		
Coffee	*Coffea arabica*	seeds
Tea	*Camellia sinensis*	leaves and leaf buds
Kola	*Cola nitida*	cotyledons (seed leaves)
Cacao	*Theobroma cacao*	seeds
Guarana	*Paullinia cupana*	seeds
Maté	*Ilex paraguariensis*	leaves
Ephedra (Ma Huang)	*Ephedra*	stems
Licorice	*Glycyrrhiza glabra*	rhizome and roots
Mistletoe, American	*Phoradendron leucarpum*	leaves
Rosemary	*Rosmarinus officinalis*	leaves and/or tops

Remember, high blood pressure is a serious condition. Do not self-medicate with herbs without consulting your doctor.

Use	Considered Effective*	Considered Safe*
Stimulant	Yes	Maybe, in moderate amounts for people with normal blood pressure
Antiasthmatic, nasal decongestant	Yes	Maybe, for people with normal blood pressure No, for people with high blood pressure
Treats coughs and colds	Maybe	Maybe, in moderate amounts for people with normal blood pressure No, for people with high blood pressure
Increases blood pressure	Maybe	No
Stimulant, increases blood pressure	Yes	No

*by herbal expert Varro E. Tyler, PhD

Diuretic Herbs

Many herbal remedy books recommend herbs with diuretic properties to help lower your blood pressure. However, herbal diuretics don't have the same effects on your body that the manufactured diuretics have.

Just like diuretic drugs, they increase blood flow in your kidneys and cause you to urinate more. But unlike diuretic drugs, they don't help your body get rid of sodium and chloride along with the water. They are more properly called

Herb	Source	Part Used
Borage	*Borago officinalis*	leaves and tops
Buchu	*Barosma*	leaves
Hibiscus	*Hibiscus sabdariffa*	flowers
Horsetail	*Equisetum arvense*	overground plant
Juniper	*Juniperus communis*	fruits (berries)
Lovage Root	*Levisticum officinale*	rhizome and roots
Mormon Tea	*Ephedra nevadensis*	stems
Parsley	*Petroselinum crispum*	leaves, seeds and stems
Sarsaparilla	*Smilax*	roots
Saw Palmetto	*Serenoa repens*	ripe fruits

Remember, high blood pressure is a serious condition. Do not self-medicate with herbs without consulting your doctor.

"aquaretics" instead of diuretics. As herbal expert Dr. Varro E. Tyler writes, "This means that the herbal aquaretics are not suited for the treatment of edema and especially not for hypertension."

The herbs are still useful in helping prevent bladder infections and kidney stones. Urinating more can help you avoid these problems. Some of the herbs are useful in other ways as well. The following chart lists the diuretic herbs you may see advertised as blood-pressure reducers.

Use	Considered Effective*	Considered Safe*
Diuretic, astringent (for diarrhea)	Yes	Maybe
Diuretic, urinary antiseptic	Yes	Yes
Diuretic, laxative	Yes	Yes
Diuretic and astringent in kidney and bladder ailments	Maybe	Yes
Diuretic	Yes	Probably
Diuretic, helps digestion	Yes	Yes
Diuretic, treats diarrhea	Yes	Yes
Diuretic, helps digestion	Yes	Yes
Diuretic, flavoring	Yes	Yes
Diuretic, treats prostatic hypertrophy	Yes	Yes

*by herbal expert Varro E. Tyler, PhD

Growing an Herb Garden

Herb	Site	Soil	Propagating
Chamomile	Full sun.	Light and well-drained.	Sow in spring. These are perennials. Divide in spring or autumn. Take 3-inch cuttings from side shoots in summer.
Chicory	Sunny and open.	Light, preferably alkaline. Dig deeply for good roots.	Sow in early summer.
Catnip	Sun or light shade.	Well-drained.	Sow or divide whole plant in spring. Take softwood cuttings in late spring.
Garlic	Sun or partial shade.	Rich, moist and well-drained. Tolerates poorer soil.	Take offsets or divide bulb in autumn or spring. Plant garlic cloves 1 1/2 inches deep. Sow seed in spring.
Ginseng	Shade.	Cool, humus-rich soil.	Sow seed in early spring in a heated greenhouse.
Valerian	Full sun or light shade. Ideally prefers cool roots and warm foliage.	Rich, moist loam.	Sow in spring, pressing seed into soil. But don't cover. Divide roots in spring or autumn.

Remember, high blood pressure is a serious condition.

Growing	Harvesting	Preserving
Plant 4 to 6 inches apart. For *M. recutita*, plant 9 inches apart. For *A. tinctoria*, plant 18 inches apart.	Gather leaves at any time. Pick flowers when they are fully opened.	Dry the leaves and flowers.
Thin or transplant to 18 inches apart.	Gather leaves when young. Dig up roots in first autumn.	Dry the leaves and root.
Thin or transplant to 12 inches apart. Cut back in autumn. A bruised leaf or root will need protection because it will attract cats.	Gather young and flowering tops.	Dry whole plant.
Transplant or thin to 6 inches apart. Water in dry spells and enrich soil annually. Remove flowers for better flavor. Divide and replant clumps every three to four years. For indoor supply, pot in autumn.	Dig bulbs in late summer.	Make garlic oil and garlic vinegar.
Transplant outside.	Harvest after three to nine years.	Dry the root.
Transplant or thin to two feet apart. Can be grown indoors.	Dig complete root in second season in late autumn. Remove pale, fibrous roots, leaving edible rhizome.	Slice rhizome to dry.

Do not self-medicate with herbs without consulting your doctor.

Making an Herb Tea

You can buy an herbal tea in tea bags or in loose form. Tea bags are the easiest method. Loose teas can be made by infusion or decoction.

An infusion is the simplest method. You steep the leaves and flowers in hot water for five to 10 minutes. Decoctions are for hard and woody herbs, and for denser materials like roots and barks. You let them come to a rolling boil for 15 or 20 minutes.

Making an Infusion

- ❑ Use either fresh or dried herbs. Fresh herbs contain more water, so three parts fresh herb replace one part of the dried herb.
- ❑ Place one teaspoon of the dried herb or three teaspoons of fresh herb for each cup of tea into the teapot.
- ❑ Add boiling water. Cover. Let steep about five minutes, or leave overnight.
- ❑ Sweeten to taste. You can use honey or raw brown sugar.
- ❑ Infusions work best for leaves, flowers and green stems. To infuse bark, root, seeds or resin, you'll need to powder them before adding them to the water.
- ❑ Remember to use a teapot with a well-fitting lid so you won't lose any of the volatile oils through evaporation.

Making a Decoction

- ❑ Put one teaspoon of the dried herb or three teaspoons of fresh herb for each cup of water into a pot. Powder or cut herbs into small pieces. Add desired amount of water.
- ❑ Bring to a boil. Simmer for 15 minutes, or until one

quarter of original volume.
- ❑ Turn off heat and steep with the lid on for three minutes, or until cool.
- ❑ Sweeten to taste. You can use honey or raw brown sugar.
- ❑ Will keep fresh in refrigerator for up to three days.

How to Learn More About Herbs

Herbs and herbal remedies are becoming more and more popular these days. They can be an effective, inexpensive addition to your regular medical treatment. If you want more information on herbal medicine and high blood pressure, try contacting these groups:

American Association of Acupuncture and
    Oriental Medicine
4101 Lake Boone Trail, Suite 201
Raleigh, North Carolina 27607
(919) 787-5181

American Association of Naturopathic Physicians
2366 Eastlake Avenue, Suite 322
Seattle, Washington 98102
(206) 323-7610

American Botanical Council
P.O. Box 201660
Austin, Texas 78720
(512) 331-8868

Herb Research Foundation
1007 Pearl Street, Suite 200
Boulder, Colorado 80302
(303) 449-2265

The American Herbalists Guild
P.O. Box 1683
Sequel, California 95073

Alternative Medical Association
7909 SE. Stark Street
Portland, Oregon 97215
(503) 254-7555

30 || Calories Burned Per Minute

Many charts that list calories burned during exercise don't take your weight into account. That means they aren't very accurate. A 180-pound man can burn twice as many calories doing the same exercise as a 100-pound woman.

To use our chart, simply find your weight and your favorite exercise, then multiply by the number of minutes you work out. That will give you how many calories you burn during exercise.

If the number of calories you burn seems low, don't be discouraged. The chart doesn't take into account the extra calories you burn for hours after exercise and the extra calories your lean muscles use when you are just sitting around.

Exercise Activity	Calories Burned Per Minute Of Exercise							
Your weight in lbs. ➡	100	110	120	130	140	150	160	170
Aerobics, low impact	5	6	6	7	7	8	8	9
Aerobics, high impact	11	12	13	14	15	16	17	18
Bicycling, 6 mph	3	3	3	4	4	4	5	5
Bicycling, 12 mph	5	6	6	7	7	8	8	9
Bowling	2	2	3	3	3	3	3	4
Calisthenics, light	3	3	3	3	4	4	4	4
Stair climbing, machine	8	9	10	11	12	13	13	14
Stair climbing, 100 p/min.	11	12	13	14	15	16	17	18
Crosscountry skiing	11	12	13	14	15	16	17	18
Golf, riding cart	2	2	2	2	3	3	3	3
Golf, walking	3	3	3	3	4	4	4	4
Racketball, light intensity	5	6	6	7	7	8	8	9
Racketball, competitive	11	12	13	14	15	16	17	18
Rowing, light intensity	3	3	3	3	4	4	4	4
Rowing, 18 strokes p/min.	5	6	6	7	7	8	8	9
Rowing, 30 strokes p/min.	11	12	13	14	15	16	17	18
Rowing machine	6	7	7	8	8	9	10	10
Running, 6-7 mph	5	6	6	7	7	8	8	9
Running, 8-10 mph	11	12	13	14	15	16	17	18
Skating, 5 mph	3	3	3	3	4	4	4	4
Skating, 10 mph	5	6	6	7	7	8	8	9
Skiing, water or downhill	5	6	6	7	7	8	8	9
Skiing, ski machine	7	7	8	9	9	10	11	11
Swimming, slow	6	6	7	8	8	9	9	10
Swimming, fast	7	8	9	9	10	11	11	12
Tennis, doubles	3	3	3	3	4	4	4	4
Tennis, singles	5	6	6	7	7	8	8	9
Volleyball, light intensity	3	3	3	3	4	4	4	4
Walking, 2 mph	2	2	3	3	3	3	4	4
Walking, 3-4 mph	3	3	3	3	4	4	4	4
Walking, 5 mph	5	6	6	7	7	8	8	9
Weight lifting	5	6	6	7	7	8	8	9

Exercise Activity	Calories Burned Per Minute Of Exercise							
Your weight in lbs. ➡	180	190	200	210	220	230	240	250
Aerobics, low impact	10	10	11	11	12	12	13	13
Aerobics, high impact	19	20	21	22	23	24	25	26
Bicycling, 6 mph	5	6	6	6	6	7	7	7
Bicycling, 12 mph	10	10	11	11	12	12	13	13
Bowling	4	4	4	4	5	5	5	5
Calisthenics, light	5	5	5	6	6	6	6	7
Stair climbing, machine	15	16	17	18	18	19	20	21
Stair climbing, 100 p/min	19	20	21	22	23	24	25	26
Crosscountry skiing	19	20	21	22	23	24	25	26
Golf, riding cart	3	4	4	4	4	4	5	5
Golf, walking	5	5	5	6	6	6	6	7
Racketball, light intensity	10	10	11	11	12	12	13	13
Racketball, competitive	19	20	21	22	23	24	25	26
Rowing, light intensity	5	5	5	6	6	6	6	7
Rowing, 18 strokes p/min.	10	10	11	11	12	12	13	13
Rowing, 30 strokes p/min.	19	20	21	22	23	24	25	26
Rowing machine	11	11	12	13	13	14	14	15
Running, 6-7 mph	10	10	11	11	12	12	13	13
Running, 8-10 mph	19	20	21	22	23	24	25	26
Skating, 5 mph	5	5	5	6	6	6	6	7
Skating, 10 mph	10	10	11	11	12	12	13	13
Skiing, water or downhill	10	10	11	11	12	12	13	13
Skiing, ski machine	12	13	13	14	15	15	16	17
Swimming, slow	10	11	12	12	13	13	14	15
Swimming, fast	13	13	14	15	16	16	17	18
Tennis, doubles	5	5	5	5	6	6	6	6
Tennis, singles	9	10	10	11	11	12	12	13
Volleyball, light intensity	5	5	5	6	6	6	6	7
Walking, 2 mph	4	4	4	5	5	5	5	6
Walking, 3-4 mph	5	5	5	6	6	6	6	7
Walking, 5 mph	10	10	11	11	12	12	13	13
Weight lifting	10	10	11	11	12	12	13	13

31 || Healthy Recipes

Main Dishes

Chili with Beans
(serves 4)

   1/2 lb. lean ground beef
   15 1/2 oz. can kidney beans, drained (save liquid)
   1/3 cup bean liquid
   1 cup no-salt-added canned tomato puree
   1 tablespoon instant minced onion
   1 1/2 tablespoons chili powder

- Lightly brown beef in skillet. Drain fat.
- Stir in remaining ingredients.
- Bring to a boil. Reduce heat, cover and simmer 10 minutes.

> Nutritional information per serving:
> Serving size: 3/4 cup
> Calories: 230
> Total fat: 9 grams
> Saturated fatty acids: 3 grams
> Cholesterol: 34 milligrams
> Sodium: 390 milligrams

No-bake Tamale Pie
(serves 4)

> **1 recipe Chili with Beans**
> **8 oz. can no-salt-added whole-kernel corn, undrained**
> **1/2 cup yellow cornmeal**
> **dash of salt**
> **1 1/4 cups cold water**
> **1/8 teaspoon chili powder**

• Place chili in a 10-inch skillet. Stir in corn. Heat thoroughly.

• As chili heats, mix cornmeal and salt with water in a saucepan. Cook over medium heat, stirring constantly until thickened, about 2 minutes.

• Spread cornmeal mixture over hot chili to form a crust. Sprinkle with chili powder.

• Cover and cook over low heat, with lid slightly open, until topping is set, about 10 minutes.

Nutritional information per serving:
Serving size: 1 cup
Calories: 330
Total fat: 9 grams
Saturated fatty acids: 3 grams
Cholesterol: 34 milligrams
Sodium: 431 milligrams

Chicken — Italian style
(serves 4)

4 chicken breast halves, skinned and boned
1 teaspoon oil
4 oz. thin spaghetti, broken into fourths
1 small onion, cut in wedges
1 small green pepper, cut in strips
1/8 teaspoon instant minced garlic
1 teaspoon oregano leaves
1/8 teaspoon salt
1/8 teaspoon pepper
1 bay leaf
16 oz. can tomatoes
1/4 cup water
1 tablespoon parsley, chopped (optional)

• Pound chicken breasts with a metal meat mallet between sheets of plastic wrap until about 1/2-inch thick.
• Heat oil in skillet. Brown chicken on each side.
• Add spaghetti, onion and green pepper strips around chicken. Sprinkle with seasonings. Break up large pieces of tomatoes. Pour tomatoes and water over top of chicken.
• Bring to a boil. Reduce heat, cover and cook until chicken and spaghetti are done, about 15 minutes.
• Remove bay leaf. Garnish with parsley if desired.

Nutritional information per serving:
Serving size: 1 chicken breast half
    and 3/4 cup spaghetti mixture
Calories: 280
Total fat: 3 grams
Saturated fatty acids: 1 gram
Cholesterol: 68 milligrams
Sodium: 341 milligrams

Fish Fillets with Dill
(serves 4)

> **1 lb. frozen haddock or cod fillets**
> **1 tablespoon lemon juice**
> **1/8 teaspoon dried dill weed**
> **1/8 teaspoon salt**
> **dash of pepper**

• Thaw frozen fish in refrigerator overnight or thaw in microwave oven. Separate into four fillets or pieces.
• Place fish in heated skillet. Sprinkle with lemon juice and seasonings.
• Cover and cook over moderate heat until fish flakes when tested with a fork, about 5 minutes.

Nutritional information per serving:
Serving size: 1 fillet
Calories: 95
Total fat: 1 gram
Saturated fatty acids: Trace
Cholesterol: 55 milligrams
Sodium: 147 milligrams

Mini Meatloaves
(serves 4)

1/3 cup wheat crackers, crushed
1 tablespoon instant minced onion
1/3 cup skim milk
1 egg
1/2 teaspoon basil leaves
1/8 teaspoon salt
3/4 lb. lean ground beef

• Preheat oven to 375°F.
• Soak crackers and onion in milk until soft and milk is absorbed.
• Add egg and seasonings. Mix well.
• Gently mix ground beef with milk mixture.
• Shape into four individual loaves, about 3 1/2 inches by 2 inches by 1 1/4 inches. Place in shallow baking pan.
• Bake 25 minutes or until done. Drain fat.

Nutritional information per serving:
Serving size: 1 loaf
Calories: 230
Total fat: 14 grams
Saturated fatty acids: 6 grams
Cholesterol: 119 milligrams
Sodium: 194 milligrams

Baked Stuffed Peppers
(serves 4)

2 green peppers, halved and seeded
1 recipe Mini Meatloaf mixture
1/4 cup tomato sauce

• Preheat oven to 375°F.
• Cook peppers in boiling water for 2 minutes. Drain well.
• Fill green pepper halves with meat mixture. Place in glass baking dish. Spread one tablespoon tomato sauce over each serving.
• Bake uncovered for 45 minutes or until meat is done.

Nutritional information per serving:
Serving size: 1/2 green pepper
Calories: 245
Total fat: 15 grams
Saturated fatty acids: 6 grams
Cholesterol: 119 milligrams
Sodium: 287 milligrams

Hawaiian Meatballs
(serves 4)

1 recipe Mini Meatloaf mixture
8 oz. can pineapple chunks, juice-pack
1 1/2 teaspoons Worcestershire sauce
1/8 teaspoon garlic powder
dash of pepper
1/2 cup green pepper, cut into 1-inch pieces
1 tablespoon cornstarch
1 tablespoon water

• Shape meat mixture into 12 balls. Brown in hot skillet about 10 minutes. Drain fat.
• Drain pineapple and save juice. Add water to juice to make 3/4 cup liquid. Add liquid and seasonings to meatballs.
• Bring to a boil, reduce heat, cover and cook for 5 minutes.
• Add pineapple chunks and green pepper. Cook 1 minute longer.
• Mix cornstarch and water until smooth. Add to mixture. Cook until thickened, about 2 minutes. Stir as needed.

Nutritional information per serving:
Serving size: 3 meatballs plus
   3/8 cup fruit and sauce
Calories: 275
Total fat: 14 grams
Saturated fatty acids: 6 grams
Cholesterol: 119 milligrams
Sodium: 219 milligrams

London Broil
(serves 4)

1 lb. top round steak
1/4 cup reduced-calorie Italian or French salad
   dressing

• Trim fat from steak and place steak in plastic food storage bag. Add salad dressing. Close bag securely. Turn bag to distribute dressing over entire surface of meat. Place on plate and refrigerate overnight.
• Remove steak from plastic bag. Place on broiler pan.
• Broil about 2 inches from heat, allowing about 7 minutes per side.
• Slice into thin slices, cutting across the grain on the diagonal from top to bottom of the steak.

Nutritional information per serving:
Serving size: about 2 3/4 oz.
Calories: 175
Total fat: 7 grams
Saturated fatty acids: 2 grams
Cholesterol: 68 milligrams
Sodium: 171 milligrams

Stovetop Sweet Potatoes and Pork
(serves 4)

4 (about 1 lb.) thin-cut pork chops
1 cup apple juice
1 medium onion, cut in 1/4-inch slices
1 tablespoon flour
1/8 teaspoon ground allspice
1/8 teaspoon salt
17 oz. can sweet potatoes, vacuum-packed

• Trim fat from chops. Brown on both sides in hot skillet. Add 3/4 cup of the apple juice. Top with onion slices. Cover and cook 5 minutes at reduced heat.
• Mix flour and seasonings. Stir into remaining 1/4 cup apple juice. Stir into liquid in pan.
• Arrange sweet potatoes around and over chops. Spoon sauce over potatoes.
• Cover and cook about 10 minutes longer, until potatoes are hot and chops are done.

Nutritional information per serving:
Serving size: 1 chop and about
    3/4 cup vegetables
Calories: 270
Total fat: 6 grams
Saturated fatty acids: 2 grams
Cholesterol: 45 milligrams
Sodium: 192 milligrams

Chicken and Cabbage Stirfry

(serves 4)

   3 chicken breast halves, skinned and boned
   1 teaspoon oil
   3 cups green cabbage, cut in 1/2-inch slices
   1 tablespoon cornstarch
   1/2 teaspoon ground ginger
   1/4 teaspoon garlic powder
   1/2 cup water
   1 tablespoon soy sauce

• Cut chicken breast halves into strips.

• Heat oil in skillet. Add chicken strips and stirfry over moderately high heat, turning pieces constantly, until lightly browned, about 2 to 3 minutes.

• Add cabbage and stirfry 2 minutes until cabbage is tender-crisp.

• Mix cornstarch and seasonings. Add to water and soy sauce, mixing until smooth. Stir into chicken mixture. Cook until thickened and pieces are coated, about 1 minute.

Nutritional information per serving:
Serving size: 1 cup
Calories: 135
Total fat: 2 grams
Saturated fatty acids: Trace
Cholesterol: 51 milligrams
Sodium: 326 milligrams

Variation

Beef and Cabbage Stirfry

Use 3/4 lb. boneless beef round steak in place of chicken. Trim fat from steak. Slice steak across the grain into thin strips, about 1/8 inch wide and 3 1/2 inches long. (It is easier to slice meat thinly if it is partially frozen.)

Nutritional information per serving:
Serving size: 3/4 cup
Calories: 140
Total fat: 5 grams
Saturated fatty acids: 1 gram
Cholesterol: 44 milligrams
Sodium: 309 milligrams

Pasta Primavera
(serves 6)

1 cup broccoli flowers
1 cup snow peas
1 small zucchini, sliced
1/2 cup mushrooms, sliced
3 small tomatoes cut into wedges
1 lb. box spaghetti or linguini
2 teaspoons olive oil
1 teaspoon margarine
3 cloves garlic, crushed
1/2 cup chicken stock
1/2 cup skim milk
1/2 cup grated parmesan cheese
1 tablespoon cornstarch
1/2 cup water

• Steam broccoli, snow peas, zucchini and mushrooms until tender-crisp. Cook spaghetti or linguini to desired tenderness, drain and keep warm.
• Sauté garlic for about 2 minutes; do not brown. Add the vegetables (except tomatoes) and pasta. Toss together.
• Combine chicken stock, skim milk and parmesan cheese in a small saucepan and simmer gently. Add tomatoes.
• Mix together cornstarch and water; add to sauce.
• Combine pasta, vegetables and sauce and toss.

Nutritional information per serving:
Serving size: 1 cup
Calories: 413
Total fat: 6 grams
Saturated fatty acids: 2 grams
Cholesterol: 6 milligrams
Sodium: 283 milligrams

Meat Sauce
(4 servings)

1/2 lb. lean ground beef
1/3 cup onion, chopped
1/3 cup green pepper, chopped
Half of a 29 oz. can (about 1 3/4 cups) no-salt-added
   tomato puree
1 teaspoon oregano
1/4 teaspoon dried basil leaves
1/4 teaspoon garlic powder or 2 cloves of minced
   fresh garlic
1/2 teaspoon salt
dash of cayenne pepper
1 bay leaf

• Cook beef, onion and green pepper in a saucepan until beef
is lightly browned. Drain fat.
• Mix in remaining ingredients.
• Heat to boiling. Reduce heat, cover and cook slowly until
flavors are blended, about 30 minutes. Stir as needed.
• Remove bay leaf.
• Serve over spaghetti (cooked without salt)

Nutritional information per serving:
Serving size: 1 cup spaghetti with
   2/3 cup sauce
Calories: 315
Total fat: 9 grams
Saturated fatty acids: 3 grams
Cholesterol: 34 milligrams
Sodium: 200 milligrams

Beef and Vegetable Stirfry

12 oz. beef round steak, boneless
1 teaspoon oil
1/2 cup carrots, sliced
1/2 cup celery, sliced
1/2 cup onion, sliced
1 tablespoon soy sauce
1/8 teaspoon garlic powder
dash of pepper
2 cups zucchini squash, cut in thin strips
1 tablespoon cornstarch
1/4 cup water

• Trim all fat from steak. Slice steak across the grain into thin strips about 1/8-inch wide and 3 inches long. (Partially frozen meat is easier to slice.)
• Heat oil in skillet. Add beef strips and stirfry over high heat, turning pieces constantly, until beef is no longer red, about 3 to 5 minutes. Reduce heat.
• Add carrots, celery, onion and seasonings. Cover and cook until carrots are slightly tender, about 3 minutes. Add squash. Cook until vegetables are tender-crisp, about 3 minutes.
• Mix cornstarch and water until smooth. Add slowly to beef mixture, stirring constantly. Cook until thickened and vegetables are coated with a thin glaze.

Nutritional information per serving:
Serving size: 3/4 cup
Calories: 150
Total fat: 5 grams
Saturated fatty acids: 1 gram
Cholesterol: 44 milligrams
Sodium: 317 milligrams

Variation

Chicken and Vegetable Stirfry

Use 3 chicken breast halves without bone or skin (about 12 oz. of raw chicken) instead of beef. Slice into thin strips.

Nutritional information per serving:
Serving size: 3/4 cup
Calories: 140
Total fat: 2 grams
Saturated fatty acids: Trace
Cholesterol: 51 milligrams
Sodium: 335 milligrams

Enchilada Casserole
(serves 4)

Filling
1/2 cup onion, chopped
1/2 cup green pepper, chopped
1/4 cup celery, chopped
1/4 cup water, boiling
1 cup chicken, cooked, diced
1 cup canned pinto beans, drained
1/2 cup no-salt added tomato puree
8 corn tortillas

Sauce
1 1/2 cups no-salt-added tomato puree
3/4 cup water
1 tablespoon chili powder
1/8 teaspoon ground cumin
1/8 teaspoon garlic powder
1/8 teaspoon salt

Topping
1/4 cup Monterey Jack cheese, shredded

• Preheat oven to 350°F.
• Cook onion, green pepper and celery in boiling water until tender. Drain liquid if necessary.
• Add chicken, beans and 1/2 cup of tomato puree. Mix gently.
• Mix all sauce ingredients together thoroughly.
• In an 8-inch square baking ban, place four tortillas, the filling mixture, and one-half of the sauce. Cover with four tortillas and remaining sauce.
• Sprinkle cheese over top.

• Bake until cheese is melted and sauce is bubbly, about 30 minutes.

Nutritional information per serving:
Serving size: 4 by 4 inch piece
Calories: 300
Total fat: 7 grams
Saturated fatty acids: 2 grams
Cholesterol: 35 milligrams
Sodium: 378 milligrams

Eggs Fu-Yung
(serves 4)

Egg mixture
   3 eggs (see Note)
   2 cups bean sprouts, fresh
   2/3 cup chicken or beef, cooked, diced
   2 oz. can mushrooms, stems and pieces, drained
   1 tablespoon instant minced onion
   2 teaspoons oil

Sauce
   2/3 cup water
   2 teaspoons soy sauce
   1 tablespoon cornstarch
• Beat eggs with electric mixer until very thick and light, about 5 minutes.
• Fold in bean sprouts, chicken or beef, mushrooms and onion.
• Heat oil in skillet over moderate heat.
• Pour egg mixture by half-cupfuls into the pan. Brown on one side; turn and brown other side. Keep warm while preparing sauce.
• Mix sauce ingredients in small saucepan until smooth.
• Cook over low heat, stirring constantly, until thickened.
• Serve sauce over patties.
Note: Use only clean eggs with no cracks in the shells.

Nutritional information per serving:
Serving size: 2 patties and
   2 tablespoons sauce
Calories: 155
Total fat: 8 grams
Saturated fatty acids: 2 grams
Cholesterol: 224 milligrams
Sodium: 303 milligrams

Stuffed Baked Potato
(serves 4)

> **4 baking potatoes, about 1/2 lb. each**
> **1/2 cup low-fat cottage cheese**
> **3 tablespoons skim milk**
> **1 teaspoon chives, dried or fresh**
> **1/8 teaspoon pepper**
> **paprika as desired**

- Preheat oven to 425°F.
- Wash and dry potatoes, Prick skins with a fork. Bake potatoes until tender, 50 to 60 minutes. (Potatoes may be baked in a microwave oven. Use the directions that came with your oven.)
- Beat cottage cheese until smooth.
- Slice tops off potatoes. Scoop out insides of potatoes and add to cottage cheese. Add milk and seasonings. Beat until well-blended.
- Stuff potato skins with potato-cheese mixture. Sprinkle with paprika.
- Return potatoes to oven. Bake about 10 minutes or until heated and tops are lightly browned.

Nutritional information per serving:
Serving size: 1 potato each
Calories: 155
Total fat: Trace
Saturated fatty acids: Trace
Cholesterol: 1 milligram
Sodium: 128 milligrams

Broiled Sesame Fish
(serves 4)

1 lb. cod fillets, fresh or frozen
1 teaspoon margarine, melted
1 tablespoon lemon juice
1 teaspoon dried tarragon leaves
1/8 teaspoon salt
dash of pepper
1 tablespoon sesame seeds
1 tablespoon parsley

• Thaw frozen fish in refrigerator overnight or defrost briefly in a microwave oven. Cut fish into 4 portions.
• Place fish on a broiler pan lined with aluminum foil. Brush margarine over fish.
• Mix lemon juice, tarragon leaves, salt and pepper. Pour over fish.
• Sprinkle sesame seeds evenly over fish.
• Broil until fish flakes easily when tested with a fork, about 12 minutes.
• Garnish each serving with parsley.

Nutritional information per serving:
Serving size: 2 1/2 oz.
Calories: 110
Total fat: 3 grams
Saturated fatty acids: Trace
Cholesterol: 46 milligrams
Sodium: 155 milligrams

Pizza

(serves 4)

    1 refrigerated pizza crust, 12-inch diameter
    3/4 cup no-salt-added canned tomato puree
    1 teaspoon oregano
    1/2 teaspoon garlic powder
    1 small onion, sliced
    1/2 small green pepper, thinly sliced
    1 cup mushrooms, fresh, sliced
    1 cup Mozzarella cheese, part-skim-milk, shredded

- Preheat oven to 450°F.
- Place crust on ungreased pizza pan or baking sheet.
- Mix puree, oregano and garlic powder. Spread evenly over crust.
- Place vegetables on top of puree.
- Sprinkle with cheese.
- Bake until cheese melts and vegetables are tender, about 15 minutes.

Nutritional information per serving:
Serving size: 2 pieces
Calories: 275
Total fat: 6 grams
Saturated fatty acids: 3 grams
Cholesterol: 15 milligrams
Sodium: 404 milligrams

Chicken Vegetable Stew
(serves 4)

> **2 chicken breast halves, without skin**
> **1 1/2 cups water**
> **1/4 teaspoon salt**
> **2 whole cloves**
> **1 bay leaf**
> **2/3 cup frozen mixed vegetables**
> **2/3 cup potatoes, pared, diced**
> **1/2 cup onion, chopped**
> **1/4 cup celery, sliced**
> **1 cup tomatoes**
> **1/4 teaspoon ground thyme**
> **1/8 teaspoon pepper**
> **1/4 cup flour**
> **1/4 cup water**

• Cover and cook chicken in water with salt, cloves and bay leaf until tender, about 45 minutes.
• Remove chicken from broth. Separate meat from bones. Dice meat. Skim fat from broth. Discard cloves and bay leaf.
• Add water to make 2 cups. Cook mixed vegetables, potatoes, onion and celery in broth for 10 minutes.
• Break up tomatoes. Add tomatoes, thyme and pepper to broth mixture. Cook slowly for 15 minutes. Add chicken.
• Mix flour and water until smooth. Stir into chicken mixture. Cook, stirring constantly, until thickened, about 1 minute.

Nutritional information per serving:
Serving size: 1 cup
Calories: 175
Total fat: 2 grams
Saturated fatty acids: 1 gram
Cholesterol: 37 milligrams
Sodium: 303 milligrams

Side Dishes

Vegetable Medley
(serves 4)

 2 tablespoons water
 5 cups (1 lb.) mixed vegetables (see Note)
 1/2 teaspoon marjoram leaves
 2 tablespoons reduced-calorie French or Italian
   salad dressing

• Heat water in skillet. Add vegetables. Sprinkle with marjoram.

• Cover and cook 5 minutes or until vegetables are tender-crisp. Drain, if necessary.

• Toss vegetables with salad dressing.

Note: Choose vegetable pieces that are similar in size, such as broccoli and cauliflower florets, carrot slices, green pepper strips, sliced celery, mushrooms, zucchini slices, etc.

Nutritional information per serving:
Serving size: 3/4 cup
Calories: 40
Total fat: 1 gram
Saturated fatty acids: Trace
Cholesterol: Trace
Sodium: 86 milligrams

Herbed Vegetable Combo

2 tablespoons water
1 cup zucchini squash, thinly sliced
1 1/4 cups yellow squash, thinly sliced
1/2 cup green pepper, cut into 2-inch strips
1/4 cup celery, cut into 2-inch strips
1/4 cup onion, chopped
1/2 teaspoon caraway seed
1/8 teaspoon garlic powder
1 medium tomato, cut into 8 wedges

• Heat water in large skillet.
• Add squash, green pepper, celery and onion.
• Cover and cook over moderate heat until vegetables are tender-crisp, about 4 minutes.
• Sprinkle seasonings over vegetables. Top with tomato wedges. Cover and cook over low heat until tomato wedges are just heated, about 2 minutes.

Nutritional information per serving:
Serving size: 3/4 cup
Calories: 25
Total fat: Trace
Saturated fatty acids: Trace
Cholesterol: 0
Sodium: 11 milligrams

Rice and Pasta Pilaf
(serves 4)

1/3 cup uncooked brown rice
1 1/2 cups chicken broth, unsalted
1/3 cup thin spaghetti, broken into 1/2- to 1-inch
  pieces
2 teaspoons margarine
2 tablespoons green onions, chopped
2 tablespoons green pepper, chopped
2 tablespoons fresh mushrooms, chopped
1/2 clove garlic, minced
1/2 teaspoon savory
1/4 teaspoon salt
1/8 teaspoon pepper

• Cook rice in 1 cup of the broth in a covered saucepan until almost tender, about 35 minutes.
• Cook spaghetti in margarine over low heat until golden brown, about 2 minutes. Stir frequently.
• Add browned spaghetti, vegetables, remaining 1/2 cup of chicken broth and seasonings to rice.
• Bring to boil, reduce heat, cover and cook over medium heat until liquid is absorbed, about 10 minutes.
• Remove from heat. Let stand 2 minutes.

Nutritional information per serving:
Serving size: 1/2 cup
Calories: 125
Total fat: 3 grams
Saturated fatty acids: 1 gram
Cholesterol: 0
Sodium: 177 milligrams

Sweet Potato Custard
(serves 6)

> **1 cup mashed cooked sweet potato**
> **1/2 cup mashed banana (about 2 small)**
> **1 cup evaporated skim milk**
> **2 tablespoons packed brown sugar**
> **2 beaten egg yolks (or 1/3 cup egg substitute)**
> **1/2 teaspoon salt**
> **1/4 cup raisins**
> **1 tablespoon sugar**
> **1 teaspoon cinnamon**

- Preheat oven to 300°F.
- In a medium bowl stir together sweet potato and banana.
- Add milk, blending well.
- Add brown sugar, egg yolks and salt, mixing thoroughly.
- Spray a 1-quart casserole with nonstick spray coating.
- Put sweet potato mixture in casserole.
- Combine raisins, sugar and cinnamon. Sprinkle over top of sweet potato mixture
- Bake for about 45 minutes or until a knife inserted near center comes out clean.

Note: If made with egg substitute, the amount of cholesterol will be 2 mg.

Nutritional information per serving:
Serving size: 1/2 cup
Calories: 144
Total fat: 2 grams
Saturated fatty acids: less than 1 gram
Cholesterol: 92 milligrams
Sodium: 235 milligrams

Garlic Mashed Potatoes
(serves 4)

1 lb. potatoes (2 large)
2 cups skim milk
2 large cloves garlic, chopped
1/2 teaspoon white pepper

• Peel potatoes; cut in quarters.
• Cook, covered, in a small amount of boiling water for about 20 minutes or until tender. Remove from heat. Drain. Recover the pot with potatoes.
• In a small saucepan over low heat, cook garlic in milk until garlic is soft, about 30 minutes.
• Add milk-garlic mixture and white pepper to potatoes. Beat with an electric mixer on low speed or mash with a potato masher until smooth.

Nutritional information per serving:
Serving size: 1/2 cup
Calories: 141
Total fat: less than 1 gram
Saturated fatty acids: less than 1 gram
Cholesterol: 2 milligrams
Sodium: 70 milligrams

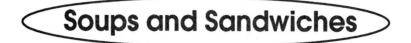

Soups and Sandwiches

Broccoli Soup
(serves 4)

1 1/2 cups broccoli, chopped (see Note)
1/4 cup celery, diced
1/4 cup onion, chopped
1 cup chicken broth, unsalted
2 cups skim milk
2 tablespoons cornstarch
1/4 teaspoon salt
dash of pepper
dash of ground thyme
1/4 cup Swiss cheese, shredded

• Place vegetables and broth in saucepan. Bring to boil, reduce heat, cover and cook until vegetables are tender, about 8 minutes.
• Mix milk, cornstarch, salt, pepper and thyme. Add to cooked vegetables. Cook, stirring constantly, until soup is slightly thickened and mixture just begins to boil.
• Remove from heat. Add cheese and stir until melted.
Note: A 10 oz. package of frozen chopped broccoli can be used instead of fresh broccoli. The soup will have about 120 calories and 260 milligrams of sodium.

Nutritional information per serving:
Serving size: 1 cup
Calories: 110
Total fat: 3 grams
Saturated fatty acids: 2 grams
Cholesterol: 9 milligrams
Sodium: 252 milligrams

Potato-Beef Soup
(serves 4)

1/3 lb. lean ground beef
3 cups water
1 cup onions, sliced
1/2 cup celery, chopped
1/2 teaspoon salt
1/8 teaspoon pepper
1 bay leaf
2 whole cloves
1 1/2 cups potatoes, sliced
1/2 cup carrots, shredded
2 teaspoons parsley, chopped

• Brown beef in hot 2-quart saucepan. Turn carefully as needed to brown on all sides. Keep meat in chunks. Drain fat.

• Add water, onions, celery and seasonings to beef. Bring to boil, reduce heat and cook slowly for 30 minutes.

• Add potatoes, carrots and parsley. Cook until potatoes are tender, about 15 minutes.

• Remove bay leaf and cloves before serving.

Nutritional information per serving:
Serving size: 1 1/4 cups
Calories: 140
Total fat: 5 grams
Saturated fatty acids: 2 grams
Cholesterol: 23 milligrams
Sodium: 334 milligrams

Vegetable Soup
(serves 4)

1 cup potatoes, diced
1 cup cabbage, chopped
1/2 cup onion, chopped
1/2 cup celery, diced
1/2 cup carrots, sliced
1/2 cup frozen green beans
1/4 teaspoon oregano
1/4 teaspoon marjoram
1/4 teaspoon salt
1 bay leaf
dash of pepper
2 cups water
1 cup tomatoes

• Place all ingredients except tomatoes in a saucepan. Cover and boil gently for 10 minutes.
• Break up tomatoes. Add to vegetable mixture and continue cooking until vegetables are tender, about 20 minutes.
• Remove bay leaf before serving.

Nutritional information per serving:
Serving size: 1 cup
Calories: 70
Total fat: Trace
Saturated fatty acids: Trace
Cholesterol: 0
Sodium: 269 milligrams

Vegetable Beef Soup
(serves 4)

   10 1/2 oz. can unsalted chicken broth
   1/2 cup water
   2 cups frozen mixed vegetables for soup
   16 oz. can tomatoes, broken up
   1 cup beef, cooked and diced
   1 teaspoon thyme leaves, crushed
   dash of pepper
   1/4 teaspoon salt
   1 bay leaf
   2 oz. (about 1 1/4 cups) narrow-width noodles, uncooked

• Heat broth and water. Add vegetables, meat and seasonings. Bring to a boil, reduce heat and boil gently, uncovered, for 15 minutes.
• Add noodles. Cook until noodles are tender, about 10 minutes.
• Remove bay leaf.

Nutritional information per serving:
Serving size: 1 cup
Calories: 200
Total fat: 4 grams
Saturated fatty acids: 1 gram
Cholesterol: 42 milligrams
Sodium: 391 milligrams

Beef and Coleslaw Pita
(serves 4)

1 cup lean beef, cooked, cut in thin strips
1 cup coleslaw
1 medium tomato, sliced into 8 slices
2 whole-wheat pita bread loaves

- Drain coleslaw.
- Toss coleslaw with beef strips in a bowl.
- Cut pita bread in halves.
- Place one-fourth of filling in each bread half.
- Top with tomato slices.

Nutritional information per serving:
Serving size: 1 sandwich
Calories: 175
Total fat: 6 grams
Saturated fatty acids: 1 gram
Cholesterol: 25 milligrams
Sodium: 69 milligrams

Tuna and Sprouts Sandwich
(serves 4)

> 2 tablespoons salad dressing, mayonnaise-type
> 1/4 teaspoon celery seed
> 1/4 teaspoon onion powder
> 6 1/2 oz. can tuna, water-packed, unsalted, undrained
> 1/2 cup alfalfa sprouts
> 4 whole-wheat hamburger rolls

• Mix salad dressing and seasonings in a bowl. Add tuna and sprouts. Mix well.

• Use about one-fourth of filling per sandwich.

```
Nutritional information per serving:
Serving size: 1 sandwich
Calories: 200
Total fat: 4 grams
Saturated fatty acids: 1 gram
Cholesterol: 32 milligrams
Sodium: 313 milligrams
```

Variation

Chicken and Sprouts Sandwich

Use a 5 oz. can of chicken, undrained, instead of tuna.

Note: One cup of finely diced cooked chicken and 1 tablespoon of unsalted chicken broth can be used instead of the canned chicken. The sodium will be 320 milligrams.

Nutritional information per serving:
Serving size: 1 sandwich
Calories: 200
Total fat: 6 grams
Saturated fatty acids: 2 grams
Cholesterol: 25 milligrams
Sodium: 473 milligrams

Chicken Salad Sandwich
(serves 4)

> **2 tablespoons salad dressing, mayonnaise-type**
> **1/8 teaspoon onion powder**
> **1/8 teaspoon dried tarragon, crushed**
> **dash of garlic powder**
> **1 cup chicken, without skin, cooked, chopped**
> **1/2 cup celery, chopped**
> **8 slices whole-wheat bread**
> **4 lettuce leaves**

• Mix salad dressing and seasonings in a bowl. Stir in chicken and celery. Mix well.

• Spread about 1/3 cup of the filling on each of four bread slices. Top with lettuce and remaining bread.

> Nutritional information per serving:
> Serving size: 1 sandwich
> Calories: 230
> Total fat: 6 grams
> Saturated fatty acids: 1 gram
> Cholesterol: 33 milligrams
> Sodium: 387 milligrams

Variation

Beef Salad Sandwich

Use 1 cup chopped, cooked lean beef instead of chicken.

```
Nutritional information per serving:
Serving size: 1 sandwich
Calories: 235
Total fat: 7 grams
Saturated fatty acids: 2 grams
Cholesterol: 32 milligrams
Sodium: 385 milligrams
```

Mexican Bean Tortilla Roll-ups
(serves 2)

1 teaspoon vinegar
1/4 to 1 teaspoon chili powder
1/8 teaspoon onion powder
2 teaspoons salad dressing, mayonnaise-type
3/4 cup pinto or kidney beans, cooked, drained, unsalted, chopped (see Note)
3 tablespoons celery, chopped
2 flour tortillas
4 slices tomato
2 lettuce leaves

• Mix vinegar, chili powder and onion powder with salad dressing in bowl. Add beans and celery. Mix well.
• Soften tortillas in heated skillet about 1 1/2 minutes. Turn, if necessary.
• Place half of bean filling onto each tortilla near one edge. Top with lettuce and tomato. Roll up.
Note: Canned, drained pinto or red kidney beans may be used instead of cooked beans. Sodium will be 318 milligrams for pinto beans and 282 milligrams for kidney beans.

Nutritional information per serving:
Serving size: 1 roll-up
Calories: 175
Total fat: 3 grams
Saturated fatty acids: 1 gram
Cholesterol: 1 milligram
Sodium: 53 milligrams

Salads

Chef's Salad
(serves 1)

1/3 cup lettuce, torn into pieces
1/3 cup spinach, torn into pieces
1/4 cup kidney beans, cooked, drained (see Note)
2 tablespoons carrots, shredded
2 green pepper rings
2 radishes, sliced
2 broccoli florets
2 tomato wedges
1/2 oz. (about 2 tablespoons) Swiss cheese strips
1 oz. (about 1/4 cup) chicken, cooked, cut in strips
1 1/2 tablespoons low-calorie Italian dressing

- Toss spinach and lettuce pieces together in serving container.
- Mix remaining vegetables and place on greens.
- Top with cheese and chicken strips.
- Pour dressing over salad just before eating.

Note: Canned kidney beans can be used instead of drained home-cooked kidney beans. Sodium will be 406 milligrams. Leftover beans can be frozen for use another time.

Nutritional information per serving:
Serving size: 1 salad
Calories: 210
Total fat: 8 grams
Saturated fatty acids: 3 grams
Cholesterol: 37 milligrams
Sodium: 257 milligrams

Tuna Macaroni Salad

(serves 4)

> 3/4 cup elbow macaroni, uncooked
> 6 1/2 oz. can tuna, packed in water, drained
> 1/2 cup celery, thinly sliced
> 1 cup seedless red grapes, halved
> 3 tablespoons salad dressing, mayonnaise-type,
>   reduced-calorie

• Cook macaroni according to package directions, omitting salt. Drain.
• Mix together macaroni, tuna, celery and grapes.
• Stir in salad dressing.
• Serve warm or cold.

Nutritional information per serving:
Serving size: 1 cup
Calories: 185
Total fat: 3 grams
Saturated fatty acids: Trace
Cholesterol: 10 milligrams
Sodium: 230 milligrams

Try these tasty variations:

Salmon Macaroni Salad

Use a 7 1/2 oz. can of drained salmon instead of tuna.

Nutritional information per serving:
Serving size: 1 cup
Calories: 185
Total fat: 5 grams
Saturated fatty acids: 1 gram
Cholesterol: 24 milligrams
Sodium: 307 milligrams

Chicken Macaroni Salad

Use 1 cup diced cooked chicken instead of tuna.

Nutritional information per serving:
Serving size: 1 cup
Calories: 195
Total fat: 5 grams
Saturated fatty acids: 1 gram
Cholesterol: 32 milligrams
Sodium: 113 milligrams

Beef Macaroni Salad

Use 1 cup diced cooked lean beef instead of tuna.

Nutritional information per serving:
Serving size: 1 cup
Calories: 200
Total fat: 5 grams
Saturated fatty acids: 1 gram
Cholesterol: 31 milligrams
Sodium: 111 milligrams

Fruit Salad
(serves 6)

1 medium-size peach, sliced
1 medium-size pear, sliced
1 medium-size apple, sliced
2 medium-size bananas, sliced
1/2 cantaloupe, sliced
Juice of 1 1/2 lemons
4 teaspoons sugar
1/4 teaspoon cinnamon (optional)
1/4 teaspoon nutmeg (optional)
1/4 teaspoon cloves (optional)

• Combine all ingredients in a large bowl and mix. Chill one hour and serve.

```
Nutritional information per serving:
Serving size: 3/4 cup
Calories: 128
Total fat: less than 1 gram
Saturated fatty acids: less than 1 gram
Cholesterol: 0
Sodium: 6 milligrams
```

Apple and Grape Salad
(serves 4)

1 envelope (about 1 tablespoon) unflavored gelatin
1/4 cup water
1 1/2 cups apple juice
1 cup apple, unpared, diced
1/2 cup red grapes, halved, seeded
1/4 cup celery, chopped

• Soften gelatin in water for 5 minutes. Heat gelatin over low heat, stirring constantly, until dissolved.
• Add apple juice. Chill until mixture begins to thicken.
• Stir in fruit and celery.
• Pour into 3-cup mold.
• Chill until set.

Nutritional information per serving:
Serving size: 1/2 cup
Calories: 80
Total fat: Trace
Saturated fatty acids: Trace
Cholesterol: 0
Sodium: 11 milligrams

Waldorf Salad
(serves 6)

> 4 apples, cored and cubed
> 1/4 cup celery, finely chopped
> 1/2 cup raisins
> Juice of 1 lemon
> 1 tablespoon low-fat mayonnaise
> 2 teaspoons sugar
> 1/8 teaspoon cinnamon
> 1/8 teaspoon nutmeg
> 1/8 teaspoon cloves

- Combine all ingredients in a large bowl and mix.
- Chill for one hour and serve.

Nutritional information per serving:
Serving size: 3/4 cup
Calories: 110
Total fat: less than 1 gram
Saturated fatty acids: less than 1 gram
Cholesterol: 1 milligram
Sodium: 19 milligrams

Snacks and Desserts

Orange-Apricot Cookies
(makes about 4 dozen cookies)

1 cup all-purpose flour
3/4 cup whole-wheat flour
1/4 cup sugar
2 teaspoons baking powder
1/2 teaspoon ground cinnamon
1/4 teaspoon salt
3/4 cup dried apricots, chopped
1/2 cup orange juice, fresh
1/4 cup oil
1 teaspoon orange rind, grated
1 egg, beaten

- Preheat oven to 375°F.
- Mix dry ingredients thoroughly.
- Add remaining ingredients. Mix well.
- Drop dough by teaspoonfuls onto ungreased baking sheet, about 1 inch apart.
- Bake about 11 minutes or until lightly browned.
- Remove from baking sheet while still warm.
- Cool on rack.

Nutritional information per serving:
Serving size: 2 cookies
Calories: 80
Total fat: 2 grams
Saturated fatty acids: Trace
Cholesterol: 12 milligrams
Sodium: 58 milligrams

Oatmeal Applesauce Cookies
(makes about 5 dozen cookies)

1 cup all-purpose flour
1 teaspoon baking powder
1 teaspoon ground allspice
1/4 teaspoon salt
1/2 cup margarine
1/2 cup sugar
2 egg whites
2 cups rolled oats, quick-cooking
1 cup unsweetened applesauce
1/2 cup raisins, chopped

- Preheat oven to 375°F.
- Grease baking sheet.
- Mix flour, baking powder, allspice and salt.
- Beat margarine and sugar until creamy. Add egg whites; beat well.
- Add dry ingredients.
- Stir in oats, applesauce and raisins. Mix well.
- Drop by level tablespoonfuls onto baking sheet.
- Bake 11 minutes or until edges are lightly browned.
- Cool on rack.

Nutritional information per serving:
Serving size: 2 cookies
Calories: 90
Total fat: 4 grams
Saturated fatty acids: Trace
Cholesterol: 0
Sodium: 72 milligrams

Pumpkin Cupcakes
(makes 24 cupcakes)

1 1/2 cups whole-wheat flour
1 cup all-purpose flour
3/4 cup sugar
2 tablespoons baking powder
2 teaspoons ground cinnamon
1/2 teaspoon ground nutmeg
1/4 teaspoon salt
3 eggs, slightly beaten
1 cup skim milk
1/2 cup oil
1 cup canned pumpkin
3/4 cup raisins, chopped
1 tablespoon vanilla

- Preheat oven to 350°F.
- Place 24 paper baking cups in muffin tins.
- Mix dry ingredients thoroughly.
- Mix remaining ingredients; add to dry ingredients. Stir until dry ingredients are barely moistened.
- Fill paper cups two-thirds full.
- Bake about 20 minutes or until toothpick inserted in center comes out clean. Remove from muffin tins and cool on rack.
- Freeze cupcakes that will not be eaten in the next few days.

Nutritional information per serving:
Serving size: 1 cupcake
Calories: 140
Total fat: 6 grams
Saturated fatty acids: 1 gram
Cholesterol: 34 milligrams
Sodium: 132 milligrams

Mixed Fruit

(serves 2)

1/2 cup apple, unpared, diced
1/2 cup banana, sliced
1/2 cup grapefruit sections, cut up
2 tablespoons juice from grapefruit or pineapple
1/3 cup grapes, halved
1/3 cup pineapple tidbits, juice-packed, drained

• Mix apple, banana, and grapefruit sections with juice
prevent darkening of apple and banana.
• Add grapes and pineapple.
• Chill.
Note: Fresh fruits in season may be substituted, as desire
Use peaches, nectarines, melon, berries or apricots.

Nutritional information per serving:
Serving size: 1 cup
Calories: 110
Total fat: 1 gram
Saturated fatty acids: Trace
Cholesterol: 0
Sodium: 1 milligram

Fruit Juice Cubes
(makes 45 cubes)

1 1/2 tablespoons (1 1/2 envelopes) unflavored gelatin
3/4 cup water
6 oz. can frozen grape or apple juice concentrate

• Very lightly grease 9- by 5-inch loaf pan or plastic ice cube trays.
• Soften gelatin in water in a small saucepan for 5 minutes.
• Heat over low heat, stirring constantly, until gelatin dissolves. Remove from heat.
• Add fruit juice concentrate; mix well. Pour into pan.
• Cover and refrigerate. Chill until set.
• Cut into 1-inch cubes. Keep covered during refrigerator storage.

> Nutritional information per serving:
> Serving size: 4 cubes
> Calories: 40
> Total fat: Trace
> Saturated fatty acids: Trace
> Cholesterol: 0
> Sodium: 4 milligrams

Crunchy Snack Mix
(serves 12)

1 cup pretzels, unsalted
1 cup roasted peanuts, unsalted
1 cup raisins
1/2 cup sunflower seeds, unsalted

- Break pretzels into bite-size pieces.
- Mix ingredients together.
- Store in airtight container.

Nutritional information per serving:
Serving size: 1/4 cup
Calories: 150
Total fat: 9 grams
Saturated fatty acids: 1 gram
Cholesterol: 0
Sodium: 12 milligrams

Chili Popcorn
(serves 4)

4 cups popped popcorn
1 tablespoon margarine, melted
1 1/4 teaspoons chili powder
1/4 teaspoon ground cumin
dash of garlic powder

- Mix hot popcorn and margarine
- Mix seasonings thoroughly; sprinkle over popcorn. Mix well.
- Serve immediately.

```
Nutritional information per serving:
Serving size: 1 cup
Calories: 50
Total fat: 3 grams
Saturated fatty acids: 1 gram
Cholesterol: 0
Sodium: 42 milligrams
```

Mexican Snack Pizzas
(serves 4)

> 2 whole-wheat English muffins
> 1/4 cup tomato puree
> 1/4 cup kidney beans, canned, drained, chopped
> 1 tablespoon onion, chopped
> 1 tablespoon green pepper, chopped
> 1/2 teaspoon oregano leaves
> 1/4 cup Mozzarella cheese, part skim milk, shredded
> 1/4 cup lettuce, shredded

- Split muffins; toast lightly.
- Mix puree, beans, onion, green pepper and oregano. Spread on muffin halves. Sprinkle with cheese.
- Broil until cheese is bubbly, about 2 minutes.
- Garnish with shredded lettuce.

> Nutritional information per serving:
> Serving size: 1/2 English muffin
> Calories: 95
> Total fat: 2 grams
> Saturated fatty acids: 1 gram
> Cholesterol: 4 milligrams
> Sodium: 300 milligrams

Salsa

(makes about 1 cup)

8 oz. can no-salt-added tomato sauce
1 tablespoon chili peppers, canned, drained, finely chopped
1/4 cup green pepper, finely chopped
2 tablespoons onion, finely chopped
1 clove garlic, minced
1/4 teaspoon oregano
1/8 teaspoon ground cumin

• Mix all ingredients thoroughly.
• Chill before serving to blend flavors.
• Serve with toasted pita bread, breadsticks or raw vegetable pieces.

Nutritional information per serving:
Serving size: 1/2 cup
Calories: 40
Total fat: Trace
Saturated fatty acids: Trace
Cholesterol: 0
Sodium: 120 milligrams

Bran Apple Bars
(makes 16 bars)

> 1 cup whole-bran cereal (see Note)
> 1/2 cup skim milk
> 1 cup flour
> 1 teaspoon baking powder
> 1/2 teaspoon cinnamon
> 1/4 teaspoon nutmeg
> 1/3 cup margarine
> 1/2 cup brown sugar, packed
> 2 egg whites
> 1 cup apple, pared, chopped

- Preheat oven to 350°F.
- Lightly grease 9- by 9-inch baking pan.
- Soak bran in milk until milk is absorbed
- Mix dry ingredients thoroughly.
- Beat margarine and sugar until creamy. Add egg whites; beat well. Stir in apples and bran mixture. Add dry ingredients; mix well. Pour into pan.
- Bake 30 minutes or until a toothpick inserted in center comes out clean. Cool on rack. Cut into 16 bars.

Note: Check the nutrition label of cereals for sodium content. Some whole-bran cereals contain almost twice as much sodium as others.

> Nutritional information per serving:
> Serving size: 1 bar
> Calories: 110
> Total fat: 4 grams
> Saturated fatty acids: 1 gram
> Cholesterol: Trace
> Sodium: 109 milligrams

Curry Vegetable Dip
(makes about 1 cup)

8 oz. carton plain low-fat yogurt
1/4 cup carrots, shredded
2 teaspoons green onions, minced
1 tablespoon salad dressing, mayonnaise-type
1 teaspoon sugar
1/4 teaspoon curry powder
dash of pepper

• Mix ingredients in a bowl.
• Chill.
• Serve with crisp raw vegetable pieces, such as celery, carrot or summer squash.

Nutritional information per serving:
Serving size: 1/2 cup
Calories: 120
Total fat: 8 grams
Saturated fatty acids: Trace
Cholesterol: 8 milligrams
Sodium: 136 milligrams

Pineapple-Apricot Pie
(8-inch pie, 8 servings)

Graham cracker crust
  1 cup graham crackers, crushed
  3 tablespoons margarine

Filling
  15 1/4 oz. can crushed pineapple, juice-packed
  16 oz. can apricot halves, juice-packed
  1/4 cup sugar
  3 tablespoons cornstarch
  1/2 teaspoon cinnamon
  1 cup juice from pineapple and apricots
  2 teaspoons lemon juice

To make crust:
• Preheat oven to 375°F.
• Mix graham cracker crumbs and margarine thoroughly. Save 1/4 cup of crumb mixture for top of pie.
• Press remaining crumb mixture into 8-inch pie pan so the bottom and sides are completely covered.
• Bake until crust is firm, about 5 minutes. Cool.

To make filling:
• Drain pineapple and apricots; save 1 cup juice. Coarsely chop apricots.
• Mix sugar, cornstarch and cinnamon in saucepan. Stir in fruit juice.
• Cook over low heat, stirring constantly, until thickened. Remove from heat.
• Add pineapple, apricots and lemon juice. Mix well.
• Spoon filling into crust. Sprinkle remaining crumb mixture over top of filling.

• Chill until set.

Nutritional information per serving:
Serving size: 1 slice (divide pie
    evenly into 8 slices)
Calories: 170
Total fat: 5 grams
Saturated fatty acids: 1 gram
Cholesterol: 0
Sodium: 125 milligrams

Banana-Spice Snack Cake
(serves 9)

3/4 cup whole-wheat flour
3/4 cup all-purpose flour
1/2 cup sugar
1 teaspoon baking powder
1/2 teaspoon baking soda
1 teaspoon cinnamon
1/2 teaspoon nutmeg
1/4 teaspoon ground cloves
1/4 teaspoon salt
1 cup bananas, ripe, mashed
1/4 cup yogurt, plain, low-fat
1/4 cup oil
1 egg, slightly beaten
1 teaspoon vanilla

• Preheat oven to 350°F.
• Lightly grease 9- by 9-inch baking pan.
• Mix dry ingredients thoroughly.
• Mix remaining ingredients; add to dry ingredients. Stir until dry ingredients are barely moistened. Pour into baking pan.
• Bake 20 minutes or until toothpick inserted in center comes out clean.

Nutritional information per serving:
Serving size: 1 piece (divide cake
    evenly into 9 pieces)
Calories: 205
Total fat: 7 grams
Saturated fatty acids: 1 gram
Cholesterol: 31 milligrams
Sodium: 165 milligrams

Raisin Whole-Wheat Bread Pudding
(serves 4)

1 1/2 cups whole-wheat bread, cut in 1-inch cubes
1/3 cup raisins
2 tablespoons sugar
3/4 teaspoon cinnamon
1 egg
1/4 teaspoon vanilla
1 1/4 cups skim milk

- Preheat oven to 325°F.
- Place bread cubes in 1-quart casserole. Sprinkle with raisins.
- Mix sugar and cinnamon. Stir in egg. Add vanilla.
- Heat milk; slowly stir into egg mixture. Pour over bread.
- Bake until tip of knife inserted in center comes out clean, about 40 minutes.

Nutritional information per serving:
Serving size: 1/2 cup
Calories: 145
Total fat: 2 grams
Saturated fatty acids: Trace
Cholesterol: 70 milligrams
Sodium: 139 milligrams

Fruit Sherbet
(serves 8)

   1 envelope unflavored gelatin
   1/2 cup apricot nectar
   1/2 cup apricot halves, juice-packed, drained
   1 small banana, ripe
   2 tablespoons light corn syrup
   1 cup skim milk
   1/4 cup frozen orange juice concentrate

• Soften gelatin in apricot nectar for 5 minutes. Heat, stirring constantly, until gelatin dissolves
• Puree apricots and banana in blender.
• Add gelatin mixture and remaining ingredients. Mix well.
• Pour into an 8- by 8-inch pan.
• Cover and freeze until icy.
• Beat in a bowl until frothy. Pour into pan. Cover; refreeze.

Nutritional information per serving:
Serving size: 1/2 cup
Calories: 70
Total fat: Trace
Saturated fatty acids: Trace
Cholesterol: 1 milligram
Sodium: 22 milligrams

Breads

Baking Mix
(makes about 8 cups)

3 cups whole-wheat flour
3 cups all-purpose flour
3 tablespoons baking powder
1 1/2 teaspoons salt
3/4 cup nonfat dry milk
3/4 cup vegetable shortening

- Mix dry ingredients thoroughly.
- Cut in shortening with pastry blender or mixer until fine crumbs are obtained and shortening is evenly dispersed.
- Store, tightly covered, in refrigerator. Use within 3 months.
- Use for biscuits or muffins.

Biscuits
(makes 8 biscuits)

> **1 1/2 cups Baking Mix**
> **1/3 cup water**

- Preheat oven to 425°F.
- Stir most of the water into mix. Add rest of water as needed to make a dough that is soft but not sticky. Shape dough into a ball.
- Pat or roll dough into a rectangle about 8 by 4 inches. Cut into eight pieces.
- Place on ungreased baking sheet.
- Bake until lightly browned, about 15 minutes.

Nutritional information per serving:
Serving size: 1 biscuit
Calories: 90
Total fat: 3 grams
Saturated fatty acids: 1 gram
Cholesterol: Trace
Sodium: 149 milligrams

Zucchini Bread
(1 loaf)

1 cup whole-wheat flour
1 cup all-purpose flour
1 1/2 teaspoons baking powder
1 teaspoon cinnamon
1/4 teaspoon baking soda
1/4 teaspoon salt
3 egg whites
1/2 cup sugar
1/3 cup oil
1 1/2 teaspoons vanilla
2 cups zucchini squash, coarsely shredded, lightly packed

- Preheat oven to 350°F.
- Grease 9- by 5- by 3-inch loaf pan.
- Mix dry ingredients, except sugar. Beat egg whites until frothy. Add sugar, oil and vanilla. Continue beating for 3 minutes. Stir in zucchini; mix lightly.
- Add dry ingredients. Mix just until dry ingredients are moistened. Pour into loaf pan. Bake 40 minutes or until toothpick inserted in center comes out clean.
- Cool on rack. Remove from pan after 10 minutes.
- To serve, cut into 18 slices about 1/2-inch thick.

Nutritional information per serving:
Serving size: 1 slice
Calories: 110
Total fat: 4 grams
Saturated fatty acids: 1 gram
Cholesterol: 0
Sodium: 87 milligrams

Applesauce Muffins
(makes 8 muffins)

> 1 1/2 cups Baking Mix
> 1 tablespoon sugar
> 1/2 teaspoon ground cinnamon
> 1 egg white, slightly beaten
> 1/2 cup applesauce, unsweetened
> 1/4 cup water

- Preheat oven to 400°F.
- Grease muffin tins.
- Stir Baking Mix, sugar and cinnamon together.
- Mix egg white, applesauce and water thoroughly. Add to dry ingredients. Stir until dry ingredients are barely moistened. Batter will be lumpy.
- Fill muffin tins two-thirds full.
- Bake until lightly browned, about 20 minutes.

Nutritional information per serving:
Serving size: 1 muffin
Calories: 105
Total fat: 4 grams
Saturated fatty acids: 1 gram
Cholesterol: Trace
Sodium: 156 milligrams

Whole-Wheat Cornmeal Muffins
(makes 8 muffins)

2/3 cup yellow cornmeal, degerminated
2/3 cup whole-wheat flour
1 tablespoon sugar
2 teaspoons baking powder
1/8 teaspoon salt
2/3 cup skim milk
1 egg, beaten
2 tablespoons oil

- Preheat oven to 400°F.
- Grease 8 muffin tins or use paper liners.
- Mix dry ingredients thoroughly.
- Mix milk, egg and oil. Add to dry ingredients. Stir until dry ingredients are barely moistened. Batter will be lumpy.
- Fill muffin tins two-thirds full.
- Bake until lightly browned, about 20 minutes.

Nutritional information per serving:
Serving size: 1 muffin
Calories: 135
Total fat: 4 grams
Saturated fatty acids: 1 gram
Cholesterol: 35 milligrams
Sodium: 146 milligrams

32 | Menus Designed to Lower High Cholesterol

Taking control of your eating habits is the cornerstone of lowering your cholesterol. Three dietary factors send your cholesterol soaring: Eating too much saturated fat, eating too much cholesterol, and taking in more calories than you use up.

As part of the National Cholesterol Education Program (NCEP), the Expert Panel on Detection, Evaluation, and Treatment of High Blood Cholesterol designed the one·day menus on the following pages to lower your LDL cholesterol levels.

The menus are in pairs. The first menu of each pair supplies 8 to 10 percent of calories from saturated fat, 30 percent or less of calories from total fat, and less than 300 mg/day of cholesterol. The NCEP recommends that everyone adopt an eating plan based on these guidelines. The second menu of each pair reduces saturated fat to less than 7 percent of calories and cholesterol to less than 200 mg/day.

You may already follow an eating plan similar to the first menu in the pair. If you have followed this low-fat, low-cholesterol plan for at least three months and you still have high cholesterol, you should move to the lower-fat, lower-cholesterol second menu plan.

Of course, you would never follow the same menu day after day. But these typical eating plans can help you develop your own menus that will work for a lifetime of healthy eating.

Before you drastically alter your eating habits, discuss your plans with your doctor. Through regular visits, he can check your progress toward healthier cholesterol and blood pressure levels.

Low-fat, Low-cholesterol, Nutritionally Balanced
Sample Menus
Traditional American Cuisine
Males 25-49 Years

Breakfast
Bagel, plain (1 medium)
   Cream Cheese, low-fat (2 tsp)
Cereal, shredded wheat (1 1/2 cups)
Banana (1 small)
Milk, **1%** (1 cup)
Orange Juice (3/4 cup)
Coffee (1 cup)
Milk, **1%** (1 oz)

Lunch
Minestrone Soup, canned, low sodium (1 cup)
Roast Beef Sandwich
      Whole Wheat Bread (2 slices)
   * Lean Roast Beef, unseasoned (**3 oz**)
      American Cheese, low-fat and low sodium (3/4 oz)
      Lettuce (1 leaf)
      Tomato (3 slices)
      Mayonnaise, low-fat and low sodium (2 tsp)
Fruit and Cottage Cheese Salad
      Cottage Cheese, **2%** and low sodium (1/2 cup)
      Peaches, canned in juice (1/2 cup)
Apple Juice, unsweetened (1 cup)

Dinner
   * **Salmon** (3 oz)
      Vegetable Oil (1 tsp)
   * Baked Potato (1 medium)

Margarine (2 tsp)
* Green Beans (1/2 cup), seasoned with margarine (1/2 tsp)
* Carrots (1/2 cup), seasoned with margarine (1/2 tsp)
White Dinner Roll (1 medium)
Margarine (1 tsp)
Ice Milk (1 cup)
Iced Tea, unsweetened (1 cup)

Snack
* Popcorn (3 cups)
Margarine (1 T)

Calories	2,518
Total Carbohydrates, % kcals	53
Total Fat, % kcals:	29
Simple Carbohydrates, % kcals	36
Saturated Fatty Acids, % kcals	8.6
Complex Carbohydrates, % kcals	64
Cholesterol, mg	181
* Sodium, mg	1,821
Protein, % kcals	18

100% RDA met for all nutrients except: Zinc 90%

Boldface food items are different in the following menu.

* No salt is added in recipe preparation or as seasoning. All margarine is low sodium.

Low-fat, Low-cholesterol, Nutritionally Balanced
Sample Menus
Traditional American Cuisine
Males 25-49 Years
Saturated Fat and Cholesterol Further Reduced

Breakfast
    Bagel, plain (1 medium)
        Margarine (2 tsp)
        Jelly (2 tsp)
    Cereal, shredded wheat (1 1/2 cups)
    Banana (1 small)
    Milk, **skim** (1 cup)
    Orange Juice (3/4 cup)
    Coffee (1 cup)
        Milk, **skim** (1 oz)

Lunch
    Minestrone Soup, canned, low sodium (1 cup)
    Roast Beef Sandwich
        Whole Wheat Bread (2 slices)
     * Lean Roast Beef, unseasoned (**2 oz**)
        American Cheese, low-fat and low sodium (3/4 oz)
        Lettuce (1 leaf)
        Tomato (3 slices)
        Margarine (2 tsp)
    Fruit and Cottage Cheese Salad
        Cottage Cheese, **1%** and low sodium (1/2 cup)
        Peaches, canned in juice (1/2 cup)
        Apple Juice, unsweetened (1 cup)

Dinner

* **Flounder** (3 oz)
    Vegetable Oil (1 tsp)
* Baked Potato (1 medium)
    Margarine (2 tsp)
* Green Beans (1/2 cup), seasoned with margarine (1/2 tsp)
* Carrots (1/2 cup), seasoned with margarine (1/2 tsp)
  White Dinner Roll (1 medium)
    Margarine (1 tsp)
  Frozen Yogurt (1 cup)
  Iced Tea, unsweetened (1 cup)

Snack

* Popcorn (3 cups)
    Margarine (1 T)

Calories	2,533
Total Carbohydrates, % kcals	55
Total Fat, % kcals:	28
Simple Carbohydrates, % kcals	36
Saturated Fatty Acids, % kcals	6.6
Complex Carbohydrates, % kcals	64
Cholesterol, mg	150
* Sodium, mg	1,803
Protein, % kcals	17

100% RDA met for all nutrients except: Zinc 90%

Boldface food items are different from the previous menu.

*** No salt is added in recipe preparation or as seasoning. All margarine is low sodium.**

Low-fat, Low-cholesterol, Nutritionally Balanced
Sample Menus
Traditional American Cuisine
Females 25-49 Years

Breakfast
Bagel, plain (1/2 medium)
    Cream Cheese, low-fat (1 tsp)
Cereal, shredded wheat (1 cup)
Banana (1 small)
Milk, **1%** (1 cup)
Orange Juice (**3/4 cup**)
Coffee (1 cup)
    Milk, **1%** (1 oz)

Lunch
Minestrone Soup, canned, low sodium (1/2 cup)
Roast Beef Sandwich
    Whole Wheat Bread (2 slices)
  * Lean Roast Beef, unseasoned (**3 oz**)
    American Cheese, low-fat and low sodium (3/4 oz)
    Lettuce (1 leaf)
    Tomato (3 slices)
    Mayonnaise, low-fat and low sodium (2 tsp)
Apple (1 medium)
Water (1 cup)

Dinner
 * **Salmon** (3 oz)
        Vegetable Oil (1 tsp)
 * Baked Potato (1/2 medium)
        Margarine (1 tsp)
 * Green Beans (1/2 cup), seasoned with margarine (1/2 tsp)
 * Carrots (1/2 cup), seasoned with margarine (1/2 tsp)
   White Dinner Roll (1 medium)
        Margarine (1 tsp)
   Ice Milk (1/2 cup)
   Iced Tea, unsweetened (1 cup)

Snack
 * Popcorn (**2 cups**)
        Margarine (**1 tsp**)

Calories	1,831
Total Carbohydrates, % kcals	52
Total Fat, % kcals:	30
Simple Carbohydrates, % kcals	37
Saturated Fatty Acids, % kcals	8.7
Complex Carbohydrates, % kcals	63
Cholesterol, mg	156
* Sodium, mg	1,415
Protein, % kcals	18

100% RDA met for all nutrients except: Zinc 90%

Boldface food items are different in the following menu.

*** No salt is added in recipe preparation or as seasoning. All margarine is low sodium.**

Low-fat, Low-cholesterol, Nutritionally Balanced Sample Menus Traditional American Cuisine Females 25-49 Years Fat and Cholesterol Further Reduced

Breakfast
    Bagel, plain (1/2 medium)
        Margarine (1 tsp)
        Jelly (1 tsp)
    Cereal, shredded wheat (1 cup)
    Banana (1 small)
      Milk, **skim** (1 cup)
      Orange Juice (**1 cup**)
      Coffee (1 cup)
          Milk, **skim** (1 oz)

Lunch
    Minestrone Soup, canned, low sodium (1/2 cup)
    Roast Beef Sandwich
        Whole Wheat Bread (2 slices)
      *   Lean Roast Beef, unseasoned (**2 oz**)
        American Cheese, low-fat and low sodium (3/4 oz)
        Lettuce (1 leaf)
        Tomato (3 slices)
        Margarine (2 tsp)
    Apple (1 medium)
    Water (1 cup)

Dinner
    *   **Flounder** (3 oz)
         Vegetable Oil (1 tsp)
    *   Baked Potato (1/2 medium)
         Margarine (1 tsp)
    *   Green Beans (1/2 cup), seasoned with margarine (1/2 tsp)
    *   Carrots (1/2 cup), seasoned with margarine (1/2 tsp)
         White Dinner Roll (1 medium)
         Margarine (1 tsp)
         Frozen Yogurt (1/2 cup)
         Iced Tea, unsweetened (1 cup)

Snack
    *   Popcorn (**3 cups**)
         Margarine (**2 tsp**)

Calories	1,867
Total Carbohydrates, % kcals	55
Total Fat, % kcals:	29
Simple Carbohydrates, % kcals	38
Saturated Fatty Acids, % kcals	6.8
Complex Carbohydrates, % kcals	62
Cholesterol, mg	134
* Sodium, mg	1,417
Protein, % kcals	16

100% RDA met for all nutrients except: Zinc 90%

Boldface food items are different from the previous menu.

* No salt is added in recipe preparation or as seasoning. All margarine is low sodium.

Low-fat, Low-cholesterol, Nutritionally Balanced
Sample Menus
Asian-American Cuisine
Males 25-49 Years

Breakfast
> Banana (1 medium)
> Whole Wheat Bread (2 slices)
> > Margarine (2 tsp)
> Orange Juice (1 cup)
> Milk, **1%** (1 cup)

Lunch
> Beef Noodle Soup, canned, low sodium (1 cup)
> Chinese Noodle and Beef Salad
> > * **Lean Roast Beef** (3 oz)
> > Peanut Oil (**2 tsp**)
> > Soy Sauce, low sodium (1 tsp)
> > Peanuts, unsalted (**1 T**)
> > Carrots (1/2 cup)
> > Squash (1/2 cup)
> > Onion (1/2 cup)
> > Chinese Noodles, soft type (1/4 cup)
> * Steamed White Rice (1 cup)
> Apple (1 medium)
> Tea, unsweetened (1 cup)

Dinner
> Pork Stirfry with Vegetables
> > Pork Cutlet (**3 oz**)
> > Peanut Oil (**2 tsp**)
> > Soy Sauce, low sodium (1 tsp)
> > Peanuts, unsalted (**1 T**)

Broccoli (1/2 cup)
Carrots (1/2 cup)
Mushrooms (1/4 cup)
* Steamed White Rice (1 cup)
* Wonton Soup, prepared with low-sodium broth (1/2 cup)
Milk, **1%** (1 cup)
Tea, unsweetened (1 cup)

Snack

Egg roll, vegetarian, baked with peanut oil and low-sodium soy sauce (1 medium)
Chinese Mustard (1 tsp)
Sweet and Sour Sauce (1 tsp)
Tea, unsweetened (1 cup)

Calories	2,494
Total Carbohydrates, % kcals	53
Total Fat, % kcals:	30
Simple Carbohydrates, % kcals	30
Saturated Fatty Acids, % kcals	8.1
Complex Carbohydrates, % kcals	70
Cholesterol, mg	238
* Sodium, mg	1,663
Protein, % kcals	17

100% RDA met for all nutrients except: Zinc 90%

Boldface food items are different in the following menu.

* No salt is added in recipe preparation or as seasoning. All margarine is low sodium

Low-fat, Low-cholesterol, Nutritionally Balanced
Sample Menus
Asian-American Cuisine
Males 25-49 Years
Fat and Cholesterol Further Reduced

Breakfast
    Banana (1 medium)
    Whole Wheat Bread (2 slices)
        Margarine (2 tsp)
    Orange Juice (1 cup)
    Milk, **skim** (1 cup)

Lunch
    Beef Noodle Soup, canned, low sodium (1 cup)
    Chinese Noodle and Beef Salad
      * **Sirloin Steak** (3 oz)
        Peanut Oil (**2 1/2 tsp**)
        Soy Sauce, low sodium (1 tsp)
        Peanuts, unsalted (**2 T**)
        Carrots (1/2 cup)
        Squash (1/2 cup)
        Onion (1/4 cup)
        Chinese Noodles, soft type (1/4 cup)
    * Steamed White Rice (1 cup)
    Apple (1 medium)
    Tea, unsweetened (1 cup)

Dinner
    Pork Stirfry with Vegetables
        Pork Cutlet (**2 oz**)
        Peanut Oil (**2 1/2 tsp**)
        Soy Sauce, low sodium (1 tsp)

Peanuts, unsalted (**2 T**)
Broccoli (1/2 cup)
Carrots (1/2 cup)
Mushrooms (1/4 cup)
* Steamed White Rice (1 cup)
* Wonton Soup, prepared with low-sodium broth (1/2 cup)
Milk, **skim** (1 cup)
Tea, unsweetened (1 cup)

Snack

Egg roll, vegetarian, baked with peanut oil and low-sodium soy sauce (1 medium)
Chinese Mustard (1 tsp)
Sweet and Sour Sauce (1 tsp)
Tea, unsweetened (1 cup)

Calories	2,480
Total Carbohydrates, % kcals	54
Total Fat, % kcals:	29
Simple Carbohydrates, % kcals	29
Saturated Fatty Acids, % kcals	6.2
Complex Carbohydrates, % kcals	71
Cholesterol mg	205
* Sodium, mg	1,649
Protein, % kcals	17

100% RDA met for all nutrients except: Zinc 90%

Boldface food items are different from the previous menu.

* No salt is added in recipe preparation or as seasoning. All margarine is low sodium.

Low-fat, Low-cholesterol, Nutritionally Balanced
Sample Menus
Asian-American Cuisine
Females 25-49 Years

Breakfast
  Banana (**1 medium**)
  Whole Wheat Bread (2 slices)
      Margarine (2 tsp)
  Orange Juice (3/4 cup)
  Milk, **1%** (1 cup)

Lunch
  Beef Noodle Soup, canned, low sodium (1 cup)
  Chinese Noodle and Beef Salad
      * **Lean Roast Beef** (3 oz)
      Peanut Oil (**1 1/2 tsp**)
      Soy Sauce, low sodium (1 tsp)
      Carrots (1/2 cup)
      Squash (1/2 cup)
      Onion (1/4 cup)
      Chinese Noodles, soft type (1/4 cup)
  * Steamed White Rice (1/2 cup)
  Apple (1 medium)
  Tea, unsweetened (1 cup)

Dinner

Pork Stirfry with Vegetables
    Pork Cutlet (**3 oz**)
    Peanut Oil (**1 1/2 tsp**)
    Soy Sauce, low sodium (1 tsp)
    Broccoli (1/2 cup)
    Carrots (1/2 cup)
    Mushrooms (1/4 cup)
Steamed White Rice (1/2 cup)
Milk, **1%** (3/4 cup)
Tea, unsweetened (1 cup)

Snack

Wonton Soup, prepared with low-sodium broth (1/2 cup)
Tea, unsweetened (1 cup)

Calories	1,853
Total Carbohydrates, % kcals	51
Total Fat, % kcals:	30
Simple Carbohydrates, % kcals	34
Saturated Fatty Acids, % kcals	9.0
Complex Carbohydrates, % kcals	66
Cholesterol, mg	207
* Sodium, mg	1,323
Protein, % kcals	19

100% RDA met for all nutrients except: Zinc 90%

Boldface food items are different in the following menu.

*** No salt is added in recipe preparation or as seasoning. All margarine is low sodium.**

Low-fat, Low-cholesterol, Nutritionally Balanced
Sample Menus
Asian-American Cuisine
Females 25-49 Years
Fat and Cholesterol Further Reduced

Breakfast
    Banana (**1/2 medium**)
    Whole Wheat Bread (2 slices)
        Margarine (2 tsp)
    Orange Juice (3/4 cup)
    Milk, **skim** (1 cup)

Lunch
    Beef Noodle Soup, canned, low sodium (1 cup)
    Chinese Noodle and Beef Salad
      * **Sirloin Steak** (3 oz)
        Peanut Oil (**1 T**)
        Soy Sauce, low sodium (1 tsp)
        Carrots (1/2 cup)
        Squash (1/2 cup)
        Onion (1/4 cup)
        Chinese Noodles, soft type (1/4 cup)
    * Steamed White Rice (1/2 cup)
    Apple (1 medium)
    Tea, unsweetened (1 cup)

Dinner

Pork Stirfry with Vegetables
>> Pork Cutlet (**2 oz**)
>> Peanut Oil (**1 T**)
>> Soy Sauce, low sodium (1 tsp)
>> Broccoli (1/2 cup)
>> Carrots (1/2 cup)
>> Mushrooms (1/4 cup)
* Steamed White Rice (1/2 cup)
Milk, **skim** (3/4 cup)
Tea, unsweetened (1 cup)

Snack

Wonton Soup, prepared with low-sodium broth (1/2 cup)
Tea, unsweetened (1 cup)

Calories	1,815
Total Carbohydrates, % kcals	52
Total Fat, % kcals:	29
Simple Carbohydrates, % kcals	33
Saturated Fatty Acids, % kcals	6.8
Complex Carbohydrates, % kcals	67
Cholesterol, mg	176
* Sodium, mg	1,300
Protein, % kcals	19

100% RDA met for all nutrients except: Zinc 90%

Boldface food items are different from the previous menu.

**** No salt is added in recipe preparation or as season-
ing. All margarine is low sodium.***

Low-fat, Low-cholesterol, Nutritionally Balanced
Sample Menus
Mexican-American Cuisine
Males 25-49 Years

Breakfast
>   Cantaloupe (1/2 cup)
> *   Farina, prepared with **1%** milk (1 cup)
>   White Bread (2 slices)
> >   Margarine (2 tsp)
> >   Jelly (2 tsp)
>   Orange Juice (3/4 cup)
>   Hot Cocoa, prepared with **1%** milk (1 cup)

Lunch
>   Beef Enchilada
> >   Tortilla, corn (2 tortillas)
> >   *   Lean Roast Beef (**3 oz**)
> >   Vegetable Oil (**1 tsp**)
> >   Cheddar Cheese, low-fat and low sodium (1 oz)
> >   Onion (1/8 cup)
> >   Tomato (1/8 cup)
> >   Lettuce (1/4 cup)
> >   Chili Peppers (2 tsp)
> *   Refried Beans (3/4 cup), prepared with vegetable oil
>   Carrots (6 sticks), Celery (6 sticks)
>   Milk, **1%** (1/2 cup)

Dinner

    Chicken Taco
        Tortilla, corn (2 tortillas)
     *   Chicken Breast, without skin (3 oz)
        Vegetable Oil (**1 tsp**)
        Cheddar Cheese, low-fat and low sodium (1 oz)
        Guacamole (2 T)
        Salsa (2 T)
   * Corn (**1/2 cup**), seasoned with margarine (**1/2 tsp**)
   * Spanish Rice (1 cup), prepared with margarine
     Banana (1 medium)
     Coffee (1 cup)
        Milk, **1%** (1 oz)

Snack

    Ice Milk (3/4 cup)

Calories	2,557
Total Carbohydrates, % kcals	52
Total Fat, % kcals:	29
Simple Carbohydrates, % kcals	40
Saturated Fatty Acids, % kcals	8.3
Complex Carbohydrates, % kcals	60
Cholesterol, mg	185
* Sodium, mg	1,801
Protein, % kcals	19

100% RDA met for all nutrients except: Zinc 90%

Boldface food items are different in the following menu.

*** No salt is added in recipe preparation or as seasoning. All margarine is low sodium**

Low-fat, Low-cholesterol, Nutritionally Balanced
Sample Menus
Mexican-American Cuisine
Males 25-49 Years
Fat and Cholesterol Further Reduced

Breakfast

    Cantaloupe (1/2 cup)
*   Farina, prepared with **skim** milk (1 cup)
    White Bread (2 slices)
        Margarine (2 tsp)
        Jelly (2 tsp)
    Orange Juice (3/4 cup)
    Hot Cocoa, prepared with **skim** milk (1 cup)

Lunch

    Beef Enchilada
        Tortilla, corn (2 tortillas)
   *   Lean Roast Beef (**2 oz**)
        Vegetable Oil (**1/2 tsp**)
        Cheddar Cheese, low-fat and low sodium (1 oz)
        Onion (1/8 cup)
        Tomato (1/8 cup)
        Lettuce (1/4 cup)
        Chili Peppers (2 tsp)
* Refried Beans (3/4 cup), prepared with vegetable oil
    Carrots (6 sticks), Celery (6 sticks)
    Milk, **skim** (1/2 cup)

Dinner

Chicken Taco
    Tortilla, corn (2 tortillas)
*   Chicken Breast, without skin (3 oz)
    Vegetable Oil (**1/2 tsp**)
    Cheddar Cheese, low-fat and low sodium (1 oz)
    Guacamole (2 T)
    Salsa (2 T)
* Corn (**1 cup**), seasoned with margarine (**1 tsp**)
* Spanish Rice (1 cup), prepared with margarine
Banana (1 medium)
Coffee (1 cup)
    Milk, **skim** (1 oz)

Snack

* **Popcorn** (3 cups)
    Margarine (1 T)

Calories	2,574
Total Carbohydrates, % kcals	55
Total Fat, % kcals:	28
Simple Carbohydrates, % kcals	36
Saturated Fatty Acids, % kcals	6.2
Complex Carbohydrates, % kcals	64
Cholesterol, mg	136
* Sodium, mg	1,921
Protein, % kcals	17

100% RDA met for all nutrients except: Zinc 90%

Boldface food items are different in the previous menu.

* No salt is added in recipe preparation or as seasoning. All margarine is low sodium.

Low-fat, Low-cholesterol, Nutritionally Balanced
Sample Menus
Mexican-American Cuisine
Females 25-49 Years

Breakfast
Cantaloupe (1/2 cup)
* Farina, prepared with **1%** milk (3/4 cup)
White Bread (1 slice)
    Margarine (1 tsp)
    Jelly (1 tsp)
Orange Juice (3/4 cup)
Hot Cocoa, prepared with **1%** milk (1 cup)

Lunch
Beef Enchilada
    Tortilla, corn (2 tortillas)
  * Lean Roast Beef (**3 oz**)
    Vegetable Oil (2/3 tsp)
    Cheddar Cheese, low-fat and low sodium (1/2 oz)
    Onion (1/8 cup)
    Tomato (1/8 cup)
    Lettuce (1/4 cup)
    Chili Peppers (2 tsp)
* Refried Beans (**1/2 cup**), prepared with vegetable oil
Carrots (4 sticks), Celery (4 sticks)
Milk, **1%** (1/2 cup)

Dinner
Chicken Taco
> Tortilla, corn (1 tortilla)
> * Chicken Breast, without skin (3 oz)
> Vegetable Oil (2/3 tsp)
> Cheddar Cheese, low-fat and low sodium (1/2 oz)
> Guacamole (1 T)
> Salsa (1 T)

* Corn (1/2 cup), seasoned with margarine (1/2 tsp)
* Spanish Rice (1/2 cup), prepared with margarine
Banana (**1/2 medium**)
Coffee (1 cup)
> Milk, **1%** (1 oz)

Snack
Ice Milk (1/2 cup)

Calories	1,852
Total Carbohydrates, % kcals	51
Total Fat, % kcals:	29
Simple Carbohydrates, % kcals	41
Saturated Fatty Acids, % kcals	8.5
Complex Carbohydrates, % kcals	59
Cholesterol, mg	169
* Sodium, mg	1,429
Protein, % kcals	20

100% RDA met for all nutrients except: Zinc 90%

Boldface food items are different in the following menu.

* No salt is added in recipe preparation or as seasoning. All margarine is low sodium.

Low-fat, Low-cholesterol, Nutritionally Balanced
Sample Menus
Mexican-American Cuisine
Females 25-49 Years
Fat and Cholesterol Further Reduced

Breakfast
> Cantaloupe (1/2 cup)
> * Farina, prepared with **skim** milk (3/4 cup)
> White Bread (1 slice)
>> Margarine (1 tsp)
>> Jelly (1 tsp)
> Orange Juice (3/4 cup)
> Hot Cocoa, prepared with **skim** milk (1 cup)

Lunch
> Beef Enchilada
>> Tortilla, corn (2 tortillas)
>> * Lean Roast Beef (**2 oz**)
>> Vegetable Oil (2/3 tsp)
>> Cheddar Cheese, low-fat and low sodium (1/2 oz)
>> Onion (1/8 cup)
>> Tomato (1/8 cup)
>> Lettuce (1/4 cup)
>> Chili Peppers (2 tsp)
> * Refried Beans (**2/3 cup**), prepared with vegetable oil
> Carrots (4 sticks), Celery (4 sticks)
> Milk, **skim** (1/2 cup)

Dinner

Chicken Taco
>   Tortilla, corn (1 tortilla)
> * Chicken Breast, without skin (3 oz)
>   Vegetable Oil (2/3 tsp)
>   Cheddar Cheese, low-fat and low sodium (1/2 oz)
>   Guacamole (1 T)
>   Salsa (1 T)

* Corn (1/2 cup), seasoned with margarine (1/2 tsp)
* Spanish Rice (1/2 cup), prepared with margarine
> Banana (**1 medium**)
> Coffee (1 cup)
>> Milk, **skim** (1 oz)

Snack

Popcorn (1 cup)
> **Margarine** (1 tsp)

Calories	1,860
Total Carbohydrates, % kcals	53
Total Fat, % kcals:	28
Simple Carbohydrates, % kcals	36
Saturated Fatty Acids, % kcals	6.2
Complex Carbohydrates, % kcals	64
Cholesterol, mg	127
* Sodium, mg	1,450
Protein, % kcals	19

100% RDA met for all nutrients except: Zinc 90%

Boldface food items are different in the previous menu.

* No salt is added in recipe preparation or as seasoning. All margarine is low sodium.

Low-fat, Low-cholesterol, Nutritionally Balanced
Sample Menus
Southern Cuisine
Males 25-49 Years

Breakfast
Oatmeal (1 cup), prepared with **1%** milk
Milk, **1%** (1 cup)
English Muffin (1 medium)
    Cream Cheese, low-fat (2 T)
Orange Juice (1 cup)
Coffee (1 cup)
    Milk, **1%** (1 oz)

Lunch
 * Baked Chicken Breast, without skin (3 oz)
        Vegetable Oil (1 tsp)
Salad
        Lettuce (1/2 cup)
        Tomato (1/2 cup)
        Cucumber (1/2 cup)
        Oil and Vinegar Dressing, regular calorie (1 T)
 * White Rice (**1 cup**), seasoned with margarine (**1 tsp**)
 * Baking Powder Biscuit, prepared with vegetable oil (1 medium)
        Margarine (2 tsp)
Water (1 cup)

Dinner
 * Lean Roast Beef (**3 oz**)
        Onion (1/4 cup)
        Beef Gravy (1 T), **1% milk based**

* Turnip Greens (1/2 cup), seasoned with margarine (1/2 tsp)
Sweet Potato (1 medium)
    Brown Sugar (1 tsp)
Cornbread (1 medium slice), prepared with margarine
    Margarine (1 tsp)
Honeydew Melon (1/4 medium)
Pumpkin Cookies (2 medium), prepared with vegetable oil
Iced Tea (1 cup), sweetened with sugar

Snack

Saltine Crackers, unsalted tops (8 crackers)
Mozzarella Cheese, made with part skim milk (**1 1/2 oz**)
Dried Prunes (2 medium)

Calories	2,560
Total Carbohydrates, % kcals	52
Total Fat, % kcals:	30
Simple Carbohydrates, % kcals	36
Saturated Fatty Acids, % kcals	9.4
Complex Carbohydrates, % kcals	64
Cholesterol, mg	241
* Sodium, mg	1,790
Protein, % kcals	18

100% RDA met for all nutrients except: Zinc 90%

Boldface food items are different in the following menu.

*** No salt is added in recipe preparation or as seasoning. All margarine is low sodium.**

Low-fat, Low-cholesterol, Nutritionally Balanced
Sample Menus
Southern Cuisine
Males 25-49 Years
Fat and Cholesterol Further Reduced

Breakfast
    Oatmeal (1 cup), prepared with **skim** milk
    Milk, **skim** (1 cup)
    English Muffin (1 medium)
        Margarine (2 tsp)
        Jelly (2 tsp)
    Orange Juice (1 cup)
    Coffee (1 cup)
        Milk, **skim** (1 oz)

Lunch
  * Baked Chicken Breast, without skin (3 oz)
        Vegetable Oil (1 tsp)
    Salad
        Lettuce (1/2 cup)
        Tomato (1/2 cup)
        Cucumber (1/2 cup)
        Oil and Vinegar Dressing, regular calorie (1 T)
  * White Rice (**1 1/4 cup**), seasoned with margarine (**1 1/4 tsp**)
  * Baking Powder Biscuit, prepared with vegetable oil (1 medium)
        Margarine (2 tsp)
    Water (1 cup)

Dinner
  * Lean Roast Beef (**2 oz**)

Onion (1/4 cup)

Beef Gravy (1 T), **water based**

* Turnip Greens (1/2 cup), seasoned with margarine (1/2 tsp)

Sweet Potato (1 medium)

Brown Sugar (1 tsp)

Cornbread (1 medium slice), prepared with margarine

Margarine (1 tsp)

Honeydew Melon (1/4 medium)

Pumpkin Cookies (2 medium), prepared with vegetable oil

Iced Tea (1 cup), sweetened with sugar

Snack

Saltine Crackers, unsalted tops (8 crackers)

Mozzarella Cheese, made with part skim milk (**3/4 oz**)

Dried Prunes (2 medium)

Calories	2,536
Total Carbohydrates, % kcals	55
Total Fat, % kcals:	29
Simple Carbohydrates, % kcals	35
Saturated Fatty Acids, % kcals	6.7
Complex Carbohydrates, % kcals	65
Cholesterol, mg	177
* Sodium, mg	1,538
Protein, % kcals	16

100% RDA met for all nutrients except: Zinc 90%

Boldface food items are different in the previous menu.

* No salt is added in recipe preparation or as seasoning. All margarine is low sodium.

Low-fat, Low-cholesterol, Nutritionally Balanced
Sample Menus
Southern Cuisine
Females 25-49 Years

Breakfast
>   Oatmeal (3/4 cup), prepared with **1% milk**
>   Milk, **1% (3/4 cup)**
>   English Muffin (1 medium)
>   **Cream Cheese, low-fat (2 tsp)**
>   Orange Juice (3/4 cup)
>   Coffee (1 cup)
>   Milk, **1%** (1 oz)

Lunch
>   * Baked Chicken Breast, without skin (3 oz)
>   Vegetable Oil (1 tsp)
>   Salad
>   Lettuce (1/2 cup)
>   Tomato (1/2 cup)
>   Cucumber (1/2 cup)
>   Oil and Vinegar Dressing, regular calorie (2 tsp)
>   * White Rice (1/2 cup), seasoned with margarine (1/2 tsp)
>   * Baking Powder Biscuit, prepared with vegetable oil (1/2 medium)
>   Margarine (1 tsp)
>   Water (1 cup)

Dinner
>   * Lean Roast Beef **(3 oz)**
>   Onion (1/4 cup)
>   Beef Gravy (1 T), **1% milk based**

* Turnip Greens (1/2 cup), seasoned with margarine (1/2 tsp)

Sweet Potato (1/2 medium)
   Brown Sugar (1/2 tsp)
Cornbread (1/2 medium slice), prepared with margarine
   Margarine (1/2 tsp)
Honeydew Melon (1/4 medium)
Pumpkin Cookie (1 medium), prepared with vegetable oil
Iced Tea (1 cup), sweetened with sugar

Snack

Saltine Crackers, unsalted tops (4 crackers)
Mozzarella Cheese, made with part skim milk (**3/4 oz**)
Dried Prunes (2 medium)

Calories	1,823
Total Carbohydrates, % kcals	50
Total Fat, % kcals:	30
Simple Carbohydrates, % kcals	42
Saturated Fatty Acids, % kcals	9.0
Complex Carbohydrates, % kcals	58
Cholesterol, mg	191
* Sodium, mg	1,241
Protein, % kcals	20

100% RDA met for all nutrients except: Zinc 90%

Boldface food items are different in the following menu.

* No salt is added in recipe preparation or as seasoning. All margarine is low sodium.

Low-fat, Low-cholesterol, Nutritionally Balanced
Sample Menus
Southern Cuisine
Females 25-49 Years
Fat and Cholesterol Further Reduced

Breakfast
    Oatmeal (3/4 cup), prepared with **skim** milk
    Milk, **skim (1 cup)**
    English Muffin (1 medium)
        Margarine (2 tsp)
        Jelly (2 tsp)
    Orange Juice (3/4 cup)
    Coffee (1 cup)
        Milk, **skim** (1 oz)

Lunch
  * Baked Chicken Breast, without skin (3 oz)
        Vegetable Oil (1 tsp)
    Salad
        Lettuce (1/2 cup)
        Tomato (1/2 cup)
        Cucumber (1/2 cup)
        Oil and Vinegar Dressing, regular calorie (2 tsp)
  * White Rice (1/2 cup), seasoned with margarine (1/2 tsp)
  * Baking Powder Biscuit, prepared with vegetable oil
    (1/2 medium)
        Margarine (1 tsp)
    Water (1 cup)

Dinner
  * Lean Roast Beef **(2 oz)**
        Onion (1/4 cup)

Beef Gravy (1 T), **water based**
* Turnip Greens (1/2 cup), seasoned with margarine (1/2 tsp)
Sweet Potato (1/2 medium)
    Brown Sugar (1/2 tsp)
Cornbread (1/2 medium slice), prepared with margarine
    Margarine (1/2 tsp)
Honeydew Melon (1/4 medium)
Pumpkin Cookie (1 medium), prepared with vegetable oil
Iced Tea (1 cup), sweetened with sugar

Snack

Saltine Crackers, unsalted tops (4 crackers)
Mozzarella Cheese, made with part skim milk (**1/2 oz**)
Dried Prunes (2 medium)

Calories	1,841
Total Carbohydrates, % kcals	53
Total Fat, % kcals:	29
Simple Carbohydrates, % kcals	42
Saturated Fatty Acids, % kcals	6.9
Complex Carbohydrates, % kcals	58
Cholesterol, mg	159
* Sodium, mg	1,162
Protein, % kcals	18

100% RDA met for all nutrients except: Zinc 90%

Boldface food items are different in the previous menu.

* No salt is added in recipe preparation or as seasoning. All margarine is low sodium.

Low-fat, Low-cholesterol, Nutritionally Balanced
Sample Menus
Lacto Ovo Vegetarian Cuisine
Males 25-49 Years

Breakfast
    Orange (1 medium)
* Pancakes, made with **1%** milk and egg whites (4 4-inch circles)
      Pancake Syrup (2 T)
      Margarine (2 tsp)
    Milk, **1%** (1 cup)
    Coffee (1 cup)
      Milk, **1%** (1 oz)

Lunch
    Vegetable Soup, canned, low sodium (1 cup)
    Bagel (1 medium)
      Processed American Cheese, low-fat and low sodium (1 1/2 oz)
    Spinach Salad
      Spinach (1 cup)
      Mushrooms (1/8 cup)
*   Olive Oil Dressing, regular calorie (1 T)
    Apple, 1 medium
    Iced Tea, sweetened with sugar (1 cup)

Dinner
* Omelette
      Egg Whites (4 large eggs)
      Green Pepper (2 T)
      Onion (2 T)
      Mozzarella Cheese, made from part skim milk (1 1/2 oz)

Vegetable Oil (1 T)
* Brown Rice (**1 1/4 cups**), seasoned with margarine (1 1/4 tsp)
* Carrots (1/2 cup), seasoned with margarine (1/2 tsp)
Whole Wheat Bread (2 slices)
Margarine (2 tsp)
Fig Bar Cookies (2 bars)
Tea (1 cup)
Honey (1 tsp)

Snack

Corn Flake Cereal (**1 1/4 cups**)
Milk, **1% (3/4 cup)**

Calories	2,529
Total Carbohydrates, % kcals	56
Total Fat, % kcals:	30
Simple Carbohydrates, % kcals	34
Saturated Fatty Acids, % kcals	8.3
Complex Carbohydrates, % kcals	66
Cholesterol, mg	99
* Sodium, mg	2,195
Protein, % kcals	14

100% RDA met for all nutrients except: Zinc 90%

Boldface food items are different in the following menu.

* No salt is added in recipe preparation or as seasoning. All margarine is low sodium.

Low-fat, Low-cholesterol, Nutritionally Balanced
Sample Menus
Lacto Ovo Vegetarian Cuisine
Males 25-49 Years
Fat and Cholesterol Further Reduced

Breakfast
Orange (1 medium)
* Pancakes, made with **skim** milk and egg whites
(4 4-inch circles)
    Pancake Syrup (2 T)
    Margarine (2 tsp)
Milk, **skim** (1 cup
Coffee (1 cup)
    Milk, **skim** (1 oz)

Lunch
Vegetable Soup, canned, low sodium (1 cup)
Bagel (1 medium)
    Margarine (2 tsp)
Spinach Salad
    Spinach (1 cup)
    Mushrooms (1/8 cup)
  * Olive Oil Dressing, regular calorie (1 T)
Apple, 1 medium
Iced Tea, sweetened with sugar (1 cup)

Dinner
* Omelette
    Egg Whites (4 large eggs)
    Green Pepper (2 T)
    Onion (2 T)

Mozzarella Cheese, made from part skim milk
(1 1/2 oz)
Vegetable Oil (1 T)
* Brown Rice (**1 1/2 cups**), seasoned with margarine
(1 1/4 tsp)
* Carrots (1/2 cup), seasoned with margarine (1/2 tsp)
Whole Wheat Bread (2 slices)
Margarine (2 tsp)
Fig Bar Cookies (2 bars)
Tea (1 cup)
Honey (1 tsp)

Snack

Corn Flake Cereal (**1 1/2 cups**)
Milk, **skim (1/2 cup)**

Calories	2,524
Total Carbohydrates, % kcals	58
Total Fat, % kcals:	29
Simple Carbohydrates, % kcals	31
Saturated Fatty Acids, % kcals	6.3
Complex Carbohydrates, % kcals	69
Cholesterol, mg	59
* Sodium, mg	2,059
Protein, % kcals	13

100% RDA met for all nutrients except: Zinc 90%

Boldface food items are different in the previous menu.

*** No salt is added in recipe preparation or as seasoning. All margarine is low sodium.**

Low-fat, Low-cholesterol, Nutritionally Balanced
Sample Menus
Lacto Ovo Vegetarian Cuisine
Females 25-49 Years

Breakfast
  Orange (1 medium)
* Pancakes, made with **1%** milk and egg whites (3 4-inch circles)
  Pancake Syrup (1 1/2 T)
  Margarine (1 1/2 tsp)
  Milk, **1%** (1 cup)
  Coffee (1 cup)
  Milk, **1%** (1 oz)

Lunch
  Vegetable Soup, canned, low sodium (1 cup)
  Bagel (1 medium)
  Processed American Cheese, low-fat and low sodium (3/4 oz)
  Spinach Salad
  Spinach (1 cup)
  Mushrooms (1/8 cup)
* Olive Oil Dressing, regular calorie (2 tsp)
  Apple, 1 medium
  Iced Tea, unsweetened (1 cup)

Dinner
* Omelette
  Egg Whites (4 large eggs)
  Green Pepper (2 T)
  Onion (2 T)
  Mozzarella Cheese, made from part skim milk (1 1/2 oz)

       Vegetable Oil (1 T)
*   Brown Rice (**1/2 cup**), seasoned with margarine (1/2 tsp)
*   Carrots (1/2 cup), seasoned with margarine (1/2 tsp)
       Whole Wheat Bread (1 slice)
           Margarine (1 tsp)
       Fig Bar Cookie (1 bar)
       Tea (1 cup)
           Honey (1 tsp)

Snack

       Bran Flake Cereal (1 cup)
       Milk, **1%** (3/4 cup)

Calories	1,820
Total Carbohydrates, % kcals	54
Total Fat, % kcals:	30
Simple Carbohydrates, % kcals	38
Saturated Fatty Acids, % kcals	8.7
Complex Carbohydrates, % kcals	62
Cholesterol, mg	71
* Sodium, mg	1,795
Protein, % kcals	16

100% RDA met for all nutrients except: Zinc 90%

Boldface food items are different in the following menu.

* No salt is added in recipe preparation or as seasoning. All margarine is low sodium.

Low-fat, Low-cholesterol, Nutritionally Balanced
Sample Menus
Lacto Ovo Vegetarian Cuisine
Females 25-49 Years
Fat and Cholesterol Further Reduced

Breakfast
Orange (1 medium)
* Pancakes, made with **skim** milk and egg whites
(3 4-inch circles)
Pancake Syrup (1 1/2 T)
Margarine (1 1/2 tsp)
Milk, **skim** (1 cup)
Coffee (1 cup)
Milk, **skim** (1 oz)

Lunch
Vegetable Soup, canned, low sodium (1 cup)
Bagel (1 medium)
Margarine (1 tsp)
Spinach Salad
Spinach (1 cup)
Mushrooms (1/8 cup)
* Olive Oil Dressing, regular calorie (2 tsp)
Apple, 1 medium
Iced Tea, sweetened with sugar (1 cup)

Dinner
* Omelette
Egg Whites (4 large eggs)
Green Pepper (2 T)
Onion (2 T)

      Mozzarella Cheese, made from part skim milk
         (1 1/2 oz)
      Vegetable Oil (1 T)
* Brown Rice (**3/4 cup**), seasoned with margarine (1/2 tsp)
* Carrots (1/2 cup), seasoned with margarine (1/2 tsp)
      Whole Wheat Bread (1 slice)
         Margarine (1 tsp)
     Fig Bar Cookie (1 bar)
     Tea (1 cup)
         Honey (1 tsp)

Snack

     Bran Flake Cereal (1 cup)
     Milk, **skim** (3/4 cup)

Calories	1,829
Total Carbohydrates, % kcals	56
Total Fat, % kcals:	29
Simple Carbohydrates, % kcals	35
Saturated Fatty Acids, % kcals	6.7
Complex Carbohydrates, % kcals	65
Cholesterol, mg	46
* Sodium, mg	1,739
Protein, % kcals	15

100% RDA met for all nutrients except: Zinc 90%

Boldface food items are different in the previous menu.

* No salt is added in recipe preparation or as season-ing. All margarine is low sodium.

33 | Where to Write For More Health Information

Many government and private organizations offer free or low-cost publications to help you learn more about health and nutrition matters. All you have to do is call or write to order the publications you need. Check the following list for fact sheets, pamphlets and booklets that can help you control your blood pressure.

Eat to Live, Free

Eating Smart, Free

The Good Life, Free

American Cancer Society
National Office
1599 Clifton Road, N.E.
Atlanta, GA 30329

Telephone 1–800–227–2345

Cholesterol and Your Heart, Free

Dining Out: A Guide to Restaurant Dining, Free

How to Have Your Cake and Eat it Too, Free

Nutrition Labeling: Food Selection Hints for Fat-Controlled Meals, Free

Nutrition Nibbles, Free

Recipes for Low-Fat, Low Cholesterol Meals, Free

The American Heart Association Diet: An Eating Plan for Healthy Americans, Free

**American Heart Association
National Center
7272 Greenville Avenue
Dallas, TX 75231**

Telephone (214) 706–1179

A Word About Low Sodium Diets, Booklet No. 617A, Free

Caffeine Jitters: Some Safety Questions Remain, Booklet No. 618A, Free

Dietary Guidelines for Americans, Booklet No. 314A, $0.50

Eating for Life, Booklet No. 116A, $1.00

Eating to Lower Your High Blood Cholesterol, Booklet No. 116A, $1.00

Food Facts for Older Adults, Booklet No. 118A, $4.00

Getting Fit Your Way, Booklet No. 121A, $3.25

How to Buy Canned & Frozen Fruits, Booklet No. 382A, $0.50

How to Buy Canned & Frozen Vegetables, Booklet No. 383A, $0.50

How to Buy Fresh Fruits, Booklet No. 384A, $0.50

How to Buy Fresh Vegetables, Booklet No. 385A, $0.50

How to Read the New Food Label, Booklet No. 522A, Free

Is Something Fishy Going On?, Booklet No. 599A, Free

Making Healthy Food Choices, Booklet No. 149A, $1.50

Personal Health Guide, Booklet No. 151A, $1.00

Prescriptions to Help Smokers Quit, Booklet No. 624A, Free

Secondhand Smoke, Booklet No. 315A, $0.50

The Food Guide Pyramid, Booklet No. 119A, $1.00

Vegetarian Diets, Booklet No. 627A, Free

Walking for Exercise and Pleasure, Booklet No. 124A, $1,00

If you order ONLY free booklets, mail your order to:

S. James
Consumer Information Center — 4D
P.O. Box 100
Pueblo, CO 81002

If you order BOTH sales booklets and free booklets, mail your order to:

R. Woods
Consumer Information Center — 4D
P.O. Box 100
Pueblo, CO 81002

Clearing the Air: A Guide To Quitting Smoking, NIH Pub. 92–1647, Free

Diet, Nutrition, and Cancer Prevention: The Good News, NIH Pub. No. 87–2878, Free

Easy Entertaining with Fruits & Vegetables for Better Health, NIH Pub. No. 92–3249, Free

Eat More Fruits & Vegetables, NIH Pub. No. 92–3248, Free

Eat More Salads for Better Health, NIH Pub. No. 92–3250, Free

Fast & Easy Fruits & Vegetables for Busy People, NIH Pub. No. 93–3247, Free

**National Cancer Institute
Public Inquiries Office
Building 31, Room 10A24
Bethesda, MD 20892**

Telephone (301) 496–5583 or 1–800–422–6237

LEAN Toward Health, Free

The Healthy Weigh: A Practical Food Guide

The New Cholesterol Countdown, Free

**National Center for Nutrition and Dietetics
American Dietetic Association
216 W. Jackson Boulevard, Suite 800
Chicago, IL 60606-6995**

Telephone 1–800–366–1655

Check Your High Blood Pressure Prevention I.Q., NIH Pub. No. 94–3671

Check Your Smoking I.Q.: An Important Quiz for the Older Smoker, NIH Pub. No. 91–3031

Check Your Weight and Heart Disease I.Q., NIH Pub. No. 93–3034

Churches as an Avenue to High Blood Pressure Control, NIH Pub. No. 92–2725

Eat Right To Help Lower Your High Blood Pressure, NIH Pub. No. 92–3289

Eat Right To Lower Your High Blood Cholesterol, NIH Pub. 92–2972

Eating To Lower Your Blood Cholesterol, NIH Pub. No. 92–2920

Exercise and Your Heart, NIH Pub. No. 93–1677

Facts About Angina, NIH Pub. No. 92–2890

Facts About Blood Cholesterol, NIH Pub. No. 90–2696

Facts About Coronary Heart Disease, NIH Pub. No. 93–2265

Facts About How to Prevent High Blood Pressure, NIH Pub. No. 94–3281

Finding Resources for Healthy Heart Programs at Work, NIH Pub. No. 92–737

Healthy Heart Handbook for Women, NIH Pub. No. 92–2720

High Blood Pressure: Treat It for Life, NIH Pub. No. 94–3312

So You Have High Blood Cholesterol, NIH Pub. No. 93–2922

Test Your Healthy Heart I.Q., NIH Pub. No. 93–2724

The Healthy Heart Handbook for Women, NIH Pub. No. 92–2720

National Heart, Lung, and Blood Institute
Public Inquiries Office
Building 31, Room 4A21
Bethesda, MD 20892

Telephone (301) 496–5343

Be Sensible About Salt

Dietary Supplements: More is Not Always Better

Don't Take It Easy — Exercise!

High Blood Pressure: A Common But Controllable Disorder

Hints for Shopping, Cooking, and Enjoying Meals

Nutrition: A Lifelong Concern

Safe Use of Medicines by Older People

Smoking: It's Never Too Late To Stop

National Institute on Aging Information Center
P.O. Box 8057
Gaithersburg, MD 20898–8057

Telephone 1–800–222–2225

1–800–222–4225 (TTY)

Obesity and Energy Metabolism, NIH Pub. No. 86–1805

Risks of Heart Disease, NIH Pub. No. 89–2985

**National Institutes of Health
Public Inquiries Office
Clinical Center — Building 10, Room 1C255
Bethesda, MD 20892**

Telephone (301) 496–2563

———————————

Know Your Brain (basic fact sheet on the anatomy and function of the human brain)

Preventing Stroke

Stroke 1994

Stroke Risk Factors and Warning Signs (bookmark)

**NIH Neurological Institute
P.O. Box 5801
Bethesda, MD 20824**

Telephone (301) 496–5751 or 1–800–352–9424

———————————

Detection, Evaluation, and Treatment of High Blood Cholesterol in Adults

Detection, Evaluation, and Treatment of High Blood Pressure

Easy Eating for Well-Seasoned Adults

Freedom from Smoking for You and Your Baby

**Primary Care Clearinghouse
8201 Greensboro Drive, Suite 600
McLean, VA 22102**

Telephone (703) 821–8955 ext. 248

———————————

✳ ‖ Glossary

aneurysm — An abnormal weakness in the wall of a blood vessel, usually an artery, that leads to ballooning. It is most often found in the aorta, which is the biggest artery in the body going from the heart through the chest and abdomen. An aneurysm can swell, enlarge and eventually rupture.

angina pectoris — A sudden pain or pressure in the chest behind the breastbone which may radiate to the shoulder, neck, arm, hand or back, usually on the left side of the body. People with angina pectoris also may feel its sensations as burning, choking or indigestion. It is caused by an insufficient supply of blood flowing through narrowed coronary arteries which supply the heart muscle.

angioplasty — A technique used to widen narrowed arteries using a balloon catheter.

angiotensin — A hormone in the blood that raises blood

pressure.

arteriosclerosis — Artery disease characterized by a loss of artery elasticity, deposits in the arteries and hardening of the walls of the arteries leading to a decreased blood flow.

artery — Any blood vessel that carries blood away from the heart to the various organs and tissues of the body.

ascites — The accumulation of fluid within the abdominal cavity, causing abdominal swelling. It can be caused by infections, heart failure, cirrhosis of the liver and some cancers.

atheromas — Small raised plaques of mushy cholesterol, fat and foam cells on the inner walls of the arteries.

atherosclerosis — A form of arteriosclerosis characterized by the deposit of cholesterol and other fatty, waxy substances on the inner walls of the arteries, often leading to narrowing and "hardening" of the arteries as scar tissue forms.

blood pressure — The force exerted on the walls of arteries, veins and capillaries as the heart pumps blood through the body.

calcium — The most abundant mineral found in the body. It is essential in the formation of teeth and bones and is necessary for the functioning of nerves and muscles. It is also important in the regulation of blood pressure.

capillaries — Minute blood vessels that connect the smallest arteries to the smallest veins.

carbohydrates — Any one of a large group of compounds, including sugars and starches, that are used as a source of energy. All carbohydrates are eventually broken down in the body to the simple sugar glucose, which can then be used in metabolic processes in the body.

cardiac — Of or relating to the heart.

cardiac arrest — A heart attack or when productive heart beating stops.

cardiovascular — Pertaining to the heart and arteries.

cholesterol — A waxy fat present in some foods of animal origin. It also is manufactured by the human body. Some cholesterol is needed by the body, but excessive amounts are associated with artery disease.

circulatory system — Also known as the cardiovascular system, it includes the heart and the network of blood vessels throughout the body. The circulatory system transports nutrients and oxygen to the tissues and removes waste products.

congestive heart failure — Occurs when the heart is unable to pump well enough to maintain good circulation. It often occurs because of a weakness in the heart muscle due to disease or a mechanical fault in the valves that control the flow of blood.

coronary heart disease or coronary artery disease — Narrowing or blockage of the coronary arteries which reduces the flow of blood to the heart muscle.

creatinine — a waste substance in the body that is excreted in the urine. Measuring the amount of creatinine in the blood allows doctors to monitor the progression of kidney disease.

diabetes mellitus — A chronic disorder characterized by high levels of glucose in the blood. It may be caused by too little insulin being produced by the pancreas or the body's resistance to insulin.

diastolic pressure — The pressure which remains in the blood vessels as the heart relaxes to allow for the flow of blood into its pumping chambers. The second number in a blood pressure reading.

diuretic — A drug that increases the flow of urine, more commonly known as a water pill.

drug interaction — One drug or other substance increasing, decreasing or changing the effects of another drug.

dyspnea — Labored or difficult breathing.

edema — Accumulation of fluid in the body.

ECG — See electrocardiogram.

electrocardiogram — A recording of the heart's electrical activity. By placing electrodes, usually with gel, on a person's arms, legs and chest, the heart's electrical activity can be monitored and recorded onto a strip of graph paper.

estrogen — The female sex hormone that is responsible for the development of secondary sexual characteristics (such as menstruation) in women.

fiber — Dietary fiber, often called roughage, is the part of food that cannot be absorbed by the body. It is essential for proper elimination of body waste because it helps food move through the body. It is found in fruits, raw vegetables and whole grains. Highly processed foods, like white flour and sugar, contain little or no fiber.

fibrosis — Thickening and scarring of connective tissue, most often a consequence of inflammation or injury.

gender — The category to which an individual is assigned on the basis of sex: male or female.

generic name — The name given to the ingredient or ingredients in a drug as distinguished from brand names for drugs which may be trademarked by manufacturers.

heart attack — Heart failure or abnormal, weak functioning of the heart after its blood supply is abruptly cut off, usually due to narrowing of the arteries or a blood clot.

heredity — The genetic transmission of a particular quality or trait from parent to offspring.

high blood pressure — See hypertension.

hormone — A substance that is produced in one part of the body (by a gland, such as the thyroid or adrenal gland). It then passes into the bloodstream and is carried to other organs or tissues, where it acts to modify their structure or function.

hypercholesterolemia — An excessive amount of cholesterol in the blood.

hyperinsulinemia — An excessive amount of insulin in the blood.

hyperplasia — The increased production and growth of normal cells in a tissue or organ. The affected part becomes larger but retains its normal form.

hypertension — Sustained high blood pressure of 140/90 or higher. The correct medical term for high blood pressure.

hypertrophy — An increase in the size of a tissue or organ brought about by the enlargement of its cells rather than by cell multiplication. Muscles undergo this change in response to increased work.

hypotension — Low blood pressure.

hypoxia — A deficiency of oxygen in the tissues.

incidence — Rate of occurrence.

infarct (infarction) — The death of part or the whole of the organ that occurs when the artery carrying its blood supply is obstructed by a blood clot or an embolus (an abnormal particle circulating in the blood). For example, a myocardial infarction affects the heart muscle when the coronary vessels are blocked.

insulin — A hormone produced by the pancreas that allows the body to regulate the amount of sugar in the bloodstream.

ischemia — An inadequate flow of blood to a part of the body, caused by constriction or blockage of the blood vessels supplying it.

kidneys — Organs located at the back of the abdomen. Kidneys are responsible for filtering the blood and removing waste materials.

lipid — A fat or fat-like substance, such as cholesterol, found in the blood.

lumen — The space within the blood vessel.

monounsaturated fats — Fatty acids that have one double or triple bond per molecule. They are easily split and other substances can join them. Found in olive oil, chicken, almonds and some other nuts.

myocardial — Refers to the heart muscle.

nephrology — The study of the kidneys.

nicotine — A poisonous, addictive substance derived from tobacco. In small doses, nicotine has a stimulating effect on the nervous system, which increases blood pressure and pulse rate.

obesity — Being 20 to 40 percent heavier than your ideal weight.

oral contraceptive — A drug containing female hormones usually synthetic estrogen and progesterone, which provides birth control by preventing ovulation or the release of eggs.

pediatrician — A doctor who specializes in the treatment of children and childhood development and illnesses.

polyunsaturated fats — Fatty acids that have more than one double or triple bond per molecule. Found in fish, soybean, safflower and corn oil. Polyunsaturated fats are usually soft or liquid at room temperature.

potassium — An essential mineral found in meat, potatoes, raisins, nuts, tomatoes, bananas, milk and other fruits. It serves as an electrolyte in the body and is important in the regulation of blood pressure.

renin — A substance released into the blood by the kidneys in response to stress. Renin levels are elevated in some types of high blood pressure.

salt — A common name for sodium chloride. It is used as a flavoring and a preservative. In the body, salt maintains fluid levels between the cells and the blood system and acts as an electrolyte to help chemical and electrical reactions.

saturated fat — A type of fat that raises blood cholesterol and triglyceride levels. Saturated fat is found in animal and dairy products such as beef, pork, lamb, veal, egg yolks, milk, butter, cheese, cream and a few vegetable fats, including coconut oil. Saturated fats are generally hard or solid at room temperature.

sedentary — Refers to an inactive lifestyle.

sphygmomanometer — An arm pressure cuff used to measure blood pressure.

stroke — An interruption of blood flow to an area of the brain. This can cause loss of function in the damaged part of the brain. Strokes can be caused by a blockage of a blood vessel in the brain or by bleeding from a blood vessel or an aneurysm into the brain. High blood pressure and smoking are the leading risk factors for stroke.

sympathetic nervous system — The division of the autonomic nervous system that is responsible for the "fight or flight" response. Activation of this division of the nervous system causes rapid heart rate, increased blood pressure, dilated pupils and sweaty palms.

systolic pressure — The pressure which is produced as the heart contracts to pump blood out into the body. The first number in a blood pressure reading.

triglycerides — A type of fat carried throughout the body by the bloodstream. High triglyceride levels are associated with overeating, obesity, high-fat or high-sugar diets, diabetes and coronary artery disease.

uremia — The buildup of waste products in the blood, often associated with the progressive narrowing of the kidneys' blood vessels.

vein — Any blood vessel that carries blood back to the heart from various parts of the body.

vitamin — Organic chemical which is essential for normal chemical reactions in the body.

vitamin supplement — Extra vitamins used to supplement or add to those found in the diet.

water pill — see diuretic.

Medical Sources

About High Blood Pressure in African-Americans,
American Heart Association

About Your Heart and Blood Pressure, American
Heart Association

American Family Physician
   Vol. 39, No. 6, p. 214
   Vol. 47, No. 1, p. 210
       No. 2, pp. 335, 526
       No. 3, p. 575
       No. 4, pp. 896, 898
       No. 5, pp. 1187, 1253, 1262
       No. 8, p. 1866
   Vol. 50, No. 1, p. 138

American Heart Association News Release
June 5, 1992
Nov. 18, 1992
April 12, 1993
May 12, 1993
Sept. 29, 1993

American Institute for Cancer Research, 1759 R Street N.W., Washington, D.C. 20069

American Journal of Cardiology
Vol. 53, p. 918
Vol. 71, No. 4, p. 263

The American Journal of Clinical Nutrition
Vol. 36, No. 3, p. 444
Vol. 39, p. 598
Vol. 49, p. 290
No. 2, p. 372
No. 3, p. 409
Vol. 50, No. 2, p. 280
No. 6, p. 1303
Vol. 51, No. 3, p. 428
Vol. 52, No. 1, p. 120
Vol. 53, p. 322S
Vol. 56, No. 1, p. 77
Vol. 57, No. 3, p. 446
No. 6, p. 868
Vol. 58, No. 3, p. 398
Vol. 59, No. 1, p. 66
No. 3, p. 667
Vol. 60, No. 4, p. 592

American Journal of Critical Care
Vol. 2, No. 4, p. 272

American Journal of Epidemiology
    Vol. 118, p. 497
    Vol. 123, p. 818
    Vol. 138, No. 11, p. 973

American Journal of Hypertension
    Vol. 6, No. 1, p. 66

American Journal of Medicine
    Vol. 94, No. 6, p. 623

Annals of Internal Medicine
    Vol. 98, p. 846
    Vol. 115, No. 10, p. 753
       No. 12, p. 917
    Vol. 118, No. 12, p. 964
    Vol. 152, No. 8, p. 1649
    Vol. 153, No. 2, p. 154

Archives of Family Medicine
    Vol. 2, No. 2, p. 130
       No. 7, p. 778

Archives of Internal Medicine
    Vol. 144, p. 1045
    Vol. 148, p. 788
    Vol. 152, No. 8, pp. 1573, 1698
    Vol. 153, No. 2, pp. 154, 186
       No. 5, p. 598
       No. 12, p. 1429
       No. 17, p. 2050
       No. 18, p. 2093

The Atlanta Journal and Constitution
March 29, 1993 (D5)
May 14, 1993 (B6)
June 16, 1993
Sept. 22, 1993 (B4)
Nov. 11, 1993
Jan. 6, 1994 (H9)
May 19, 1994 (C8)
Sept. 14, 1994 (D6)
Nov. 21, 1994 (C4)

Aviation Medical Bulletin
May 1992
January 1993
March 1993

Better Health
Vol. 5, No. 8

Blood Pressure: Take Control!, **Baylor College of Medicine, One Baylor Plaza, Room 176B, Houston, Texas 77030**

Bottom Line Personal
Vol. 14, No. 7, p. 6

Bowes and Church's Food Values of Portions Commonly Used, **15th Edition, Harper Collins Publishers Inc., New York**

British Journal of Urology
Vol. 58, p. 592

British Medical Journal
    Vol. 285, p. 1691
    Vol. 298, No. 6681, p. 1147
       No. 6688, p. 1616
    Vol. 301, No. 6751, p. 521
    Vol. 303, No. 6805, p. 785
    Vol. 304, No. 6824, p. 405
    Vol. 306, No. 6870, p. 83

Cancer
    Vol. 59, No. 7, p. 1386

Cardiac Alert
    Vol. 9, p. 5
    Vol. 14, No. 12, p. 5
    Vol. 15, No. 2, pp. 6, 7

Cardiology in the Elderly
    Vol. 1, No. 1, p. 87

Cereal Foods World
    Vol. 32, No. 8, p. 538

Cholesterol and Your Heart, **American Heart Association**

Cholesterol in Children: Healthy Eating Is a Family Affair, **National Institutes of Health, Bethesda, Md. 20892**

Circulation
    Vol. 79, p. 304
    Vol. 79, No. 5, p. 1007
    Vol. 85, No. 4, p. 1265
    Vol. 88, No. 2, p. 523
    Vol. 88, No. 6, p. 2794

The Complete and Up-to-Date Fat Book, Avery
 Publishing Group, Garden City Park, N.Y., 1993

Consumer Reports on Health
 Vol. 5, No. 6, p. 64
 Vol. 6, No. 3, p. 24
 Vol. 6, No. 11, p. 130

Controlling Your Fat Tooth, Workman Publishing,
 New York, 1991

Dairy Council Digest
 Vol. 63, No. 5, p. 25

Diet and Health, National Academy Press,
 Washington, D.C., 1989

Dietary Guidelines and Your Diet, U.S.
 Department of Agriculture
 HG - 232 - 8 through 11

Down Home Healthy, National Institutes of Health

Drug Therapy
 Vol. 23, No. 3, p. 88

Eating to Lower Your High Blood Cholesterol, U.S.
 Department on Health and Human Services

Eat Smart for a Healthy Heart Cookbook, Baron's
 Educational Series, Inc., Hauppauge, N.Y., 1987

Emergency Medicine
 Vol. 24, No. 14, p. 26
 Vol. 25, No. 12, p. 52

ESHA Research Issues
 Vol. 8, No. 4, p. 5

European Journal of Clinical Nutrition
   Vol. 42, p. 857

FDA Consumer
   Vol. 26, No. 10, p. 16

The Food Guide Pyramid, United States
   Department of Agriculture

Food Safety Notebook
   Vol. 4, No. 9, p. 88

Food, Nutrition and Health
   Vol. 16, No. 12, p. 1
   Vol. 18, No. 2, p. 1

Geriatrics
   Vol. 35, p.34
   Vol. 44, No. 6, p. 13
   Vol. 47, No. 8, p. 33
      No. 11, p. 24
      No. 12, pp. 16, 57
   Vol. 48, No. 4, pp. 47, 83
      No. 6, pp. 18, 73
      No. 9, p. 88
      No. 11, p. 26

Harvard Health Letter
   Vol. 17, No. 7, p. 1
   Vol. 18, No. 3, p. 3

Harvard Heart Letter
   Vol. 4, No. 3, pp. 7, 8

Health & Healing
   Vol. 3, No. 2, p. 1

Health Confidential
   Vol. 7, No. 11, p. 3

The Health Letter
Vol. 2, p. 1

The Healthy Heart Cookbook, Tactical Air Command
Medical Services

Heartstyle
Vol. 2, No. 4, pp. 1, 4, 6
Vol. 4, No. 1, p. 4

HerbalGram
Vol. 30, p. 11

High Blood Pressure and Cardiovascular Prevention
Vol. 1, No. 2, p. 93

High Blood Pressure in Teenagers, American Heart
Association

Human Nutrition Information Service, U.S.
Department of Agriculture

Hypertension
Vol. 6, p. 574
Vol. 13, No. 1, p. 1
Vol. 19, No. 2, p. 175
No. 6, p. 749
Vol. 21, No. 2, p. 248
No. 3, pp. 267, 301, 308, 380
No. 4, pp. 391, 406, 439, 510, 525
No. 5, p. 714
Vol. 22, No, 3, pp. 292, 371
No. 6, p. 826
Vol. 23, No. 4, p. 531
Vol. 24, No. 1, p. 83

The Johns Hopkins Medical Letter
    Vol. 4, No. 3, p. 12
    Vol. 5, No. 8, p. 8

The Johns Hopkins Medical Letter, Health After 50
    Vol. 5, No. 8, p. 1

Journal of General Internal Medicine
    June 1993

Journal of Human Hypertension
    Vol. 7, p. 403

Journal of Hypertension
    Vol. 4, p. 5182
    Vol. 11, No. 11, p. 1267

The Journal of Nutrition
    Vol. 120, No. 4, p. 325
    Vol. 124, No. 1, p. 78

Journal of Nutrition for the Elderly
    Vol. 13, No. 2, p. 66

Journal of Nutritional Science Vitaminology
    Vol. 32, p. 581

Journal of Optimal Nutrition
    Vol. 3, No. 1, p. 32

Journal of the American College of Nutrition
    Vol. 8, No. 6, p. 567
    Vol. 9, No. 4, p. 352

The Journal of the American Dietetic Association
    Vol. 93, No. 9, p. 1007
    Vol. 94, No. 4, p. 425

The Journal of the American Medical Association
Vol. 201, No. 918, p. 22
Vol. 212, p. 2267
Vol. 229, p. 1068
Vol. 247, p. 992
Vol. 253, p. 3263
Vol. 257, pp. 1772, 3251
Vol. 258, p. 214
Vol. 259, pp. 225, 2553, 2561
Vol. 261, No. 23, p. 3419
Vol. 262, No. 13, p. 1801
    No. 17, p. 2395
Vol. 263, No. 14, p. 1929
    No. 20, p. 2766
Vol. 264, No. 6, p. 707
Vol. 265, No. 14, p. 1833
Vol. 266, No. 8, p. 1070
Vol. 267, No. 6, p. 811
    No. 13, p. 1857
Vol. 269, No. 3, p. 323
Vol. 270, No. 20, pp. 2439, 2494
Vol. 272, No. 10, p. 781

Journal of the National Cancer Institute
Vol. 84, No. 24, p. 1887

Journal of Urology
Vol. 132, p. 1140

JR College of Physicians
Vol. 9, p. 138

The Lancet
    Vol. 339, No. 8789, p. 342
    Vol. 341, No. 8843, p. 454
    Vol. 341, No. 8836, p. 27
    Vol. 341, No. 8846, p. 695
    Vol. 341, No. 8855, p. 1248
    Vol. 342, No. 8885, p. 1455

Less Stress in 30 Days, New American Library, New York, 1986

Lipids
    Vol. 21, p. 715

Mayo Clinic Health Letter
    Vol. 11, No. 5, p. 1

Medical Abstracts Newsletter
    Vol. 12, No. 3, p. 2
    Vol. 13, No. 1, p. 3
        No. 5, p. 3
        No. 8, p. 3
        No. 11, p. 3

Medical Tribune
    Vol. 30, No. 6, p. 14
    Vol. 31, No. 20, p. 15
    Vol. 33, No. 5, p. 19
        No. 22, p. 2
    Vol. 34, No. 2, pp. 4, 13
        No. 7, p. 21
        No. 8, p. 1
        No. 13, pp. 1, 14
        No. 20, p. 7
    Vol. 35, No. 2, p. 12

Medical Tribune for the Internist & Cardiologist
Vol. 35, No. 13, p. 5
No. 14, p. 18

Medical World News
Vol. 30, No. 11, p. 30
No, 16, p. 14
Vol. 31, No. 5, p. 20
No. 6, p. 11
Vol. 33, No. 11, p. 9
Vol. 34, No. 5, p. 23

Men's Confidential
Vol. 9, No. 1, p. 6
No. 2, p. 3
No. 10, p. 5

Metabolism
Vol. 33, No. 2, p. 164

Modern Medicine
Vol. 57, No. 11, pp. 22, 103

National Cholesterol Education Program's Report of the Expert Panel on Blood Cholesterol Levels in Children and Adolescents, U.S. Department of Health and Human Services

National Institutes of Health News Release
June 8, 1994

The New England Journal of Medicine
    Vol. 278, p. 1381
    Vol. 312, p. 1548
    Vol. 313, p. 582
    Vol. 318, pp. 17, 1127
    Vol. 319, No. 7, p. 385
    Vol. 320, No. 16, p. 1037
        No. 17, p. 1148
    Vol. 322, No. 12, p. 849
    Vol. 327, No. 4, p. 242
        No. 10, p. 669
        No. 14, p. 998
        No. 19, p. 1350
        No. 27, pp. 1893, 1947
    Vol. 328, No. 9, p. 603
        No. 20, p. 1494
    Vol. 329, No. 26, p. 1912
    Vol. 330, No. 25, p. 1776

Nutrition
    Vol. 55, No. 3, p. 4

Nutrition Action Health Letter
    Vol. 20, No. 2, p. 8
        No. 3, p. 13
        No. 8, pp. 4, 13
    Vol. 21, No. 9, p. 10

Nutrition and Your Health: Dietary Guidelines for Americans, U.S. Department of Agriculture

Nutrition Forum
    Vol. 10, No. 3, p. 22

Nutrition Prescription, Crown Publishers, Inc., New York, 1987

Nutrition Research Newsletter
Vol. 11, p. 405
No. 9, p. 961
Vol. 12, No. 6, p. 69
No. 11/12, p. 122

Nutrition Today
Vol. 27, No. 4, p. 27
Vol. 28, No. 2, p. 4
No. 3, p. 30

Nutritive Value of Foods, **U.S. Department of Agriculture**

The Physician and Sportsmedicine
Vol. 14, No. 5, p. 181
Vol. 20, No. 8, p. 15
No. 12, p. 123
Vol. 21, No. 1, p. 125
No. 2, pp. 55, 124
No. 3, pp. 204, 227
No. 6, p. 45
No. 10, p. 103
No. 11, p. 89
Vol. 22, No. 3, p. 28
No. 7, pp. 15, 23
No. 10, p. 11

Physician Assistant
Vol. 17, No. 4, p. 37

Physiological Behavior
Vol. 38, No. 4, p. 459
Vol. 42, No. 4, p. 389

Postgraduate Medicine
   Vol. 79, No 4, p. 352
   Vol. 85, No. 4, p. 406
      No. 6, p. 243
   Vol. 91, No. 8, p. 225
   Vol. 92, No. 2, p. 265
   Vol. 93, No. 1, p. 082
      No. 6, p. 199

Psychosomatic Medicine
   Vol. 43, p. 25

The Real Vitamin and Mineral Book: Going Beyond the RDA for Optimum Health, Avery Publishing, Garden City Park, N.Y., 1990

Recommended Dietary Allowances, 10th Edition, National Academy Press, Washington, D.C., 1989

Salt, Sodium and Blood Pressure. Piecing Together the Puzzle, American Heart Association

Science
   Vol. 144, No. 23, p. 380

Science and Education Administration, U.S. Department of Agriculture

Science News
- Vol. 133 p. 356
- Vol. 134, p. 228
  - No. 20, p. 308
- Vol. 135, No. 12, p. 183
  - No. 16, p. 250
- Vol. 136, No. 12, p. 184
- Vol. 137, No. 19, p. 292
  - No. 23, p. 367
  - No. 25, p. 398
- Vol. 138, No. 12, p. 177
- Vol. 140, No. 18, p. 285
- Vol. 142, No. 20, p. 326
- Vol. 143, No. 12, p. 186
- Vol. 144, No. 10, p. 153
  - No. 13, p. 196
  - No. 23, p. 380
- Vol. 145, No. 25, p. 390

So You Have High Blood Cholesterol, **U.S. Department of Health and Human Services**

Southern Medical Journal
- Vol. 83, No. 10, p. 1131

Stay Healthy
- Vol. 6, No. 12, p. 47

Stroke
- Vol. 24, No. 5, p. 639

Tufts University Diet & Nutrition Letter
- Vol. 10, No. 12, p. 3

U.S. Pharmacist
Vol. 14, No. 6, p. 28
Vol. 17, No. 12, p. 34
Vol. 18, No. 9, p. 100
Supplement March 1993
Supplement March 1994

University of California at Berkeley Wellness Letter
Vol. 9, No. 6, p. 3
    No. 7, p. 7
Vol. 10, No. 1, p. 4
    No. 11, p. 8
Vol. 11, No. 1, p. 2

The Wall Street Journal
March 2, 1994, B9

Western Journal of Medicine
Vol. 141, p. 193
Vol. 150, No. 3, p. 562
Vol. 160, No. 5, pp. 465, 483

Working Group Report on High Blood Pressure in Pregnancy, National High Blood Pressure Education Program, U.S. Dept. of Health and Human Services, August 1991

Working Group Report on Primary Prevention of Hypertension, National High Blood Pressure Education Program, National Institutes of Health, May 1993

Chart Sources ────────────────────

Agricultural Handbook Number 8, 1989 Supplement, USDA, 1989

Agricultural Handbook Number 8, 1990 Supplement, USDA, 1991

Agricultural Handbook Number 8-10, USDA, 1992

Agricultural Handbook Number 8-12, USDA, 1984

Agricultural Handbook Number 8-13, USDA, 1990

Agricultural Handbook Number 8-17, USDA, 1989

Agricultural Handbook Number 8-18, USDA, 1992

Agricultural Handbook Number 8-19, USDA, 1991

Agricultural Handbook Number 8-21, USDA, 1988

Agricultural Handbook Number 8-6, USDA, 1980

American Family Physician
Vol. 50, No. 1, p. 138

Archives of Internal Medicine
Vol. 153, No. 2, p. 154

Aviation Medical Bulletin
April 1993 (p. 3)

Controlling Your Fat Tooth, **Workman Publishing, New York, 1991**

Centers for Disease Control, National Center for Health Statistics, Third National Health and Nutrition Examinations Survey (1988-91), as reported in the National Institutes of Health's Working Report on Primary Prevention of Hypertension

Convenience Food Facts by Arlene Monk, R.D., C.D.E., DCI/Chronimed Publishing, Minneapolis, MN, 1991

Food Values by Jean A.T. Pennington, Harper Collins Publishers, Inc., N.Y., 1989

MasterCook Mac by Arion Software, Austin, Texas, 1994

Nutritionist IV software by N-Squared Computing, First DataBank Division, The Hearst Corporation, 1994 (415) 588-5454

The Fifth Report of the Joint National Committee on Detection, Evaluation and Treatment of High Blood Pressure, Jan. 25, 1993

U.S. Department of Agriculture / Department of Health and Human Services, 1990

U.S. Department of Agriculture, Human Nutrition Information Service

Herbal Sources

Alternative Medicine: The Definitive Guide, Future Medicine Publishing Inc., Puyallup, Wash., 1993

Alternative Medicine Yellow Pages, Future
Medicine Publishing Inc., Puyallup, Wash.,
1994

*Heinerman's Encyclopedia of Fruits, Vegetables
and Herbs* by John Heinerman, Parker
Publishing Co., West Nyack, N.Y., 1988

Herbs of Choice by Varro E. Tyler, PhD., ScD., The
Haworth Press Inc., Binghamton, N.Y., 1994

Herbs, RD Home Handbook, The Reader's Digest
Association Inc., Pleasantville, N.Y., 1990

The Honest Herbal by Varro E. Tyler, PhD., The
Haworth Press Inc., Binghamton, N.Y., 1993

Graphic Sources ────────────────

Geriatrics
Vol. 47, No. 8, p. 40

LifeArt Collections

Medical Illustration Library

The Physician and Sportsmedicine
Vol. 22, No. 10, p. 111

**U.S. Department of Agriculture / Department of
Health and Human Services**

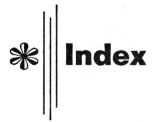 **Index**

Cardizem 284
Cardizem SR 284
Cardizem CD 284
Cardura 283
Carrots 91, 159, 181, 189
Carteolol 280
Cartrol 280
Catapres 281
Catheter 18, 268, 507
Catnip 376, 382
Cauliflower 91, 159, 181, 189,
    202
Cavity 42, 508
Celery 91, 159
Cellulose 88
Cena-K 290
Cereal(s), *see also* Breakfast
    125, 134, 135, 168-170, 177,
    200, 224
Cerebral arteries 25
Cerebral infarction 36
Chamomiles 374, 382
Checkup(s) 1, 44, 66
Cheese(s) 94, 132, 134-135,
    137, 143, 149-150, 177-178,
    194, 222, 514
Cherries 178, 189
Chest pain 28-30, 64, 127, 279,
    293
Chicken 94, 151, 175, 179, 181,
    223, 513
Chickpeas 159, 168, 189
Chicory 376, 382
Chili 223
Chills 270
Chinese-Americans 201
Chinook 211

Chives 180
Chlorothiazide 287-288
Chlorthalidone 287-288
Chocolate 150-151, 177, 206,
    224-225
Choking 29, 507
Cholesterol 2, 4-6, 10, 14, 64, 89,
    106-107, 129-130, 137-145,
    149-152, 157-166, 169,
    186-187, 197-198, 210,
    217-227, 231-232, 279,
    282-283, 508-509, 511-512,
    514
  and Exercise 106-107,
    226-227
  and Fiber 140, 157-160,
    164-166, 226
  and Magnesium 197-198
  and Saturated fats 137, 149
Chromium 279
Cider 180
Cigarette(s), *see also* Smoking
    48, 65, 249-257
Cimetidine 206
Cinnamon 90, 181
Circadian rhythm(s) 73
Cirrhosis 508
Citrus 202
Clonidine 281-282, 288
Clot(s) 124, 187, 225, 239, 263,
    511-512
Cloves 225
Cocaine 56
Cocktails 180
Cocoa butter 151, 222
Coconut oil 149, 151, 222, 514
Cod 211

H

Halcion 207
Halibut 211
Ham 93
Hamstrings 117
Hangover 250
Hawthorn 374
Hazelnuts 224
HDL cholesterol 107, 150, 162, 165, 218, 220-221, 225-227, 231, 279
Headache(s) 15, 38, 64, 197, 205, 216, 255, 270, 277, 281
Heart attack(s), *see also* Myocardial infarction 2, 25, 27-30, 36, 64, 84, 105-106, 156, 161, 165, 188, 199, 218, 221-222, 238-239, 249, 251, 263, 272, 276, 279, 284, 509, 511
Heart attack warning signs 28
Heart disease 2, 4, 23, 36, 49, 52, 55, 57, 64, 79, 89, 97, 99-100, 107, 121, 124, 141, 155, 158, 160, 166, 169, 210, 215, 218-220, 225, 230-233, 240, 252, 279, 287, 509
Heart failure, *see also* Congestive heart failure 2, 25, 30-36, 48, 58, 276-277, 280, 284, 508-509, 511
Heartbeat, irregular, *see also* Arrythmia 204, 277
Heartburn 30
Hemorrhage, Hemorrhagic stroke 36-37, 250

Hemorrhoids 155-156
Heparin 188
Herbs 94, 179, 216, 223, 373-386
Herb tea 384
Heredity 14, 47, 55, 57, 231, 511
Herring 211-212
H-H-R 288
Hibiscus 380
High density lipoprotein, *see* HDL cholesterol
Home monitoring 66-67
Honey 88, 179, 376
Honeydew 202
Hormone(s) 13-14, 52, 55, 89, 104, 185, 191, 198, 207, 217, 224, 229, 235, 241, 260, 269, 275, 507, 510-513
Horsetail 380
Human Nutrition Information Service 146
Hybridization 53
Hydra-Zide 288
Hydralazine 281, 288
Hydrex 287
Hydro-Chlor 287
Hydro-D 287
Hydro-Serp 288
Hydrochlorothiazide 287-289
HydroDIURIL 287
Hydroflumethiazide 287, 289
Hydrogenated 149, 152, 223
Hydrolysates 140
Hydromox 287, 289
Hydromox R 289
Hydropine 289
Hydropres 288

Y

Z